Health and Well-Being among Older Adults: Current Trends and Future Challenges

Health and Well-Being among Older Adults: Current Trends and Future Challenges

Guest Editors

Paulo Santos-Costa
Manuela Vilar
Liliana B. Sousa

MDPI

Basel • Beijing • Wuhan • Barcelona • Belgrade • Novi Sad • Cluj • Manchester

Guest Editors
Paulo Santos-Costa
Gerontogeriatric Nursing
Nursing School of the
University of Coimbra
Coimbra
Portugal

Manuela Vilar
Center for Research in
Neuropsychology and
Cognitive and Behavioral
Intervention (CINEICC)
University of Coimbra
Coimbra
Portugal

Liliana B. Sousa
The Health Sciences
Research Unit:
Nursing (UICISA: E)
University of Coimbra
Coimbra
Portugal

Editorial Office
MDPI AG
Grosspeteranlage 5
4052 Basel, Switzerland

This is a reprint of the Special Issue, published open access by the journal *European Journal of Investigation in Health, Psychology and Education* (ISSN 2254-9625), freely accessible at: https://www.mdpi.com/journal/ejihpe/special_issues/8I78E26T7B.

For citation purposes, cite each article independently as indicated on the article page online and as indicated below:

Lastname, A.A.; Lastname, B.B. Article Title. *Journal Name* **Year**, *Volume Number*, Page Range.

ISBN 978-3-7258-8281-6 (Hbk)
ISBN 978-3-7258-8282-3 (PDF)
https://doi.org/10.3390/books978-3-7258-8282-3

Contents

About the Editors

Paulo Santos-Costa

Paulo Santos-Costa is a Professor in the Gerontogeriatric Nursing Department at the Nursing School of the University of Coimbra, where he contributes to teaching, research, and innovation in nursing science. He holds a PhD in Nursing from the Universidade Católica Portuguesa and a master's degree in Nursing with a specialization in Ward Management from the Nursing School of Coimbra. His academic training also includes a post-degree specialization in Community Nursing from the Red Cross Northern Health School and postgraduate studies in Gerontogeriatrics and Clinical Supervision. He collaborates with professional and scientific organizations, including service on the boards of the Phi Xi Chapter of Sigma Theta Tau International and the Portuguese Association of Vascular Access. His editorial activity includes serving as Academic Editor and Guest Editor for international journals, as well as frequent peer review. His research spans vascular access, infection control, aging, and the development of innovative health technologies, resulting in publications, book chapters, and intellectual property. His work has been recognized through national and international distinctions that reflect sustained engagement in advancing nursing practice and research.

Manuela Vilar

Manuela Vilar holds a PhD in Psychology, specializing in Psychological Assessment, from the Faculty of Psychology and Educational Sciences of the University of Coimbra, where she is an Assistant Professor. She is a member of the Laboratory of Psychological Assessment and Psychometrics at the same institution. Her teaching covers several curricular units in the fields of Psychological and Neuropsychological Assessment, including Psychological Assessment I, Neuropsychological Assessment, Assessment Instruments and Psychological Reports, and Assessment and Rehabilitation Programs for Older Adults. Her research includes publications in national and international journals and conference presentations, particularly on the assessment of quality of life and functional capacity in older adults, as well as on neuropsychological assessment of children and adolescents.

Liliana B. Sousa

Liliana B. Sousa is an Auxiliary Researcher at the Nursing School of the University of Coimbra, where she contributes to research and development activities in the Health Sciences Research Unit: Nursing (UICISA: E). She holds a PhD in Psychology from the Faculty of Psychology and Educational Sciences of the University of Coimbra, and previously completed a master's degree in Psychological Assessment, Counseling, and Rehabilitation at the same institution. Her early work in psychometrics involved adapting and validating psychological assessment instruments. Her subsequent research has focused on innovation in health technologies, including the design of preclinical and clinical study protocols, the preparation of regulatory documentation for medical device development, and the supervision of biomedical engineering theses. She has contributed to national and institutional innovation initiatives, participated in capacity-building and research project submissions, authored scientific publications, and is listed as an inventor on patents associated with her work. She has also collaborated in editorial and scientific revision processes for academic publications in nursing management.

Preface

This reprint gathers a set of recent studies on the theme of Health and Well-Being among Older Adults: Current Trends and Future Challenges. It reflects ongoing efforts across several disciplines to document and analyze the conditions shaping later life, with attention to physical, psychological, social, and cultural dimensions of aging. The contributions address topics such as cognitive functioning, emotional well-being, digital engagement, sexuality, spirituality, and experiences of isolation, each offering focused evidence from specific national or community contexts.

The motivation for assembling this collection stems from demographic changes affecting many societies and the need to better understand how older adults navigate evolving health and social environments. Responding to the original call, the authors situate their work within broader discussions linked to the Sustainable Development Goals and consider how various aspects of resilience, mental health, community connectedness, care practices, and cultural perspectives influence well-being in later life. Although the studies differ in design and scope, they share a commitment to examining concrete challenges and opportunities encountered by older adults.

This reprint is intended for researchers, practitioners, educators, students, and policymakers seeking up-to-date examples of empirical work in the field. While the contributions are necessarily limited to their respective contexts and methodological choices, together they provide a useful snapshot of current research directions and highlight areas that warrant further investigation.

We invite you to read the contributions closely and consider how each study illuminates particular aspects of aging in contemporary contexts. The findings are not exhaustive, nor do they settle the broader questions in the field. Still, they offer grounded observations and analyses that can inform reflection, stimulate dialogue, and support the gradual development of more responsive approaches to aging.

Paulo Santos-Costa, Manuela Vilar, and Liliana B. Sousa
Guest Editors

European Journal of
Investigation in Health, Psychology and Education

MDPI

Editorial

Aging with Purpose and Justice: What Recent Evidence from the Special Issue Tells Us and What It Leaves Unsaid

Paulo Santos-Costa [1,*], Liliana B. Sousa [2] and Manuela Vilar [2]

1 The Health Sciences Research Unit: Nursing (UICISA: E), Nursing School of the University of Coimbra, 3004-011 Coimbra, Portugal
2 Neuropsychological Assessment and Ageing Processes (NAAP) Group, Center for Research in Neuropsychology and Cognitive and Behavioral Intervention (CINEICC), Faculty of Psychology and Educational Sciences, University of Coimbra, 3000-115 Coimbra, Portugal
* Correspondence: paulocosta@esenfc.pt

Introduction

While population aging may be celebrated as a public health and social progress success story, it is a more nuanced experience than this, and aging without well-being is a hollow victory. As the United Nations' 2030 Agenda for Sustainable Development states, "leaving no one behind" requires that older people are not simply included in health and social systems; it refers to the recognition of older people as rights bearing citizens who can contribute to society, make meaning, and grow.

Similarly, the Decade of Healthy Ageing (2021–2030) led by the World Health Organization (WHO, 2020) calls for courageous action in four areas: (i) transforming the way we think about age and aging; (ii) creating communities that support and optimize the unique contributions and capabilities of older persons; (iii) delivering integrated care; and (iv) ensuring access to long term care when needed. This Special Issue, called "Health and Well-Being among Older Adults: Current Trends and Future Challenges", includes nine contributions from over a dozen European and Asian countries and provides practical accounts of both what has been achieved as well as questions still to be answered.

One clear contribution is the recognition that digital inclusion is now inseparable from social inclusion. Eto and Yamatsu in Japan showed that eHealth literacy strengthens older adults' social activity, while Parra-Sánchez et al. in Spain revealed how geography and gender shape the perceived benefits of technology among elders living with visual impairment. Fernández-Piqueras et al., also in Spain, highlighted how uneven digital competence generates new vulnerabilities and proposed intergenerational learning as a pathway to inclusion. These studies speak directly to Sustainable Development Goal (SDG) 10 (Reduced Inequalities) by confronting a new form of inequity, the "digital divide", and to the WHO Decade's call to foster environments that support older people's abilities (WHO, 2020). However, one key issue still unanswered is the role of the digital infrastructure, platform design, accessibility considerations, or affordability, in creating systematic exclusion. For there to be equitable aging, future research and policy must work to support older adults' digital skills but also pay attention to the systemic biases embedded in the technologies they are asked to use.

A second thread concerns cognitive health and prevention, aligning closely with SDG 3 (Good Health and Well-Being). Bouhaben et al. in Spain provided evidence that olfactory identification may serve as a cost-effective biomarker for early cognitive decline, while Tsiakiri et al. in Greece demonstrated that computerized cognitive training can stabilize decline in older adults with minor neurocognitive disorders. Tomás et al., drawing on data from more than 61,000 older adults, confirmed that loneliness, pain, and frailty are decisive predictors of quality of life, with loneliness emerging as the most consistent determinant. These studies contribute to the Decade's call for integrated, person-centered care (WHO, 2020) and align with the Global Coalition on Aging (GCOA, 2022) framework's insistence that age-related conditions, whether frailty or cognitive decline, should not be passively accepted as inevitable, but proactively managed with preventive strategies. Yet, here again, questions remain. How can low-cost biomarkers like olfactory testing be embedded in public health systems that often underfund geriatric care? What forms of cognitive training are scalable and culturally adaptable beyond research contexts? And why do health systems continue to privilege frailty and pain over loneliness, despite robust evidence of its corrosive effects within this cohort?

The Special Issue also insists that well-being in later life extends beyond health to questions of sexuality, meaning, and spirituality. Von Humboldt et al. studying older adults in Portugal and Spain, showed that sexual well-being remains diverse and culturally shaped, challenging the persistent ageist assumption that sexuality fades into irrelevance in later life. Cojocaru et al. in Romania highlighted the sources of meaning for institutionalized elders, from spirituality to intergenerational value transmission, underscoring that existential and relational needs remain vital even in contexts of dependency. A study by Volkos et al. conducted in Greece further demonstrated the links between loneliness, health behaviors, and biological markers, reinforcing that emotional and physical dimensions of aging cannot be separated. These contributions directly advance SDG 5 (Gender Equality) by recognizing sexuality and intimacy as ongoing in later life, and they align with SDG 16 (Peace, Justice, and Strong Institutions) by exposing how institutional settings often neglect the psychosocial dimensions of aging. Yet, they raise uncomfortable questions. If sexuality and spirituality are empirically shown to matter, why are they absent from most health and social care models? Are they taught in-depth during formal training of healthcare professionals such as nurses and doctors? How long can policymakers and practitioners ignore these dimensions without reproducing ageism in subtler forms?

Geographically, the scope of this Special Issue is notable. It encompasses local studies from Japan, Greece, Spain, Portugal, and Romania, alongside cross-national analysis of 28 European countries and Israel conducted by Tomás et al. This diversity responds to SDG 17 (Partnerships for the Goals) by demonstrating how comparative and collaborative research can generate insights that no single country could produce alone. At the same time, it underscores how unevenly the research map is populated. We hear little about aging in Africa, Latin America, or the Global South, despite these regions experiencing some of the fastest demographic transitions. If the 2030 Agenda is truly global, then scholarship must urgently extend beyond high-income and European contexts to capture the plurality of aging experiences.

Across themes, the contributions collected here affirm two central points. First, that aging is irreducibly multidimensional, requiring integrated approaches across health, psychology, education, and social policy. Second, that progress is possible, but only if research findings are translated into bold policies that align with global agendas. Digital literacy must be embedded as a citizenship right, cognitive health interventions must be scaled and equitably funded, loneliness must be recognized as a health condition, and sexuality and spirituality must be legitimized in care frameworks.

At the same time, this Special Issue reveals blind spots; namely, the economic dimensions of aging, the intersections of ethnicity and migration, and the voices of the oldest-old remain underexplored. These omissions should not be seen as shortcomings but as an invitation for further scholarship that continues to push the boundaries of how we understand aging.

Finally, the contributions to this Special Issue are not only empirical studies but responses to the global call for action on aging. They align with specific Sustainable Development Goals, advance the priorities of the WHO Decade of Healthy Ageing (WHO, 2020), and reinforce the International Council on Active Aging (ICAA, 2016) and GCOA (2022) insistence that ageism, neglect, and inequity cannot be tolerated in aging societies.

They also leave us with critical challenges; namely, to broaden the geographies of research, to take seriously the non-biomedical dimensions of aging, and to build policies that match the complexity of older adults lived experiences. In highlighting both contributions and unanswered questions, this Special Issue demonstrates that healthy aging is not simply a technical or clinical challenge, but a profound societal project, and one that demands courage, imagination, and above all, justice.

Author Contributions: Conceptualization, P.S.-C.; validation, P.S.-C., L.B.S. and M.V.; writing—original draft preparation, P.S.-C., L.B.S. and M.V.; writing—review and editing, P.S.-C., L.B.S. and M.V.; project administration, P.S.-C., L.B.S. and M.V. All authors have read and agreed to the published version of the manuscript.

Conflicts of Interest: The authors declare no conflicts of interest.

Abbreviations

The following abbreviations are used in this manuscript:

GCOA	Global Coalition on Aging
ICAA	International Council on Active Aging
SDG	Sustainable Development Goal
WHO	World Health Organization

List of Contributions:

1. Eto, M., & Yamatsu, K. (2024). Associations of eHealth literacy with social activity among community-dwelling older adults: A cross-sectional study. *European Journal of Investigation in Health, Psychology and Education*, *14*(5), 1279–1294. https://doi.org/10.3390/ejihpe14050084.
2. Parra-Sánchez, A., Zorrilla-Muñoz, V., Martinez-Navarrete, G., & Fernandez, E. (2024). Technological perception with rural and urban differentiation and its influence on the quality of life of older people with age-related macular degeneration. *European Journal of Investigation in Health, Psychology and Education*, *14*(5), 1470–1488. https://doi.org/10.3390/ejihpe14050097.
3. Fernández-Piqueras, R., González-García, R. J., Sanz-Ponce, R., & Calero-Plaza, J. (2025). Digital divides in older people: Assessment of digital competencies and proposals for meaningful inclusion. *European Journal of Investigation in Health, Psychology and Education*, *15*(10), 196. https://doi.org/10.3390/ejihpe15100196.
4. Bouhaben, J., Delgado-Lima, A. H., & Delgado-Losada, M. L. (2024). Olfactory identification as a biomarker for cognitive impairment: Insights from healthy aging, subjective cognitive decline, and mild cognitive impairment. *European Journal of Investigation in Health, Psychology and Education*, *14*(12), 2978–3000. https://doi.org/10.3390/ejihpe14120196.
5. Tsiakiri, A., Plakias, S., Vlotinou, P., Athanasouli, P., Terzoudi, A., Kyriazidou, S., Serdari, A., Karakitsiou, G., Megari, K., Aggelousis, N., Vadikolias, K., & Christidi, F. (2025). Innovative health promotion strategies: A 6-month longitudinal study on computerized cognitive training for older adults with minor neurocognitive disorders. *European Journal of Investigation in Health, Psychology and Education*, *15*(3), 34. https://doi.org/10.3390/ejihpe15030034.
6. Tomás, J. M., Sanz, A., & Torres, Z. (2025). A Bayesian structural equation model to predict quality of life in European older adults. *European Journal of Investigation in Health, Psychology and Education*, *15*(7), 127. https://doi.org/10.3390/ejihpe15070127.
7. Von Humboldt, S., Cabras, E., Low, G., & Leal, I. (2024). Sexual well-being and aging patterns: Findings of a cluster analysis among older adults in Portugal and Spain. *European Journal of*

Investigation in Health, Psychology and Education, *14*(7), 2013–2028. https://doi.org/10.3390/ejihpe14070134.

8. Cojocaru, L., Soponaru, C., Muntele-Hendreș, D., & Ceobanu, C. (2025). Meaning in life among aged people: A qualitative study of an institutionalized elderly sample. *European Journal of Investigation in Health, Psychology and Education*, *15*(6), 91. https://doi.org/10.3390/ejihpe15060091.
9. Volkos, P., Linardakis, M., Stachteas, P., Anastasiou, F., Tatsioni, A., Kampa, M., & Symvoulakis, E. K. (2024). Association between levels of loneliness, laboratory measurements, and behavioral aspects in a primary care setting in Crete, Greece. *European Journal of Investigation in Health, Psychology and Education*, *14*(4), 1055–1067. https://doi.org/10.3390/ejihpe14040069.

References

Global Coalition on Aging, & Nutricia. (2022). *Fighting ageism to empower older persons to age in good health: A call to action*. Global Coalition on Aging/Nutricia.

International Council on Active Aging. (2016). *Preparing for the decade of healthy aging, 2020–2030: A call to action*. International Council on Active Aging.

World Health Organization. (2020). *Decade of healthy ageing: Baseline report*. World Health Organization.

European Journal of
Investigation in Health, Psychology and Education

MDPI

Article

Digital Divides in Older People: Assessment of Digital Competencies and Proposals for Meaningful Inclusion

Rocío Fernández-Piqueras [1], Rómulo J. González-García [2], Roberto Sanz-Ponce [1,*] and Joana Calero-Plaza [2]

[1] Faculty of Education and Educational Sciences, Catholic University of Valencia, C/Sagrado Corazón, 5, 46110 Godella, Valencia, Spain; rocio@ucv.es
[2] Campus Capacitas, Catholic University of Valencia, 46110 Godella, Valencia, Spain; rj.gonzalez@ucv.es (R.J.G.-G.); joana.calero@ucv.es (J.C.-P.)
* Correspondence: roberto.sanz@ucv.es

Abstract

Background: Currently, population aging and the growing incorporation of digital technologies into everyday life highlight the need to ensure the digital inclusion of older adults. This is due to the existence of a significant digital divide that affects this population group, limiting not only their access to services and opportunities but also their emotional well-being and quality of life. The lack of digital skills can generate feelings of exclusion, frustration, and dependence, negatively impacting their mental health and autonomy. Methods: The objective of this study is to assess the level of basic digital competence in 404 older adults using the Scale of Basic Digital Competence in Older Adults (DigCompB_PM) in order to identify existing digital divides and provide empirical evidence for the design of educational interventions that promote the digital inclusion of this population group. To this end, we start with the following research question: Are older adults prepared to face the digital and knowledge society, taking into account personal variables such as age, gender, geographical location, place of residence, and type of cohabitation? Results: The findings reveal that participants scored highest in the dimension related to safety and digital device usage while scoring lowest in online collaboration, indicating a disparity between basic digital skills and collaborative competencies. Cluster analysis further demonstrates that age and previous occupational experience significantly influence digital literacy levels. These results highlight the heterogeneity of digital competence among older adults. Conclusions: The study concludes by emphasising the importance of implementing tailored policies that enhance digital literacy in this population. Key factors such as accessibility, training, and motivation should guide such efforts. Additionally, intergenerational learning emerges as a promising strategy, facilitating the development of digital skills through knowledge exchange and sustained support from younger cohorts.

Keywords: digital inclusion; older people; digital literacy; digital competence; digital divide; technological literacy

1. Introduction

Population ageing is a global phenomenon that is reshaping our societies. Increasing life expectancy, together with advances in medicine and improved living conditions, have led to a significant increase in the number of older people worldwide. As the United Nations (2017) points out, by 2050, a quarter or more of the world's population, except in Africa, will belong to this age group. This demographic shift poses new challenges and opportunities and requires an adaptation of our social and political structures. However, it is important to remember that ageing is not just a statistical fact but a biological and social process that implies new demands, relationships and interests, as Urrutia (2018) argues.

In this context, life satisfaction is a multifactorial construct that is influenced by various aspects, from individual characteristics to socio-environmental factors. Numerous studies have shown that life satisfaction is influenced by a wide range of factors, such as educational level, physical or mental health, economic status and psychosocial factors (Papi & Cheraghi, 2021; Phulkerd et al., 2021; Zhang et al., 2022; Banjare et al., 2015). Social support also emerges as a key factor. The presence of a partner or a strong family network is related to higher levels of life satisfaction. According to Chen (2022), geographical context significantly influences levels of well-being, finding significant differences between urban and rural areas and even within apparently homogeneous environments.

In this sense, in the case of older people, digital competence, understood as the ability to effectively use digital technologies to access information, communicate, carry out procedures and participate in the digital society, could emerge as a relevant factor in improving their overall well-being by facilitating access to information, fostering social connection and allowing greater autonomy in daily life. However, the digital divide, or the difficulty this group faces in accessing, using and benefiting from digital technologies compared to younger generations has been associated with inequalities in various aspects of life, such as fear and distrust of lack of digital skills, social isolation, limited access to essential services, communication opportunities or digital citizen participation, among others (Vizconde et al., 2025).

In the ageing process, the transition to retirement, children leaving home and the gradual reduction in interpersonal support networks often lead to substantial changes in the relational sphere of older people. These changes in the social structure increase the likelihood of experiencing adverse emotional states, such as loneliness, depression or anxiety, which are risk factors for overall well-being at this stage of life. The specialised literature has highlighted the need to address these psychosocial dimensions as a fundamental condition for promoting healthy ageing (Colombo & Gónzalez-Gónzalez, 2024). In this context, the potential of digital technologies as tools capable of promoting autonomy, delaying cognitive or functional decline, and contributing to the management of chronic diseases that are highly prevalent in this age group is recognised (Manheim et al., 2019; Peek et al., 2014). However, the health emergency resulting from the COVID-19 pandemic highlighted the heightened vulnerability of the population over 60 years of age, associated with both greater exposure to infection and comorbidities (Banerjee, 2020; Hwang et al., 2020) and an increase in psychosocial problems (isolation, stress, and feelings of loneliness) linked to lockdown and social distancing measures (Conroy et al., 2020).

Moreover, the COVID-19 pandemic has challenged traditional models of ageing, highlighting the importance of social participation and autonomy in older people. The adoption of digital technologies has been presented as a key strategy to promote active and healthy ageing. However, the existing digital divide has limited the access of many older people to technologies, which has had a negative impact on their quality of life and psychosocial well-being (Martínez-Alcalá et al., 2021; Ammar et al., 2021). Social distancing measures implemented during the pandemic have exacerbated this situation by restricting opportunities for social interaction and access to services for this population group. Previous research findings (Martins Van Jaarsveld, 2020; Seifert et al., 2020; Tsamakis et al., 2021) corroborate the relationship between digital inclusion and quality of life. According to Singh and Bajorek (2014), the restrictions faced by older people in the use of digital technologies cannot be understood in isolation but rather as the result of a network of biopsychosocial and sociodemographic factors, including health status, age, lifestyle habits, and gender differences. Therefore, the lack of digital skills in older people significantly reduces their ability to take advantage of the benefits offered by information and communication technologies. This situation limits their autonomy and can have a negative impact on their quality of life by restricting their access to services, information, and opportunities for social interaction.

The insufficient digital literacy of older people, coupled with the accelerating digitisation of society, has led to a situation where many feel forced to adopt technologies that they do not master. This forced adoption, far from being empowering, generates resistance and, in many cases, leads to frustration. As Martínez-Alcalá et al. (2021) and Ammar et al. (2021) point out, this tension between technological demands and the digital capabilities of older people has led to a feeling of exclusion and has hindered their full participation in the digital society. On the other hand, the perspective on ageing has evolved significantly in recent decades, moving from a negative view focused on decline to a more positive perspective that promotes active and fulfilling ageing (Triadó, 2018). In this sense, technologies offer great potential, allowing older people to stay connected, active and participative. However, for digital technologies to be truly beneficial to older people, they need to be adapted to their specific needs and capabilities. Digital inclusion, which involves designing technological solutions that are accessible and easy to use, is essential for them to be able to make the most of the opportunities offered by these technologies (Vizconde et al., 2025).

Therefore, the aim of this study is to assess the digital competence of older people according to the European DigComp 2.2 framework (Vuorikari & Holmes, 2022). Such an assessment is crucial because public policies and programmes delivered by governmental agencies and NGOs frequently rely on frameworks like DigComp to design inclusive digital literacy initiatives. For example, EU policy programmes seek to ensure that older people acquire basic digital skills as part of the Digital Decade goals, and civil society organisations often implement training tailored to seniors' needs in line with these standards (European Commission, 2023). By examining older adults' competence via DigComp 2.2, this research can provide evidence to improve the alignment of policy and NGO interventions with actual competence gaps, thereby enhancing digital inclusion in later life.

Based on the above, the following research question arises: Are older people prepared to face the digital and knowledge society, taking into account personal variables such as age and gender, geographical location, place of residence and type of cohabitation? To answer this question, this study assesses the digital competence levels of older people in order to identify the digital divides that impede the digital inclusion of this population group. To achieve this objective, the level of digital competence will be measured in a typical population sample of older people, and the existence of significant differences between the socio-demographic characteristics and the digital level of older people will be analysed.

2. Materials and Methods

This is quantitative research with a non-experimental cross-sectional design and a descriptive-comparative scope. The data were collected by means of surveys, using the questionnaire technique, applied to older people in their institutions of reference (day centres or residences) at a single point in time, with the aim of finding out the reality of their level of digital competence and analysing significant differences between groups of elderly people according to their age ranges. The analysis techniques used included descriptive statistics and cluster analysis for the segmented study of the sample, allowing us to examine these differences according to their digital competence and socio-demographic traits.

2.1. Participants

This research was carried out in eastern Spain, specifically in the province of Valencia (in its capital and some nearby towns) with people over 65 years of age. Valencia is one of the most populated cities in Spain, with a population of 176,838 older people, whose gender distribution is 40.7% men and 59.3% women, according to data published by the Statistics Office of the Valencia City Council in 2024 (Valencia City Council, 2024). Therefore, based on the sample size calculation for finite populations, with a confidence level of 95% and a margin of error of 5%, a sample of at least 384 subjects is necessary. To obtain the sample, day centres and residences for the elderly in certain neighbourhoods of Valencia and nearby towns were strategically and intentionally selected (rather than randomly). The study was presented to the relevant person in charge of each centre in order to request their voluntary collaboration. As a consequence of this sampling strategy, the sample is biased in terms of socioeconomic level, with a predominance of middle-class profiles. This limitation is mainly due to the geographical location of the participating institutions, which prevents full representation of existing socioeconomic diversity. Nevertheless, efforts were made to include participants with diverse profiles in terms of age, gender, and pre-retirement employment status to increase representativeness in these areas. Finally, there was a non-probabilistic purposive sample of 404 people over 65 years of age, of whom 35.71% were men and 64.29% were women, who freely participated in the study by means of a structured, self-administered survey.

2.2. Procedure

To carry out this study, a non-experimental and sectional research design was chosen, supervised and approved by the Ethics Committee of the Catholic University of Valencia (permit number UCV/2021-2022/155). This Committee reviewed and certified the necessary procedures on consent and voluntary participation, information on the purpose of the study, protection of personal data, as well as the guarantee of confidentiality and non-discrimination. Data were collected by means of a paper questionnaire, and an online pass was discarded due to the specific characteristics of the population analysed. Data collection took place between October 2023 and December 2024. To obtain a higher response rate, the sampling points were strategically selected in institutions for the elderly (residences and day centres). In these centres, in small groups and in different shifts, the criteria and purpose of the study were explained beforehand, so that the participants could better understand it and thus complete the questionnaire.

2.3. Instrument

The Basic Digital Competence Scale for Older People (DigCompB_PM) (Calero-Plaza et al., 2025) was used to collect the information. This scale is structured into four factors or dimensions and 16 items distributed as follows: F1-Online collaboration through digital devices (6 items), F2-Digital content creation, participation and simple searches (4 items), F3-Basic problem solving and networking training (3 items) and F4-Safety and knowledge of device use (3 items). It measures the digital competence of older adults at a basic level of acquisition of the specific sub-competences that comprise it, in accordance with the Digital Competence Framework for Citizens (Vuorikari & Holmes, 2022). As shown in Calero-Plaza et al. (2025), it has adequate psychometric properties both in terms of internal consistency with Cronbach's alpha above 0. 70 in the four factors (F1 $\alpha = 0.78$, F2 $\alpha = 0.79$, F3 $\alpha = 0.76$ and F4 $\alpha = 0.72$), as well as convergent and discriminant validity (with correlations above 0.85 in each of the four dimensions). The instrument has been validated for a specific sample of older people, so the items are numbered consecutively; their descriptions are simple and contain meaningful examples. Finally, there are three possible response options,

'I don't know how to do it', 'With assistant I can', 'I do it with a certain autonomy', which are appropriate to the context of the participant's profile. The instrument also includes an initial section to determine the socio-demographic characteristics of the elderly, which will be considered of crucial importance to contrast the digital profiles according to their typical characteristics. This section includes as intervening variables the place of residence (town or city), whether the elderly live alone, accompanied or in a residence, and the professional level of qualification they had before retirement.

2.4. Statistical Analysis

In terms of the statistical analyses carried out, an initial descriptive analysis was applied by calculating means, standard deviations, asymmetries, and kurtosis, which allowed an overall characterisation of the variables evaluated. In turn, for the segmentation of the sample, cluster analysis was used using the K-means method (K-means), a consolidated technique for classifying individuals into homogeneous groups according to various variables (Everitt et al., 2011). The selection of the optimal number of clusters was made by evaluating various solutions (between 2 and 5 clusters) based on specific statistical criteria such as the coefficient of determination (R^2), which reflects the percentage of variance explained by the segmentation obtained; the Akaike information index (AIC) and Bayesian information index (BIC), commonly used to determine the parsimony of the model (Burnham & Anderson, 2004); as well as the Silhouette index, which assesses the quality of separation and internal cohesion of the clusters (Rousseeuw, 1987). The final selection of three clusters was based on the convergence of multiple indicators ($R^2 = 0.64$, BIC = 651.88, Silhouette = 0.35, Dunn's index = 0.07, Calinski-Harabasz index = 356.89). Taken together, these values reflect an adequate balance between model parsimony and classification quality, justifying the three-group solution over other alternatives. Finally, to ensure the robustness of the chosen solution, the Dunn and Calinski-Harabasz indices were additionally calculated to validate the results of the cluster analysis (Dunn, 1974; Calinski & Harabasz, 1974).

In addition, to analyse differences based on categorical variables, a contingency analysis was performed using the chi-squared test (χ^2), which allows for the detection of associations between nominal or categorical variables (Agresti, 2013). Finally, in order to determine the existence of statistically significant differences between the clusters identified using K-means, a one-way analysis of variance (ANOVA) was carried out, a statistical procedure recommended for comparing means of three or more independent groups (Hair et al., 2014). All statistical analyses performed in this study were carried out using the JASP statistical package (version 0.19.1).

3. Results

3.1. Characteristics of Participating Users and Levels of Digital Competence According to the Scale of Basic Digital Competence in Older Adults (DigCompB_PM) Administered

The results obtained allow us to identify a general profile of the elderly participant. It is observed that it is a female person, thus fulfilling the general rule that indicates that life expectancy among women is higher than among men (National Institute of Statistics (INE) (2024)), with an average age of 75.97 years (SD = 6.83) and 65 years being the minimum age and 99 the maximum. 28.71% reside in the city of Valencia, while 71.28% come from nearby towns; 30% live alone, 56.67% live with a partner or family, and 13.33% live in nursing homes. Lastly, in terms of the level of qualification in the profession they exercised before retirement, 49.04% of the sample had no qualifications at all, compared with the remaining 50.96% who exercised some kind of management position in their respective jobs, whether senior, intermediate or technical.

Looking at the descriptive analysis of the results for each of the dimensions assessed, as shown in Figure 1, the dimension with the highest mean score was 'Safety and knowledge of device use (F4 SA)', with an mean of M = 2.13 (SD = 0.74) and a reliability index of $\alpha = 0.72$. Next, the dimension 'Digital content creation, participation and simple searches (F2 DC)' had an average rating of M = 2.11 (SD = 0.73) and a reliability index of $\alpha = 0.82$. Regarding the other dimensions, 'Basic problem solving and network training (F3 BT)' had a lower average rating of M = 1.69 (SD = 0.72) and, finally, the dimension with the lowest score was 'Online collaboration using digital devices (F1 OC)', with an average rating of M = 1.57 (SD = 0.59).

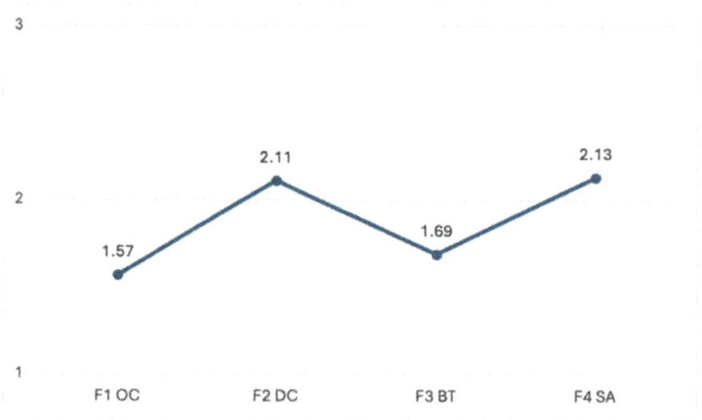

Figure 1. Average level of Digital Competence in Older People according to the Scale of Basic Digital Competence in Older Adults (DigCompB_PM). Note: Axis X: F1 OC: Online collaboration through digital devices; F2 DC: Digital content creation, participation and simple searches; F3 BT: Basic troubleshooting and networking training; F4 SA: Safety and knowledge of use of the devices. Axis Y: 1: I don't know how to do it 2: With assistance I can 3: I do it with a certain autonomy.

In terms of distribution, all scales showed moderate skewness (between −0.26 and 0.90) and negative kurtosis (from −1.32 to −0.22). These results indicate that the four dimensions provide consistent and reliable measures of the digital competencies assessed in the sample. These results can be seen in Table 1.

Table 1. Descriptive and reliability statistics for digital competence dimensions.

	Mean	**SD**	**Skewness**	**Kurtosis**
F1 OC: Online collaboration through digital devices (α Cronbach = 0.82)				
OC1—I can collaborate online with other people (e.g., with Google Drive, Dropbox...).	1.40	0.73	1.48	0.51
OC2—I am aware of the data privacy policy of Internet programs (e.g., WhatsApp).	1.58	0.85	0.91	−0.99
OC3—I know how to participate in online citizen surveys (e.g., via WhatsApp, email, social networks...).	1.58	0.79	0.89	−0.83
OC4—I know how to detect inappropriate behavior in the use of cell phones or other devices.	1.72	0.87	0.57	−1.43
OC5—I know how to add text and tags to other people's videos or photos with my cell phone.	1.64	0.84	0.75	−1.17
OC6—I know how to search for (Internet) images without copyright (without CopyRight).	1.49	0.78	1.16	−0.35
Total	1.57	0.59	0.90	−0.22

Table 1. *Cont.*

	Mean	SD	Skewness	Kurtosis
F2 DC: Digital content creation, participation and simple searches (α Cronbach = 0.84)				
DC1—I know how to send photos, videos or messages over the Internet, e.g., WhatsApp messages).	2.28	0.86	−0.57	−1.42
DC2—I can participate in Internet groups, video calls, networks. . . (e.g., through WhatsApp).	2.17	0.87	−0.34	−1.61
DC3—I know how to detect if the information that comes to me through the Internet (e.g., WhatsApp, Google, Mail. . .), is true or not.	1.87	0.90	0.26	−1.72
DC4—I know how to search for information on the Internet (e.g., through Google).	2.10	0.88	−0.19	−1.68
Total	2.11	0.73	−0.26	−1.32
F3 BT: Basic troubleshooting and networking training (α Cronbach = 0.76)				
BT1—I know how to change font sizes, change language, adapt screens, . . .	1.64	0.84	0.76	−1.15
BT2—I know how to solve simple technical problems (e.g., connect wifi, change battery. . .).	1.68	0.86	0.66	−1.33
BT3—I learn with the Internet (e.g., watching video tutorials, reading google pages, . . .).	1.75	0.91	0.50	−1.61
Total	1.69	0.72	0.58	−1.09
F4 SA: Safety and knowledge of use of the devices (α Cronbach = 0.72)				
SA1—I know that cell phone addiction can cause physical and psychological damage.	2.37	0.89	−0.81	−1.25
SA2—I am aware of the environmental impacts of cell phone use (e.g., carbon emissions, pollution from telecommunication towers. . .).	1.92	0.96	0.16	−1.90
SA3—I know what personal data I can and cannot send.	2.09	0.93	−0.18	−1.83
Total	2.13	0.74	−0.31	−1.28

3.2. Cluster Analysis

To identify homogeneous clusters in the sample (*n* = 404), a cluster analysis was carried out using the K-means method. The optimal solution corresponded to three clusters, determined using the Bayesian information criterion (BIC) and corroborated by an R^2 value of 0.64. The Silhouette index obtained (0.35) indicates adequate internal cohesion, although it shows moderate intergroup separation. This value suggests that the cluster structure is statistically acceptable in terms of differentiation between profiles. In conjunction with the parsimony indicators (AIC and BIC) and internal validity (Dunn and Calinski-Harabasz indices), the three-cluster solution can be considered consistent, although the delimitation between groups should be interpreted with caution. The optimal solution corresponded to three clusters, selected on the basis of the Bayesian information criterion (BIC) and supported by a Silhouette index of 0.35, reflecting adequate internal cohesion and moderate external separation. The quality indicators obtained are shown in Table 2.

Table 2. Quality indicators of the cluster model.

Clusters	*n*	R^2	AIC	BIC	Silhouette
3	404	0.64	603.86	651.88	0.35

Note. R^2 = variance; AIC = Akaike's information criterion; BIC = Bayesian information criterion; Silhouette = silhouette index.

As can be seen, this solution explains 64% of the total variance (R^2 = 0.64), indicating that the three identified clusters manage to capture a considerable proportion of the heterogeneity present in the data. Specifically, Cluster 1 (n = 95) explains 18% of the heterogeneity, Cluster 2 (n = 142) explains 30% and Cluster 3 (n = 167) 51%, thus showing a differentiated and significant distribution in the sample analysed. Furthermore, the sum of squares between clusters was 1032.14, out of a total sum of squares of 1612, reflecting an adequate separation. This solution was also supported by the Silhouette index (0.35), together with other indicators such as Dunn's index (0.07), the Calinski-Harabasz index (356.89), the maximum diameter (4.10) and the minimum separation (0.28), which endorse the statistical quality and validity of the segmentation obtained.

3.3. Cluster Profile

Looking at the profile of the clusters, Cluster 1 is characterised by positive scores on all dimensions (F1 = 1.46, F2 = 1.07, F3 = 1.27, F4 = 0.87), suggesting a group with a broader mastery of digital skills, both in online collaboration and in content creation, problem solving and device safety. In contrast, Cluster 2 shows negative or clearly lower scores (F1 = −0.80, F2 = −1.07, F3 = −0.82, F4 = −0.91). This pattern indicates lower proficiency in all four digital dimensions, suggesting lower participation in online collaboration, low initiative in content creation, difficulty in basic problem solving and lower knowledge of digital safety. Finally, Cluster 3 shows intermediate values (F1 = −0.15, F2 = 0.30, F3 = −0.03, F4 = 0.28), suggesting a hybrid profile: they handle certain collaboration and security tools in an acceptable way, although they do not show the same overall strength as Cluster 1, nor do they lag as far behind as Cluster 2.

Figure 2 shows the density graph for each of the clusters (pink: 1, green: 2 and blue: 3), with clearly differentiated distribution patterns in the four dimensions of digital competences: F1 (Online collaboration using digital devices), F2 (Digital content creation, participation and simple search), F3 (Basic problem solving and networking) and F4 (Safety and knowledge of device use). Cluster 1 (pink) is mostly concentrated in positive values, indicating a high and fairly uniform level across all dimensions, while Cluster 2 (green) shows very sharp peaks around negative values, indicating lower digital literacy, and Cluster 3 (blue) shows an intermediate profile with somewhat more dispersed distributions centred around values close to zero. These graphical differences are consistent with the statistical results, as they confirm the existence of three distinct profiles in terms of digital competences within the sample.

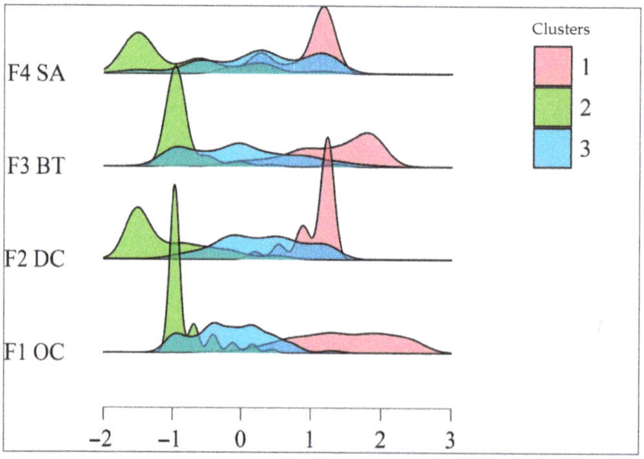

Figure 2. Graph of cluster densities. Note: F1 OC: Online collaboration through digital devices; F2 DC: Digital content creation, participation and simple searches; F3 BT: Basic troubleshooting and networking training; F4 SA: Safety and knowledge of use of the devices.

3.4. Cluster Contrast

To determine whether significant differences exist between the identified clusters, an ANOVA was conducted for each of the four factors assessed. The results (Table 3) showed high levels of significance ($p < 0.001$) in all dimensions, confirming the presence of statistically significant differences between the clusters. This analysis of variance shows that the clusters present differentiated distributions in each factor, reflecting different levels of competence in the dimensions assessed (Table 3). Thus, the segmentation obtained by means of K-means is supported by the statistical results, indicating that the identified clusters have distinctive characteristics consistent with the expected structure.

Table 3. Comparison of means in the dimensions of digital competences between clusters.

Factor	Cluster	Mean	DE	F	*p*
F1 OC: Online collaboration through digital devices	1	2.42	0.40	469.88	<0.001
	2	1.10	0.19		
	3	1.48	0.32		
F2 DC: Digital content creation, participation and simple searches	1	2.88	0.21	707.68	<0.001
	2	1.33	0.42		
	3	2.33	0.44		
F3 BT: Basic troubleshooting and networking training	1	2.60	0.45	419.79	<0.001
	2	1.11	0.30		
	3	1.67	0.54		
F4 SA: Safety and knowledge of use of the devices	1	2.78	0.33	244.81	<0.001
	2	1.46	0.58		
	3	2.33	0.57		

In terms of socio-demographic variables, the mean age of the participants varies between the groups, with Cluster 1 being the youngest (M = 72.91 years; SD = 5.87), Cluster 2 being the oldest (M = 79.50 years; SD = 7.43) and Cluster 3 being somewhere in between (M = 76.87 years; SD = 6.76). A chi-squared analysis was then calculated to determine the distribution for each of the clusters (Table 4). About the socio-demographic variables analysed, for the variable 'Sex',[1] no statistically significant associations were observed ($\chi^2 = 3.96$, gl = 2, $p = 0.14$) in the distribution between the groups, as the proportions of men and women were similarly distributed in the three groups. Likewise, neither the variable 'Do you live'[2] ($\chi^2 = 7.71$, gl = 4, $p = 0.10$) nor 'Locality'[3] ($\chi^2 = 1.13$, gl = 2, $p = 0.57$) showed significant associations with cluster membership. These results suggest that differences between clusters do not depend on gender, geographical area or where participants live. In turn, the variable 'Professional_qualification'[4] showed a significant association with cluster distribution ($\chi^2 = 71.50$, gl = 8, $p < 0.001$). It is observed that the lowest categories of professional level are mostly concentrated in Clusters 2 and 3 (48.98% and 41.33%, respectively), while in the highest professional levels there is a higher proportion of individuals belonging to Cluster 1. This result indicates that professional level is related to membership in each cluster, reflecting that those with higher professional training or experience tend to cluster in clusters with better digital competences.

Table 4. Distribution of clusters according to sociodemographic variables.

Variable	Cluster			X^2 (gl)	*p*
		Sex			
1—Male	29.41%	32.35%	38.24%	3.96 (2)	0.14
2—Female	20.52%	36.57%	42.91%		
		Do you live			
1—Alone	16.96%	38.39%	44.64%	7.71 (4)	0.10
2—Accompanied	27.92%	31.67%	40.42%		
3—Residence	17.31%	44.23%	38.46%		
		Locality			
1—Town	22.11%	35.44%	42.46%	1.13 (2)	0.57
2—City	26.89%	34.45%	38.66%		
		Professional qualification			
1—Senior management	42.11%	21.05%	36.84%	71.50 (8)	<0.001
2—Middle management	38.98%	18.64%	42.37%		
3—Senior technician	53.19%	12.77%	34.04%		
4—Middle technician	18.75%	32.81%	48.44%		
5—Unqualified	9.69%	48.98%	41.33%		

Note. X^2 = chi-squared; gl = degrees of freedom.

4. Discussion

The results obtained in this study reflect a complex reality regarding the digital competence of older people, showing the existence of significant gaps that limit their digital inclusion. In line with previous studies (Charness & Boot, 2022; Rosales & Fernández-Ardèvol, 2020; Vizconde et al., 2025), it is confirmed that the digital literacy of this age group is not homogeneous, with differences depending on various socio-demographic variables. These findings are particularly relevant in a context in which the digitisation of essential services, such as banking, health and public administration, requires older people to have a level of digital competence that they have often not acquired in a formal way.

One of the most relevant findings of this study was the identification of the dimensions with the highest scores on the Digital Competences Scale for Older People (DigCompB_PM) (Calero-Plaza et al., 2025), which were security and knowledge of the use of digital devices (M = 2.13), while the dimension with the lowest score was online collaboration using digital devices (M = 1.57). This result is consistent with previous research that has indicated that older people tend to develop basic skills for interacting with electronic devices but show difficulties in the advanced use of collaborative digital tools and in generating their own content (Gallistl et al., 2020). This situation may be due to a predominantly individual learning model in this age group, where digital interactions tend to focus on family communication and information seeking, rather than collaborative work or content production (Quan-Haase et al., 2018).

In this vein, recent studies have shown that loneliness in old age is associated with independent living, low educational levels, and other specific sociodemographic factors (Pham et al., 2021; Leukel et al., 2023; Zhao et al., 2021). To mitigate these conditions of isolation, mechanisms have been proposed to encourage social participation among older adults by improving their access to information, innovation, and health (Balboni et al., 2011). However, fear of technology can exacerbate perceptions of isolation and limit digital interaction (Conroy et al., 2020). Likewise, barriers associated with the acquisition and use of technology, such as insecurity about data protection, lack of experience, or difficulty in requesting help, directly affect the development of digital competences (Zhao et al., 2021;

Hodge et al., 2017; Reis et al., 2021). These limitations have a particularly strong impact on the areas of communication and collaboration in the DigComp framework, where there is a decline in the ability of older people to interact and actively participate in digital environments (Vuorikari & Holmes, 2022).

Despite these limitations, several authors have suggested that social media and digital platforms can become meaningful spaces for interaction that not only strengthen social ties but also contribute to the acquisition of digital skills (Falloon, 2020; Dzokoto et al., 2019; Silva et al., 2020; Tirado-Morueta et al., 2020; Ibarra et al., 2020). This social dimension of the Internet provides additional benefits, such as strengthening critical thinking and developing problem-solving strategies. Likewise, for these benefits to materialise, it is necessary to guarantee the accessibility and usability of devices (Román-García et al., 2016), as well as free and equitable access to the Internet, understood as an indispensable condition for promoting active ageing and full digital participation (Tirado-Morueta et al., 2020; Silva et al., 2020; Kim et al., 2022; Reis et al., 2021; Ibarra et al., 2020; Jin et al., 2019).

Furthermore, the results of the cluster analysis have allowed us to segment the sample into different digital competence profiles, showing that factors such as age and previous work experience significantly influence the level of digital literacy of older people. These findings are consistent with those reported by Van Deursen and Helsper (2018), who show that the lack of early exposure to technology and the absence of structured training are important barriers to the acquisition of digital skills in this population group. This reinforces the idea that digital literacy cannot be considered a spontaneous process in older people but requires specific educational interventions adapted to their learning pace.

A key aspect identified in this study is that older people show difficulties in digital problem solving and network participation, with a score close to the average (M = 1.69) in the corresponding dimension. This finding is relevant because, although some older adults manage to develop basic skills in the use of devices, many others still have difficulties in more advanced digital interaction. This reinforces the idea that lack of confidence in their own technological capabilities is one of the main obstacles to older adults' participation in complex digital environments (Rosales & Fernández-Ardèvol, 2020). Technological anxiety, understood as the fear of making mistakes or damaging devices, remains a limiting factor preventing full adoption of digital technologies in this group (Czaja et al., 2020).

Furthermore, the analysis of socio-demographic variables has identified that previous educational level and professional qualifications have a significant impact on the development of digital skills in old age. This is also in line with Czaja et al. (2020) who suggest that older people with more professional experience in sectors that have required the use of technology have higher levels of digital competence. This finding reinforces the need to develop differentiated training strategies that not only consider age as the main criterion but also integrate the educational and employment background of the participants.

On the other hand, the lack of accessibility and usability of digital tools remains a fundamental barrier to the technological inclusion of older people. This study confirms that many technological interfaces are not designed with the sensory and cognitive abilities of this age group in mind. Difficulty in using tactile devices, the absence of intuitive interfaces and the complexity of some digital processes have been identified as recurrent issues. Previous research has highlighted the need to develop more inclusive technologies, with an older user-centred design and customisation options adapted to their specific needs (Seifert & Rössel, 2022).

5. Conclusions

This research reaffirms the need for public policies that promote digital literacy in older people from an inclusive perspective and adapt to their particularities. Although there are institutional efforts to reduce the digital divide in this age group, the data obtained show that there are still significant challenges in terms of accessibility, training and motivation to use digital tools.

From a social perspective, the results obtained reinforce the idea that the digital literacy of older people should not only be understood as a question of access but also of active participation in the digital society. For these benefits to be effectively achieved, continuous support in the digital learning process is necessary. In this sense, the implementation of intergenerational training programmes can be an effective strategy for the development of digital skills in older people by facilitating learning through the exchange of knowledge with younger generations.

However, this study has some limitations that need to be considered. Firstly, the sample was selected using a non-probabilistic intentional procedure which, although adequate for statistical analysis, limits the possibility of generalising the findings to the entire elderly population. Consequently, the results should be interpreted with caution, as the size and composition of the sample may not reflect the socioeconomic and cultural diversity of this group in other contexts. Furthermore, as this is a cross-sectional study, it is not possible to analyse the evolution of digital competence over time. Secondly, the Silhouette index value reflects acceptable internal cohesion but only moderate separation between groups, which limits the clarity of the segmentation obtained. Finally, the self-administered nature of the questionnaire may have introduced bias in the responses, as some participants may have required support to understand or complete the items. Another limitation to consider is that the information was obtained through self-report questionnaires. Although the scale used has adequate validity and reliability indicators, this method of data collection may be conditioned by the subjective perceptions of the participants or by social desirability biases, which could partially affect the accuracy and objectivity of the responses. Taken together, these limitations reinforce the need to interpret the results with caution and to validate the findings through future studies with larger samples and longitudinal approaches. As for future lines of research, longitudinal studies are suggested to analyse the sustained impact of digital literacy programmes, as well as to explore in greater depth the role of emotional and motivational factors in the digital learning of older people. It would also be valuable to investigate the effectiveness of specific pedagogical methodologies, such as intergenerational learning or the use of adapted accessible technologies, in different geographical and social contexts.

In conclusion, this research contributes to the knowledge on digital competence in the elderly, highlighting the need for specific and contextualised training strategies. The evidence obtained allows for the design of more effective and personalised training programmes, according to the resulting specific groups or clusters, thus promoting greater digital autonomy in the elderly and favouring their integration in an increasingly digitalised society.

Author Contributions: Conceptualization, R.F.-P., R.J.G.-G., R.S.-P. and J.C.-P.; methodology, R.F.-P., R.J.G.-G., R.S.-P. and J.C.-P.; formal analysis, R.F.-P., R.J.G.-G., R.S.-P. and J.C.-P.; investigation, R.F.-P., R.J.G.-G., R.S.-P. and J.C.-P.; writing—original draft preparation, R.F.-P., R.J.G.-G., R.S.-P. and J.C.-P.; writing—review and editing, R.F.-P., R.J.G.-G., R.S.-P. and J.C.-P. All authors have read and agreed to the published version of the manuscript.

Funding: This research received no external funding.

Institutional Review Board Statement: The study was conducted in accordance with the Declaration of Helsinki and approved by the Institutional Review Board (or Ethics Commit-tee) of ETHICS COMMITTEE OF THE CATHOLIC UNIVERSITY OF VALENCIA (permit number UCV/2021-2022/155).

Informed Consent Statement: Informed consent was obtained from all subjects involved in the study.

Data Availability Statement: Data from this research may be requested from the authors.

Conflicts of Interest: The authors declare no conflicts of interest.

Notes

1 Sex: Male | Female | Prefer not to say.
2 Do you live: Alone | Accompanied or with family members | In residence.
3 Locality: Town | City.
4 Professional qualification: Senior management | Middle management | Senior technician | Middle technician | Unqualified.

References

Agresti, A. (2013). *Categorical data analysis* (3rd ed.). Wiley.

Ammar, A., Bouaziz, B., Trabelsi, K., Glenn, J., Zmijewski, P., Müller, P., Hamdi, C., Jmaiel, M., Chamari, K., Driss, T., & Hökelmann, A. (2021). Applying digital technology to promote active and healthy confinement lifestyle during pandemics in the elderly. *Biology of Sport, 38*(3), 391–396. [CrossRef]

Balboni, M., Rovira, S., & Vergara, S. (2011). *ICT in Latin America. A microdata analysis*. Editorial ECLAC.

Banerjee, D. (2020). The impact of COVID-19 pandemic on elderly mental health. *International Journal of Geriatric Psychiatry, 35*(12), 1466–1467. [CrossRef]

Banjare, P., Dwivedi, R., & Pradhan, J. (2015). Factors associated with the life satisfaction amongst the rural elderly in Odisha, India. *Health and Quality of Life Outcomes, 13*, 201. [CrossRef]

Burnham, K., & Anderson, D. (2004). Multimodel inference: Understanding AIC and BIC in model selection. *Sociological Methods & Research, 33*(2), 261–304. [CrossRef]

Calero-Plaza, J., González-García, R. J., & Fernández-Piqueras, R. (2025). Validation of a scale to measure digital competence in the elderly population. *International Journal of Instruction, 18*(1), 77–94. [CrossRef]

Calinski, T., & Harabasz, J. (1974). A dendrite method for cluster analysis. *Communications in Statistics-Theory and Methods, 3*(1), 1–27. [CrossRef]

Charness, N., & Boot, W. R. (2022). A grand challenge for psychology: Reducing the age-related digital divide. *Psychological Sciencei, 31*(2), 187–193. [CrossRef]

Chen, C. Y. (2022). What makes older adults happier? Urban and rural differences in the living arrangements and life satisfaction of older adults. *Journal of Housing and the Built Environment, 37*(3), 1131–1157. [CrossRef]

Colombo, L., & Gónzalez-Gónzalez, C. S. (2024). Inclusión tecnológica y competencias digitales en personas mayores: Hacia un envejecimiento activo y conectado. *Campus Virtuales, 13*(2), 199–213. [CrossRef]

Conroy, K. M., Krishnan, S., Mittelstaedt, S., & Patel, S. S. (2020). Technological advancements to address elderly loneliness: Practical considerations and community resilience implications for COVID-19 pandemic. *Working with Older People, 24*(4), 257–264. [CrossRef]

Czaja, S. J., Boot, W. R., Charness, N., & Rogers, W. A. (2020). *Designing for older adults: Principles and creative human factors approaches*. CRC Press.

Dunn, J. C. (1974). Well-separated clusters and optimal fuzzy partitions. *Journal of Cybernetics, 4*(1), 95–104. [CrossRef]

Dzokoto, G., Atiogbe, A., Agbe, A., Mensah, H., Mate-Kole, C., Dzorgbo, D.-B., & Dovie, D. (2019). Generational perspective of digital literacy among Ghanaians in the 21st century: Wither now? *Media Studies, 10*, 127–152. [CrossRef]

European Commission. (2023). *Digital decade policy programme 2030*. Shaping Europe's Digital Future. Available online: https://digital-strategy.ec.europa.eu/en/library/digital-decade-policy-programme-2030 (accessed on 10 March 2024).

Everitt, B. S., Landau, S., Leese, M., & Stahl, D. (2011). *Cluster analysis* (5th ed.). Wiley.

Falloon, G. (2020). From digital literacy to digital competence: The teacher digital competency (TdC) framework. *Educational Technology Research and Development, 68*, 2449–2472. [CrossRef]

Gallistl, V., Rohner, R., Seifert, A., & Wanka, A. (2020). Configuring the older non-user: Between research, policy and practice of digital exclusion. *Social Inclusion, 8*(2), 233–243. [CrossRef]

Hair, J. F., Black, W. C., Babin, B. J., & Anderson, R. E. (2014). *Multivariate data analysis* (7th ed.). Pearson Education Limited.

Hodge, H., Carson, D., Carson, D., Newman, L., & Garrett, J. (2017). Using internet technologies in rural communities to access services: The views of older people and service providers. *Journal of Rural Studies, 54*, 469–478. [CrossRef]

Hwang, T., Rabheru, K., Peisah, C., Reichman, W., & Ikeda, M. (2020). Loneliness and social isolation during the COVID-19 pandemic. *International Psychogeriatrics, 32*(10), 1217–1220. [CrossRef] [PubMed]

Ibarra, F., Baez, M., Cernuzzi, L., & Casati, F. (2020). A systematic review on technology-supported interventions to improve old-age social wellbeing: Loneliness, social isolation, and connectedness. *Journal of Healthcare Engineering, 2020*, 2036842. [CrossRef] [PubMed]

Jin, B., Kim, J., & Baumgartner, L. M. (2019). Informal learning of older adults in using mobile devices: A review of the literature. *Adult Education Quarterly*, *69*(2), 120–141. [CrossRef]

Kim, J., Gray, J. A., Ciesla, J. R., & Yao, P. (2022). The impact of an internet use promotion programme on communication, internet use, and the extent of social networks among low-income older adults. *Ageing* International, *47*, 348–371. [CrossRef]

Leukel, J., Schehl, B., & Sugumaran, V. (2023). Digital inequality among older adults: Explaining differences in the breadth of Internet use. *Information,* Communication & Society, *26*(1), 139–154. [CrossRef]

Manheim, I., Schwartz, E., Xi, W., Buttigieg, S. C., Mcdonnell-naughton, M., Wouters, E. J. M., & Van Zaalen, Y. (2019). Inclusion of older adults in the research and design of digital technology. *International Journal of Environmental Research and Public health*, *16*(19), 3718. [CrossRef]

Martins Van Jaarsveld, G. (2020). The effects of COVID-19 among the elderly population: A case for closing the digital divide. *Frontiers in Psychiatry*, *11*, 1211. [CrossRef]

Martínez-Alcalá, C. I., Rosales-Lagarde, A., Pérez-Pérez, Y. M., Lopez-Noguerola, J. S., Bautista-Díaz, M. L., & Agis-Juarez, R. A. (2021). The effects of Covid-19 on the digital literacy of the elderly: Norms for digital inclusion. *Frontiers in Education*, *6*, 716025. [CrossRef]

National Institute of Statistics (INE). (2024). *Mujeres y hombres en España: Salud (actualizado 20 de febrero de 2024)*. INE. Available online: https://www.ine.es/ss/Satellite?L=es_ES&c=INESeccion_C&cid=1259926380048&p=1254735110672&pagename=ProductosYServicios%2FPYSLayout&param1=PYSDetalle&param3=1259924822888 (accessed on 10 March 2024).

Papi, S., & Cheraghi, M. (2021). Multiple factors associated with life satisfaction in older adults. *Menopause Review*, *20*(1), 69–75. [CrossRef]

Peek, S. T. M., Wouters, E. J. M., Van Hoof, J., Luijkx, K. G., Boeije, H. R., & Vrijhoef, H. J. M. (2014). Factors influencing acceptance of technology for aging in place: A systematic review. *International Journal of Medical Informatics*, *83*(4), 235–248. [CrossRef] [PubMed]

Pham, M., Singh, K., & Jahnke, I. (2021). Socio-technical-pedagogical usability of online courses for older adult learners. *Interactive Learning Environments*, *31*(5), 2855–2871. [CrossRef]

Phulkerd, S., Thapsuwan, S., Chamratrithirong, A., & Gray, R. S. (2021). Influence of healthy lifestyle behaviors on life satisfaction in the aging population of Thailand: A national population-based survey. *BMC Public Health*, *21*(1), 43. [CrossRef] [PubMed]

Quan-Haase, A., Mo, G. Y., & Wellman, B. (2018). Connected seniors: How older adults in East York exchange social support online and offline. *Information, Communication & Society*, *21*(5), 680–695. [CrossRef]

Reis, L., Mercer, K., & Boger, J. (2021). Technologies for fostering intergenerational connectivity and relationships: Scoping review and emergent concepts. *Technology in Society*, *64*, 101494. [CrossRef]

Román-García, S., Almansa-Martínez, A., & Cruz-Díaz, M. (2016). Adults and elders and their use of ICTs. Media competence of digital immigrants. *Comunicar*, *49*, 101–110. [CrossRef]

Rosales, A., & Fernández-Ardèvol, M. (2020). Ageism in the era of digital platforms. *Convergence*, *26*(5–6), 1074–1087. [CrossRef]

Rousseeuw, P. J. (1987). Silhouettes: A graphical aid to the interpretation and validation of cluster analysis. *Journal of Computational and Applied Mathematics*, *20*, 53–65. [CrossRef]

Seifert, A., Cotten, S. R., & Xie, B. (2020). A double burden of exclusion? Digital and social exclusion of older adults in times of COVID-19. *Journals of Gerontology: Series B*, *76*(3), e99–e103. [CrossRef]

Seifert, A., & Rössel, J. (2022). Digital participation. In *Encyclopedia of gerontology and population aging* (pp. 1446–1450). Springer International Publishing.

Silva, P., Delerue, A., & Martínez Pecino, R. (2020). Can the internet reduce the loneliness of 50+ living alone? *Information, Communication & Society*, *25*(1), 17–33. [CrossRef]

Singh, S., & Bajorek, B. (2014). defining 'elderly' in clinical practice guidelines for pharmacotherapy. *Pharmacy Practice*, *12*(4), 489. [CrossRef] [PubMed]

Tirado-Morueta, R., Aguaded-Gómez, J. I., Ortíz-Sobrino, M. Á., Rodríguez-Martín, A., & Álvarez-Arregui, E. (2020). Determinants of social gratifications obtained by older adults moderated by public supports for internet access in Spain. *Telematics and Informatics*, *49*, 101363. [CrossRef]

Triadó, C. (2018). Active ageing, generativity and learning. *Aula Abierta*, *47*(1), 63–66. [CrossRef]

Tsamakis, K., Tsiptsios, D., Ouranidis, A., Mueller, C., Schizas, D., Terniotis, C., Nikolakakis, N., Tyros, G., Kympouropoulos, S., Lazaris, A., Spandidos, D. A., Smyrnis, N., & Rizos, E. (2021). COVID-19 and its consequences on mental health. *Experimental and Therapeutic Medicine*, *21*(3), 244. [CrossRef]

United Nations. (2017). *World population prospects: The 2017 revision—Key findings and advance tables* (Working Paper No. ESA/P/WP/248). United Nations, Department of Economic and Social Affairs, Population Division.

Urrutia, A. (2018). Envejecimiento active: Un paradigma para comprender y gobernar. *Aula Abierta*, *47*(1), 29–36. [CrossRef]

Valencia City Council. (2024). *Municipal census of inhabitants: Over 64 years old*. Available online: https://www.valencia.es/estadistica/Padron/2024/Mayores64_2024_Cast.pdf (accessed on 10 March 2024).

Van Deursen, A. J., & Helsper, E. J. (2018). Collateral benefits of Internet use: Explaining the diverse outcomes of engaging with the Internet. *New Media & Society*, *20*(7), 2333–2351. [CrossRef]

Vizconde, E., Ferreira, S., & Medina, A. (2025). Competencias digitales para la inclusión de personas mayores: Políticas, desafíos, innovaciones tecnológicas y reducción de desigualdades. *Revista Derechos Humanos y Educación*, *1*(11), 147–166.

Vuorikari, R., & Holmes, W. (2022). *DigComp 2.2. Annex 2. Citizens interacting with AI systems*. Publication Office of the European Union.

Zhang, K., Pei, J., Wang, S., Rokpelnis, K., & Yu, X. (2022). Life satisfaction in China, 2010–2018: Trends and unique determinants. *Applied Research in Quality of Life*, *17*, 2311–2348. [CrossRef]

Zhao, S., Kinshuk, Y., & Ya, N. (2021). Adoption of mobile social media for learning among Chinese older adults in senior citizen colleges. *Educational Technology Research and Development*, *69*(6), 3413–3435. [CrossRef] [PubMed]

European Journal of
Investigation in Health, Psychology and Education

MDPI

Article

A Bayesian Structural Equation Model to Predict Quality of Life in European Older Adults

José M. Tomás *, Aitana Sanz and Zaira Torres

Department of Methodology for the Behavioral Sciences, University of Valencia, 46010 Valencia, Spain; aisanzde@alumni.uv.es (A.S.); zaira.torres@uv.es (Z.T.)
* Correspondence: tomasjm@uv.es

Abstract

The ultimate goal of developed societies is to age with quality of life, but this concept is broad, and few studies have addressed which variables specifically affect its dimensions. This study aims to test a model for predicting the impact of frailty, pain, and loneliness on the four dimensions of quality of life (control, autonomy, pleasure, and self-realization). Data were drawn from a sample of 61,355 Europeans from the Wave 7 of the SHARE project, aged 60 or older (M = 71.87, SD = 8.22), from which 55.9% were females. Statistical analyses included a fully Bayesian structural equation model that evidences the significant effect of loneliness, frailty, and pain on the four dimensions of quality of life. The variables have an unequal impact on the different dimensions' loneliness was the main predictor for the dimensions control, autonomy, and pleasure, while frailty was the main predictor to self-realization. This study supports the need to address these variables to intervene on the different aspects of quality of life in old age.

Keywords: aging; frailty; loneliness; pain; quality of life; Bayesian structural equation model

1. Introduction

The World Health Organization (WHO, 2024) defines older adults as individuals aged 60 and above. This demographic group is expected to double by 2050, reaching more than 1.5 billion older adults (UN-Population, 2020). Population aging is particularly pronounced in Europe, where 21.2% of the population was 65 years or older in 2022 (Eurostat, 2023). Europeans are living longer, but with multiple health conditions or mobility limitations in their later years (Eurostat, 2020). As a result, promoting successful aging, characterized by a high quality of life (QoL) has become a central priority in Europe. To achieve this goal, we first need to understand the key factors that influence the quality of life in old age.

In this regard, the Preventive Corrective Proactive (PCP) model, developed by Kahana and Kahana, stands out for its comprehensive approach to understanding successful aging (Kahana et al., 2012; Kahana et al., 2014). The PCP model understands QoL and well-being as the last outcome of the following five components: the self-evaluation of success, life satisfaction, meaning in life, positive affect, and life-value activity (Kahana et al., 2014). The PCP model also considers preventive and corrective strategies, as well as stressors, that influence the QoL of older adults. Preventive actions include health promotion, future planning, and other proactive measures (Petretto et al., 2016). In terms of stressors, the PCP model emphasizes the impact of some geriatric symptoms, such as pain, physical frailty, or sarcopenia among others, have on QoL (Chen et al., 2021; Farrugia et al., 2021; Iglesias-López et al., 2021; Kahana & Kahana, 2003; Lee et al., 2021; Wang et al., 2021).

Geriatric symptoms are conceptualized as a non-pathological clinical condition in older adults characterized by multiple causes that lead to a unified set of manifestations (Cesari et al., 2017). These conditions arise from a complex combination of clinical, psychological, social, and environmental vulnerabilities that are extremely heterogeneous (Inouye et al., 2007). This study will focus on three common geriatric symptoms in later life—frailty, pain, and loneliness—to address the biological, psychological, and social dimensions of aging.

Frailty is considered one of the most significant geriatric symptoms, along with sarcopenia and cognitive impairment (Giné-Garriga et al., 2020). It is the most prevalent, and its main characteristic is the limited ability to cope with stressors due to a decrease in the body's homeostatic reserve, which increases the risk of falls, hospitalizations, disability, and mortality (Belenguer-Varea et al., 2023; De Luca et al., 2023; Wu et al., 2018). The likelihood of developing frailty is influenced by a range of factors, including natural physiological changes of aging, multimorbidity, malnutrition, the person's living environment, genetics, social relationships, and personal lifestyle (Belenguer-Varea et al., 2023; De Luca et al., 2023; Jenkins et al., 2023). Frailty has been negatively associated with well-being (Vestjens et al., 2018), life satisfaction (Zapata-Lamana et al., 2022), loneliness (Li et al., 2016; Hoogendijk et al., 2016), limited regular physical and social activity (De Luca et al., 2023), and worse or limited QoL (Belenguer-Varea et al., 2023; Chen et al., 2021).

Pain is a prevalent issue among older adults and affects a significant proportion of this population (Marttinen et al., 2019). In fact, many studies have examined the associations between frailty and pain (Chiou et al., 2018; Guerriero & Reid, 2020; Otones et al., 2019). Systematic reviews and meta-analyses by Saraiva et al. (2018) and Lin et al. (2020) have identified persistent pain as a significant risk factor for the development of frailty. In addition, pain has been shown to predict lower QoL and higher rates of depression (Kaye et al., 2010). In recent studies, such as Bonanni et al. (2023), pain has been associated with worsening QoL due to its strong association with depression. Pain also has been associated with loneliness (Carrasco et al., 2022; Chan et al., 2014; Smith et al., 2019).

Finally, loneliness is recognized as one of the major public health challenges of the 21st century. It is commonly defined as an unpleasant experience due to the contrast between expectations and social relationships (Bandari et al., 2019; Carrasco et al., 2022). Although loneliness can affect individuals across all age groups, it is particularly prevalent among older adults (Conacher, 2017). Several studies have related loneliness to QoL and found a negative impact of loneliness on it (Carrasco et al., 2022; Newman-Norlund et al., 2022).

Although there is a substantial body of literature that has explored the relationships among QoL, frailty, pain, and loneliness, most of the literature tends to conceptualize QoL as a single global indicator or focus on the health-related QoL concept. However, QoL is widely recognized as a complex and multidimensional construct. For that reason, our study adopts a more comprehensive approach by examining QoL through multiple dimensions. This perspective is grounded in the definition proposed by Hyde et al. (2003) and their needs satisfaction model, which incorporates both psychological and subjective well-being, encompassing hedonic and eudaimonic aspects. According to this model, four basic needs (control, autonomy, self-realization, and pleasure) must be satisfied to achieve high QoL in older age.

Control is conceptualized as the capacity to proactively influence the environment, and autonomy refers to an individual's ability to avoid external interference in their actions (Frias-Goytia et al., 2024; Patrick et al., 1993). Finally, self-realization and pleasure encompass all the dynamic and contemplative processes of being human, with the goal of experiencing a sense of purpose, fulfillment, and happiness (Frias-Goytia et al., 2024;

Giddens, 1990; Turner, 1995). The aim of this study is to test a predictive model of QoL in a large sample of Europeans. Specifically, it examines the impact of three latent variables (frailty, pain, and loneliness) on the four dimensions of QoL (control, autonomy, pleasure, and self-realization).

2. Materials and Methods

2.1. Data and Participants

This study was based on data from the 7th wave of the Survey of Aging and Retirement (SHARE-ERIC, 2024; Börsch-Supan et al., 2013). SHARE is a longitudinal study focused on the study of populations aged 50 and older from Israel and 28 European countries. The SHARE project collects data using computer-assisted personal interviewing (CAPI) and follows a probability-based sampling strategy to obtain representative samples of each participating country; further details can be found in Bergmann et al. (2019). SHARE is guided by international ethical standards, such as the Respect Code of Practice for Socio-Economic Research, and was approved by the ethics council of the Max Planck Society in Munich (Approval Code: 2021_24). The collection of SHARE data and their use are subject to the European General Data Protection Regulation. SHARE data can only be used for scientific purposes and are protected by the German Federal Statistics Act and the German Federal Data Protection Law.

Regarding the sample for this study, we included 61355 Europeans over 60 years old (M = 71.87, SD = 8.22), from which 55.9% were females, and 44.1% were males. Regarding some health indicators, this sample had a mean of 2.08 chronic diseases per person (Median = 2, SD = 1.67), and their self-perceived health, in a 1 (poor) to 5 (excellent) scale, had a mean of 2.63 (median = 3, SD = 1.03). Their economic level, measured as the ability of the household to make economic ends met, was 2.73 (Median = 3, SD = 1.01) recorded in an ordinal scale from 1 (with great difficulty) to 4 (easily).

2.2. Measures

To measure the concept and its dimensions, the CASP-12 was employed. This scale has been validated in several studies and used in international research, being the most appropriate and recommended for measuring the degree of coverage of needs and QoL of the older adults (Borrat-Besson et al., 2015; Fekete et al., 2022; Oliver et al., 2021; Pérez-Rojo et al., 2018). The CASP-12 has demonstrated robust psychometric characteristics, establishing it as a suitable multidimensional scale with four correlated factors (Hamren et al., 2015; Pérez-Rojo et al., 2018; Rodríguez-Blázquez et al., 2020). The CASP-12 encompasses the following four dimensions of QoL: control, autonomy, self-realization, and pleasure (Hyde et al., 2003). Answers are given in a Likert scale with four points, from 'never' to 'often'. The internal consistency estimates for each dimension of the scale are $\omega = 0.78$ for control, $\omega = 0.39$ for autonomy, $\omega = 0.86$ for self-realization, and $\omega = 0.81$ for pleasure. The autonomy dimension showed the weakest reliability in our study. This problem has been previously documented in relation to the CASP-12 scale (Borrat-Besson et al., 2015; Oliver et al., 2021; Rodríguez-Blázquez et al., 2020; Sim et al., 2011), and some authors have suggested item modifications or proposed bifactor or trifactor structures (Kerry, 2018; Pérez-Rojo et al., 2018). Despite these concerns about reliability, autonomy remains a key component of QoL in older age. Moreover, the four-dimensional structure of the CASP-12 scale remains widely used. So, in the present study, we opted to retain the four original dimensions of the CASP-12, to facilitate comparability across studies.

Frailty was evaluated using the established measures in SHARE (Romero-Ortuño, 2011; Santos-Eggimann et al., 2009). The assessment included the following: (a) A Mobility Index, derived from the sum of four questions regarding difficulty in activities such as walking 100 m, moving across a room, climbing stairs, and ascending a flight of stairs. Each affirmative response scored 1 point, resulting in a range of 0 to 4, with higher score indicated greater mobility limitations. (b) Appetite, assessed through a binary indicator. Individuals were asked about changes in their appetite, with a score of 1 indicating a "decreased desire for food" and a score of 0 indicating "no decrease in desire for food". (c) Fatigue, measured with a dichotomous question asking if, in the last month, individuals felt they lacked sufficient energy to engage in desired activities. (d) Vigorous physical activities, assessed by querying the frequency of engaging in vigorous physical activities, with response options ranging from 1 (more than once a week) to 4 (almost never or never). (e) Grip strength, measured twice in each hand using a dynamometer, with the higher of the two values recorded.

Loneliness was measured using the Three-Item Loneliness Scale (Hughes et al., 2004), a short version of the R-UCLA Loneliness Scale by Russell et al. (1980). The scale evaluated the frequency of feelings related to lack of companionship, exclusion, and isolation, with responses on a scale from 1 (hardly ever or never) to 3 (often). The scale showed adequate internal consistency $\omega = 0.87$.

Pain was assessed using two indicators from SHARE. A yes/no question about whether the individual took at least five different drugs per day, and the sum of two yes/no questions related to taking drugs for joint pain or other pain, resulting in a scale ranging from 0 (no pain medication) to 2 (medication for joint or other pain). In this sample, it showed an internal consistency $\omega = 0.55$.

2.3. *Statistical Analysis*

For the purposes of this study, a Bayesian Structural Equation Model (BSEM) was estimated using MPlus 8.11 (Muthén & Muthén, 2017). This model enables the analysis of latent variables or factors (where several indicators are used to measure the construct of interest), such as the dimensions of QoL, frailty, pain, and loneliness. In Bayesian estimation, parameters are treated as random, and the information about them is updated using observed data. Bayesian methods do not rely on asymptotic theory, making them suitable for non-normal data or complex models where traditional parametric methods might not be appropriate (Choi & Levy, 2017; Depaoli, 2021). In this statistical logic, based on the Bayes theorem, the data information (the likelihood function) is combined with prior distributions of the parameters to be estimated to form a posterior distribution for each parameter estimate. This procedure offers good estimates for very complex models or to address possible convergence problems (Kaplan & Depaoli, 2012; Lee & Song, 2004; Muthén & Asparouhov, 2012; Song & Lee, 2012). In Bayesian analysis, ensuring the Markov chain Monte Carlo (MCMC) algorithm converges to the target posterior distribution is crucial. In order to do so, trace plot for each parameter were examined (and showed no convergence problem), as well as R-hat calculated (largest value being 1.018). Therefore, convergence was achieved.

Standardized estimates in the Bayesian model offer the expected change in the outcome in standard deviations when the predictor changes in 1 standard deviation. These standardized estimates allow relative comparisons between estimates and can be interpreted as $\beta < 0.2$ = weak effect, $0.2 < \beta < 0.5$ = moderate, and $\beta > 0.5$ = strong effect (Acock, 2014).

3. Results

Table 1 shows the range, mean, median, and standard deviations of all observed variables involved in the model. The correlations between the observed variables included in the model are presented in the Supplementary Materials (Table S1).

Table 1. Descriptive statistics and standardized factor loadings of the variables in the model.

Factor	Indicator	Range	$\overline{X}$	*Md*	*SD*	Factor Loading	S.D.	C.I.
Control	1	1–4	2.42	2	0.99	0.658	0.003	0.652, 0.664
	2	1–4	2.76	3	0.96	0.693	0.003	0.687, 0.699
	3	1–4	3.10	3	0.96	0.678	0.003	0.672, 0.684
Autonomy	1	1–4	3.15	3	0.88	0.501	0.004	0.494, 0.509
	2	1–4	3.14	3	0.95	0.169	0.005	0.160, 0.179
	3	1–4	2.61	3	1.14	0.390	0.004	0.381, 0.399
Pleasure	1	1–4	3.45	4	0.73	0.698	0.003	0.692, 0.704
	2	1–4	3.45	4	0.70	0.732	0.003	0.727, 0.738
	3	1–4	3.35	4	0.72	0.569	0.003	0.562, 0.575
Self-realization	1	1–4	2.99	3	0.86	0.747	0.002	0.743, 0.752
	2	1–4	2.97	3	0.88	0.780	0.002	0.776, 0.784
	3	1–4	2.92	3	0.87	0.797	0.002	0.793, 0.801
Frailty	Activity	1–4	3.29	4	1.06	0.359	0.009	0.341, 0.376
	Appetite	0–1	0.11	0	0.31	0.518	0.008	0.503, 0.534
	Fatigue	0–1	0.37	0	0.48	−0.455	0.005	−0.464, −0.446
	Strength	1–98	31.54	30	10.87	0.643	0.004	0.634, 0.651
	Slowness	0–1	0.22	0	0.41	−0.595	0.007	−0.608, −0.580
Pain	5 drugs	0–1	0.32	0	0.46	0.504	0.005	0.493, 0.514
	Drugs for pain	0–2	0.33	0	0.63	0.493	0.005	0.483, 0.503
Loneliness	1	1–3	1.42	1	0.66	0.606	0.007	0.593, 0.620
	2	1–3	1.33	1	0.58	0.780	0.005	0.770, 0.790
	3	1–3	1.25	1	0.52	0.798	0.005	0.788, 0.808

Note: S.D. = posterior standard deviation, C.I. = credibility interval, *p*-values are <0.001 for all factor loadings.

The full structural model is presented in Figure 1. The model showed good data fit: RMSEA = 0.040, 90% CI [0.040–0.041]; CFI = 0.931. From a statistical point of view, the variables frailty, pain, loneliness, and the four dimensions of QoL are treated as modeled as factors (latent variables). From the theoretical point of view, the model posits frailty, pain, and loneliness as background variables and potential predictors of the QoL's dimensions.

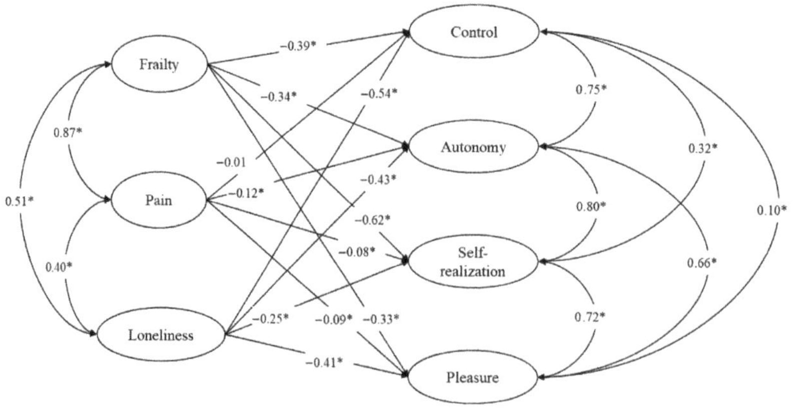

Figure 1. Standardized parameter estimates of the structural model to predict quality of life. Notes: * indicates $p < 0.05$; indicators and errors not shown for clarity.

Regarding the standardized parameter estimates. Frailty, pain, and loneliness were able to predict 64.4% of the variability of control, 59.6% of the variability of autonomy, 55.9% of the variability of self-realization, and 41.6% of the variability of pleasure. Loneliness was the main predictor for the dimensions control (β = −0.54, $p < 0.01$), autonomy (β = −0.43, $p < 0.01$), and pleasure (β = −0.41, $p < 0.01$) and exhibited a significant moderated effect in self-realization (β = −0.25, $p < 0.01$). In this turn, frailty was the main predictor to the dimension self-realization (β = −0.62, $p < 0.01$) and has significant moderate effects in control (β = −0.39, $p < 0.01$), autonomy (β = −0.34, $p < 0.01$), and pleasure (β = −0.33, $p < 0.01$). Finally, pain has a small significant effect on autonomy (β = −0.12, $p < 0.01$), self-realization (β = −0.08, $p < 0.01$), and pleasure (β = −0.09, $p < 0.01$).

All the independent variables included in the model (frailty, pain, loneliness) have significant correlations with each other, particularly demonstrating a strong positive correlation between pain and frailty (r = 0.87, $p < 0.01$). The QoL's dimensions were also correlated. The correlations that were significant and can be considered large were control with autonomy (r = 0.75, $p < 0.01$); autonomy with self-realization (r = 0.79, $p < 0.01$); self-realization with pleasure (r = 0.72, $p < 0.01$); and autonomy with pleasure (r = 0.66, $p < 0.01$). Table 2 expands on the information included in the figure and shows the prediction effects, the correlation values of the variables, and their corresponding credible intervals, posterior standard deviations, and *p*-values.

Table 2. Standardized results of the prediction effects and correlations of the variables included in the model.

Dependent Variables	Predictors	β	S.D.	*p*-Value	C.I.
Control	Frailty	−0.387	0.039	0.000	−0.464, −0.313
	Pain	−0.013	0.038	0.367	−0.085, 0.064
	Loneliness	−0.537	0.011	0.000	−0.559, −0.515
Autonomy	Frailty	−0.345	0.051	0.000	−0.448, −0.247
	Pain	−0.118	0.049	0.010	−0.211, −0.019
	Loneliness	−0.431	0.017	0.000	−0.465, −0.397
Pleasure	Frailty	−0.336	0.039	0.000	−0.415, −0.262
	Pain	0.089	0.038	0.007	0.018, 0.166
	Loneliness	−0.407	0.013	0.000	−0.432, −0.382
Self-realization	Frailty	−0.622	0.038	0.000	−0.701, −0.554
	Pain	0.076	0.037	0.012	0.010, 0.153
	Loneliness	−0.252	0.012	0.000	−0.274, −0.228
Correlated Variables		***r***	**S.D.**	***p*-Value**	**C.I.**
Control	Autonomy	0.752	0.015	0.000	0.721, 0.778
	Pleasure	0.099	0.014	0.000	0.072, 0.125
	Self-realization	0.318	0.013	0.000	0.293, 0.342
Autonomy	Pleasure	0.663	0.013	0.000	0.637, 0.688
	Self-realization	0.792	0.013	0.000	0.766, 0.817
Pleasure	Self-realization	0.717	0.006	0.000	0.705, 0.729
Frailty	Pain	0.875	0.009	0.000	0.859, 0.892
	Loneliness	0.506	0.009	0.000	0.487, 0.524
Pain	Loneliness	0.405	0.013	0.000	0.379, 0.429

Note: S.D. = posterior standard deviation, C.I. = credible interval.

4. Discussion

The present study aimed to determine the influence of frailty, pain, and loneliness on the dimensions of QoL, which are control, autonomy, pleasure, and self-realization.

Frailty, pain, and loneliness have been extensively studied in scientific literature, indicating a reciprocal relationship between them. Frailty was positively related to loneliness (Li et al., 2016; Hoogendijk et al., 2016) and pain (Guerriero & Reid, 2020; Lin et al., 2020; Otones et al., 2019; Saraiva et al., 2018), negatively with well-being (Vestjens et al., 2018), and with worse or limited QoL (Belenguer-Varea et al., 2023; Chen et al., 2021), as well as physical and social activity (De Luca et al., 2023). Similarly, there are studies associating pain with loneliness, although the results are less conclusive (Carrasco et al., 2022; Chan et al., 2014; Smith et al., 2019), and there are studies indicating a worse QoL (Bonanni et al., 2023; Kaye et al., 2010). Also, there is evidence of a negative impact of loneliness on QoL (Carrasco et al., 2022; Newman-Norlund et al., 2022), as well as on social connections (Bandari et al., 2019; Carrasco et al., 2022).

In our multivariate model, positive and generally large relationships between the four QoL's dimensions were observed, as expected in the existing literature (Pérez-Rojo et al., 2018; Towers et al., 2015). However, in our model, associations are estimated, while several predictors explain part of their variances, reinforcing QoL as a global and multidimensional construct. Furthermore, the main results obtained showed that frailty, loneliness, and pain were predictors of the different dimensions. These main variables have an unequal impact on the different dimensions of QoL; specifically, loneliness is the most important predictor of control, autonomy, and pleasure, followed by frailty, whereas in the dimension of self-realization, it was frailty that showed the strongest predictor effect. The results could be influenced by the different indicators, since the self-realization dimension asks directly about recent events, while the other dimensions assess situations that deal with both the present and the past. In other words, when faced with a state of fragility that could worsen and even become chronic, future self-realization is more affected.

Pain had a smaller effect on all dimensions, which means that having pain is considered less important when compared to physical (frailty) and social (loneliness) components. However, it is important to acknowledge that these results may be influenced by the way that pain was operationalized in our study. We assessed pain based on participants' use of pain medication; however, this is an indirect measure that may not accurately reflect the subjective experience or intensity of pain. In contrast, self-report methods are considered the most reliable means of assessing both pain presence and severity (Salaffi et al., 2015). Several validated scales are available for this aim, such as the visual analogue scale (VAS), the verbal rating scale (VRS), and the numerical rating scale (NRS) (Wood et al., 2010; Karcioglu et al., 2018). Future research could use subjective measures to determine if pain has a greater impact on QoL when it is measured with different indicators.

Our study has several strengths, such as the use of a large SHARE project sample, which uses a probabilistic sampling strategy to pick its target population. Moreover, the fact that we used a compilation of representative data from different European countries, specifically from 28 countries and Israel. However, it also has several limitations. Among the general limitations of the study, we can highlight its cross-sectional nature and the impossibility of obtaining information on causality and the direction of the variables over time. Likewise, the self-reported origin of the data contributes to the appearance of various biases, including confirmatory bias and social desirability. In addition, the results may be affected by variance-related aspects of common methods. Despite the procedures carried out to guarantee the reliability and validity of the data from SHARE, individual interviewer differences may generate a series of biases related to the data, which would affect their interpretation. Finally, future research could expand on these findings by incorporating additional variables related to loneliness, pain, frailty, and QoL, such as age, gender, educational level, marital status, and economic situation (Oliver et al., 2021; Rodríguez-Blázquez et al., 2020).

Although many factors can affect QoL in later life, this study focuses on frailty, pain, and loneliness to address the bio-psycho-social dimensions. This choice was made to address the bio-psycho-social aspects of main geriatric syndromes. It is well known that geriatric giants are prevalent and go along with the age increase in older people (Prell et al.,

2023), with those selected syndromes having the greatest impact on their functionality and autonomy (Giné-Garriga et al., 2020; Prell et al., 2023). They also have increased morbidity and mortality (Giné-Garriga et al., 2020) and a direct impact on the person's QoL (Belenguer-Varea et al., 2023; Chen et al., 2021). It is known that loneliness is a risk factor for geriatric syndromes, such as cognitive impairment (Giné-Garriga et al., 2020), and it has a negative effect on QoL (Carrasco et al., 2022; Newman-Norlund et al., 2022). Similarly, pain is a risk factor for frailty (Lin et al., 2020; Saraiva et al., 2018) and a predictor of poor QoL and depression (Bonanni et al., 2023; Kaye et al., 2010).

Regarding the implications of the results, this study highlights which specific dimensions of QoL can be targeted for intervention, considering the distinct impacts of loneliness, frailty, and pain. For instance, recognizing that loneliness significantly affects control, autonomy, and pleasure suggests that interventions should focus on reducing feelings of loneliness. In this context, several studies have implemented strategies that alleviate loneliness and enhance QoL in older adults. For example, Richards et al. (2024) demonstrated that a technology-based program designed to develop digital skills in older individuals not only reduced social isolation and loneliness but also improved quality of life by enhancing self-management and self-efficacy. Similarly, Gould et al. (2021) found that a mobile intervention supported by therapists had the potential to improve mental health-related quality of life and reduce loneliness among older adults.

Regarding frailty, it was the main predictor to the dimension self-realization, and our study highlights the importance of prevention. Evidence suggests that physical activity and nutritional interventions can modify or even reverse frailty syndrome (Woolford et al., 2020). Moreover, multicomponent prevention programs, such as the one proposed by Yu et al. (2020), have demonstrated effectiveness in reducing frailty, as well as improving physical and cognitive function and self-rated health among community-dwelling older adults with pre-frailties. Given that frailty is a modifiable condition, these prevention programs should be considered for integration into community services for older adults.

Supplementary Materials: The following supporting information can be downloaded at: https://www.mdpi.com/article/10.3390/ejihpe15070127/s1, Table S1: Correlations between the variables included in the model.

Author Contributions: Conceptualization, J.M.T. and A.S.; methodology, J.M.T. and Z.T.; formal analysis, J.M.T. and Z.T.; writing—original draft, investigation, supervision, and project administration J.M.T.; writing—review and editing Z.T. and A.S. All authors have read and agreed to the published version of the manuscript.

Funding: This research is framed in project PID2021-124418OB-I00 funded by the Spanish Ministry of Science, Innovation, and Universities MCIN/AEI/10.13039/501100011033 and by the European Regional Development Fund "ERDF A way of making Europe". Z.T. is a researcher beneficiary of the FPU program from the Spanish Ministry of Universities (FPU20/02482).

Institutional Review Board Statement: The Survey of Health, Ageing, and Retirement in Europe (SHARE) project is subject to continuous ethical review, and Wave 6 was approved by the ethics council of the Max Planck Society in Munich. Ethics Council of the Max Planck Society 2021_24 2021-06-08.

Informed Consent Statement: The sample included in our study is from the Survey on Health, Aging and Retirement in Europe (SHARE). SHARE's data collection procedures are subject to ongoing ethical review. SHARE-ERIC's activities related to human subjects research are governed by international research ethics principles, such as the Code of Respectful Practice for Socioeconomic Research (professional and ethical guidelines for the conduct of socioeconomic research) and the "Declaration of Helsinki" (a set of ethical principles regarding human experimentation developed for the medical community by the World Medical Association, last revised at the 64th WMA Meeting held in Fortalezza/Brazil in October 2013) (see https://share-eric.eu/data/search-results/result). The SHARE project obtained informed consent from all subjects involved in this study, but project users (like us) do not have access to this documentation.

Data Availability Statement: The data that support the findings of this study are available at the SHARE Research Data Center to the entire research community free of charge (www.share-project.org, accessed on 15 May 2022). Restrictions apply to the availability of these data, which were used under license for the current study and, thus, are not publicly available. Data are, however, available from the authors upon reasonable request and with permission of the SHARE Project (https://share-eric.eu/data/data-access, accessed on 17 June 2025).

Acknowledgments: This paper uses data from SHARE wave 8, (DOI: 10.6103/SHARE.w8.800). The SHARE data collection has been funded by the European Commission, DG RTD through FP5 (QLK6-CT-2001-00360), FP6 (SHARE-I3: RII-CT-2006-062193, COMPARE: CIT5-CT-2005-028857, SHARELIFE: CIT4-CT-2006-028812), FP7 (SHARE-PREP: GA N°211909, SHARE-LEAP: GA N°227822, SHARE M4: GA N°261982, DASISH: GAN°283646), and Horizon 2020 (SHARE-DEV3: GAN°676536, SHARE-COHESION: GAN°870628, SERISS: GA N°654221, SSHOC: GA N°823782, SHARE-COVID19: GA N°101015924) and by DG Employment, Social Affairs, and Inclusion through vs. 2015/0195, vs. 2016/0135, vs. 2018/0285, vs. 2019/0332, and vs. 2020/0313. Additional funding from the German Ministry of Education and Research, the Max Planck Society for the Advancement of Science, the U.S. National Institute on Aging (U01_AG09740-13S2, P01_AG005842, P01_AG08291, P30_AG12815, R21_AG025169, Y1-AG- 4553-01, IAG_BSR06-11, OGHA_04-064, HHSN271201300071C, RAG052527A), and from various national funding sources is gratefully acknowledged (see www.share-project.org, accessed on 15 May 2022).

Conflicts of Interest: The authors declare no conflicts of interest.

Abbreviations

The following abbreviations are used in this manuscript:

QoL	Quality of life

References

Acock, A. C. (2014). *A gentle introduction to stata* (4th ed.). Stata Press.

Bandari, R., Khankeh, H. R., Shahboulaghi, F. M., Ebadi, A., Keshtkar, A. A., & Montazeri, A. (2019). Defining loneliness in older adults: Protocol for a systematic review. *Systematic Reviews*, *8*, 4–9. [CrossRef]

Belenguer-Varea, A., Avellana-Zaragoza, J. A., Inglés, M., Cunha-Pérez, C., Cuesta-Peredo, D., Borrás, C., Viña, J., & Tarazona-Santabalbina, F. J. (2023). Effect of familial longevity on frailty and sarcopenia: A case-control study. *International Journal of Environmental Research and Public Health*, *20*(2), 1534. [CrossRef]

Bergmann, M., Scherpenzeel, A., & Börsch-Supan, A. (Eds.). (2019). *SHARE wave 7 methodology: Panel innovations and life histories*. MEA, Max Planck Institute for Social Law and Social Policy.

Bonanni, R., Gino Grillo, S., Cariati, I., Tranquillo, L., Iundusi, R., Gasbarra, E., Tancredi, V., & Tarantino, U. (2023). Osteosarcopenia and pain: Do we have a way out? *Biomedicines*, *11*(5), 1285. [CrossRef]

Borrat-Besson, C., Ryser, V.-A., & Gonçalves, J. (2015). *An evaluation of the CASP-12 scale used in the Survey of Ageing and Retirement in Europe (SHARE) to measure quality of life among people aged 50+*. FORS Working Paper Series, Paper 2015-4. FORS. Available online: https://forscenter.ch/wp-content/uploads/2018/07/fors_wps_2015-04_borrat-besson.pdf (accessed on 15 May 2022).

Börsch-Supan, A., Brandt, M., Hunkler, C., Kneip, T., Korbmacher, J., Malter, F., Schaan, B., Stuck, S., & Zuber, S. (2013). Data resource profile: The survey of health, ageing and retirement in Europe (SHARE). *International Journal of Epidemiology*, *42*, 992–1001. [CrossRef]

Carrasco, P. M., Crespo, D., Rubio, C., & Montenegro-Peña, M. (2022). Loneliness in the elderly: Association with health variables, pain, and cognitive performance. A population-based study. *Clínica y Salud*, *33*(2), 51–58. [CrossRef]

Cesari, M., Marzetti, E., Canevelli, M., & Guaraldi, G. (2017). Geriatric syndromes: How to treat. *Virulence*, *8*(5), 577–585. [CrossRef]

Chan, W. C. H., Kwan, C. W., Chi, I., & Chong, A. M. L. (2014). The impact of loneliness on the relationship between depression and pain of Hong Kong Chinese terminally ill patients. *Journal of Palliative Medicine*, *17*, 527–532. [CrossRef]

Chen, M. Z., Wong, M. W. K., Lim, J. Y., & Merchant, R. A. (2021). Frailty and quality of life in older adults with metabolic syndrome—Findings from the healthy older people everyday (HOPE) study. *The Journal of Nutrition, Health & Aging*, *25*(5), 637–644. [CrossRef]

Chiou, J. H., Liu, L. K., Lee, W. J., Peng, L. N., & Chen, L. K. (2018). What factors mediate the inter-relationship between frailty and pain in cognitively and functionally sound older adults? A prospective longitudinal ageing cohort study in Taiwan. *BMJ Open*, *8*, e018716.

Choi, J., & Levy, R. (2017). Markov chain monte carlo estimation methods for structural equation modeling: A comparison of subject-level data and moment-level data approaches. *Biometrics & Biostatistics International Journal*, *6*(5), 463–474. [CrossRef]

Conacher, A. (2017). *Scottish public health network social isolation & loneliness: What is the Scope for public health action?* Alison McCann Phil Mackie.

De Luca, V., Femminella, G. D., Leonardini, L., Patumi, L., Palummeri, E., Roba, I., Aronni, W., Toccoli, S., Sforzin, S., Denisi, F., Basso, A. M., Ruatta, M., Obbia, P., Rizzo, A., Borgioli, M., Eccher, C., Farina, R., Conforti, D., Mercurio, L., . . . Illario, M. (2023). Digital health service for identification of frailty risk factors in community-dwelling older adults: The SUNFRAIL+ study protocol. *International Journal of Environmental Research and Public Health*, *20*(5), 3861. [CrossRef]

Depaoli, S. (2021). *Bayesian structural equation modeling*. The Guilford Press.

Eurostat. (2020). *Ageing Europe—Looking at the lives of older people in the EU*. Publications Office of the European Union.

Eurostat. (2023). *Demography of Europe*. Publications Office of the European Union.

Farrugia, M., Erickson, K., Wendel, E., Platek, M. E., Ji, W., Attwood, K., Ma, S. J., Gu, F., Singh, A. K., & Ray, A. D. (2021). Change in physical performance correlates with decline in quality of life and frailty status in head and neck cancer patients undergoing radiation with and without chemotherapy. *Cancers*, *13*(7), 1638. [CrossRef] [PubMed]

Fekete, M., Patyán, L., Hüse, L., Huszti, E., & Takács, P. (2022). Differences of subjective well-being in European long-term care regimes. *European Journal of Mental Health*, *17*(1), 5–14. [CrossRef]

Frias-Goytia, G. L., Lojo-Seoane, C., Mallo, S. C., Nieto-Vieites, A., Juncos-Rabadán, O., & Pereiro, A. X. (2024). A systematic review of quality of life (QoL) studies using the CASP scale in older adults. *Quality of Life Research*, *33*(11), 2915–2927. [CrossRef] [PubMed]

Giddens, A. (1990). *The consequences of modernity*. Polity Press.

Giné-Garriga, M. J., Jerez-Roig, J., Coll-Planas, L., Skelton, D. A., Inzitari, M., Booth, J., & Souza, D. L. (2020). Is loneliness a predictor of the modern geriatric giants? Analysis from the survey of health, ageing, and retirement in Europe. *Maturitas*, *144*, 93–101. [CrossRef]

Gould, C. E., Carlson, C., Alfaro, A. J., Chick, C. F., Bruce, M. L., & Forman-Hoffman, V. L. (2021). Changes in quality of life and loneliness among middle-aged and older adults participating in therapist-guided digital mental health intervention. *Frontiers in Public Health*, *9*, 746904. [CrossRef]

Guerriero, F., & Reid, M. C. (2020). Linking persistent pain and frailty in older adults. *Pain Medicine*, *21*, 61–66.

Hamren, K., Chungkham, H. S., & Hyde, M. (2015). Religion, spirituality, social support and quality of life: Measurement and predictors CASP-12 (v2) amongst older Ethiopians living in Addis Ababa. *Aging & Mental Health*, *19*(7), 610–621. [CrossRef]

Hoogendijk, E. O., Suanet, B., Dent, E., Deeg, D. J., & Aartsen, M. J. (2016). Adverse effects of frailty on social functioning in older adults: Results from the longitudinal aging study amsterdam. *Maturitas*, *83*, 45–50. [CrossRef]

Hughes, M. E., Waite, L. J., Hawkley, L. C., & Cacioppo, J. T. (2004). A short scale for measuring loneliness in large surveys: Results from two population-based studies. *Research on Aging*, *26*, 655–672. [CrossRef]

Hyde, M., Wiggins, R. D., Higgs, P., & Blane, D. B. (2003). A measure of quality of life in early old age: The theory, development and properties of a needs satisfaction model (CASP-19). *Aging & Mental Health*, *7*(3), 186–194. [CrossRef]

Iglesias-López, E., García-Isidoro, S., & Castellanos-Sánchez, V. O. (2021). COVID-19 pandemic: Pain, quality of life and impact on public health in the confinement in Spain. *Annals of Palliative Medicine*, *10*, 4338–4353. [CrossRef] [PubMed]

Inouye, S. K., Studenski, S., Tinetti, M. E., & Kuchel, G. A. (2007). Geriatric syndromes: Clinical, research, and policy implications of a core geriatric concept: (See editorial comments by Dr. William Hazzard on pp 794–796). *Journal of the American Geriatrics Society*, *55*(5), 780–791. [CrossRef] [PubMed]

Jenkins, N., Welstead, M., Stirland, L., Hoogendijk, E. O., Armstrong, J., Robitaille, A., & Muñiz-Terrera, G. (2023). Frailty trajectories and associated factors in the years prior to death: Evidence from 14 countries in the Survey of Health, Aging and Retirement in Europe. *BMC Geriatrics*, *23*(1), 49. [CrossRef]

Kahana, E., & Kahana, B. (2003). Contextualizing successful aging: New directions in an age-old search. In R. Settersten, Jr. (Ed.), *Invitation to the life course* (pp. 225–255). Baywood.

Kahana, E., Kahana, B., & Lee, J. E. (2014). Proactive approaches to successful aging: One clear path through the forest. *Gerontology*, *60*, 466–474. [CrossRef]

Kahana, E., Kelley-Moore, J., & Kahana, B. (2012). Proactive aging: A longitudinal study of stress, resources, agency, and well-being in late life. *Aging & Mental Health*, *16*(4), 438–451. [CrossRef]

Kaplan, D., & Depaoli, S. (2012). Bayesian structural equation modeling. In R. H. Hoyle (Ed.), *Handbook of structural equation modeling* (pp. 650–673). The Guilford Press.

Karcioglu, O., Topacoglu, H., Dikme, O., & Dikme, O. (2018). A systematic review of the pain scales in adults: Which to use? *The American Journal of Emergency Medicine, 36*(4), 707–714. [CrossRef]

Kaye, A. D., Baluch, A., & Scott, J. T. (2010). Pain management in the elderly population: A review. *The Ochsner Journal, 10*, 179–187.

Kerry, M. J. (2018). Bifactor model of the CASP-12's general factor for measuring quality of life in older patients. *Journal of Patient-Reported Outcomes, 2*(1), 57. [CrossRef]

Lee, H., Chong, J., Jung, H. W., Baek, J. Y., Lee, E., & Jang, I. Y. (2021). Association of the FRAIL scale with geriatric syndromes and health-related outcomes in Korean older adults. *Annals of Geriatric Medicine and Research, 25*, 79–85. [CrossRef]

Lee, S. Y., & Song, X. Y. (2004). Evaluation of the bayesian and maximum likelihood approaches in analyzing structural equation models with small sample sizes. *Multivariate Behavioral Research, 39*, 653–686. [PubMed]

Li, B., Li, W., Bi, J., Meng, Q., & Fei, J. (2016). Predicting factors associated with frailty in aged patients with bone-arthrosis pain in the clinic. *The Physician and Sports Medicine, 44*, 391–396. [CrossRef]

Lin, T., Zhao, Y., Xia, X., Ge, N., & Yue, J. (2020). Association between frailty and chronic pain among older adults: A systematic review and meta-analysis. *European Geriatric Medicine, 11*(6), 945–959. [CrossRef] [PubMed]

Marttinen, M. K., Kautiainen, H., Haanpää, M., Pohjankoski, H., Vuorimaa, H., Hintikka, J., & Kauppi, M. J. (2019). Pain-related factors in older adults. *Scandinavian Journal of Pain, 9*, 987. [CrossRef]

Muthén, B. O., & Asparouhov, T. (2012). Bayesian structural equation modeling: A more flexible representation of substantive theory. *Psychological Methods, 17*, 313–335.

Muthén, L. K., & Muthén, B. O. (2017). *Mplus: Statistical analysis with latent variables: User's guide* (8th ed.). Muthén & Muthén.

Newman-Norlund, R., Newman-Norlund, S., Sayers, S., McLain, A. C., Riccardi, N., & Fridriksson, J. (2022). Effects of social isolation on quality of life in elderly adults. *PLoS ONE, 17*(11), e0276590. [CrossRef]

Oliver, A., Sentandreu-Mañó, T., Tomás, J. M., Fernández, I., & Sancho, P. (2021). Quality of life in european older adults of share wave 7: Comparing the old and the oldest-old. *Journal of Clinical Medicine, 10*(13), 2850. [CrossRef]

Otones, P., García, E., & Pedraz, A. (2019). Chronic pain and frailty in community-dwelling older adults: A systematic review. *Pain Management Nurses, 20*, 309–315.

Patrick, B. C., Skinner, E. U., & Connell, J. P. (1993). What motivate schildren' sbehaviour and emotion in theacademic domain? *Journal of Personality and Social Psychology, 65*, 781–791.

Petretto, D. R., Pili, R., Gaviano, L., & Zuddas, C. (2016). Envejecimiento activo y de éxito o saludable: Una breve historia de modelos conceptuales. *Revista Española de Geriatría y Gerontología, 51*, 229–241. [CrossRef]

Pérez-Rojo, G., Martín, N., Noriega, C., & López, J. (2018). Psychometric properties of the CASP-12 in a Spanish older community dwelling sample. *Aging & Mental Health, 22*(5), 700–708. [CrossRef]

Prell, T., Wientzek, R., & Schönenberg, A. (2023). Self-management of geriatric syndromes—An observational study. *BMC Geriatrics, 23*, 731. [CrossRef]

Richards, T. A., Oman, D., DiMartino, A., & Kotwal, A. A. (2024). A Technology-based intervention impacts quality of life for low-income older adults by reducing loneliness and improving healthcare self-efficacy and self-rated health. *Journal of Applied Gerontology, 44*(5), 825–837. [CrossRef] [PubMed]

Rodríguez-Blázquez, C., Ribeiro, O., Ayala, A., Teixeira, L., Araújo, L., & Forjaz, M. J. (2020). Psychometric properties of the CASP-12 scale in Portugal: An analysis using SHARE data. *International Journal of Environmental Research and Public Health, 17*(18), 6610. [CrossRef]

Romero-Ortuño, R. (2011). El Instrumento de Fragilidad para atención primaria de la encuesta de salud, envejecimiento y jubilación en europa (SHARE-FI): Resultados de la muestra española. *Revista Española de Geriatría y Gerontología, 46*, 243–249.

Russell, D., Peplau, L. A., & Cutrona, C. E. (1980). The Revised UCLA loneliness scale: Concurrent and discriminant validity evidence. *Journal of Personality and Social Psychology, 39*, 472–480.

Salaffi, F., Sarzi-Puttini, P., & Atzeni, F. (2015). How to measure chronic pain: New concepts. *Best Practice & Research Clinical Rheumatology, 29*(1), 164–186. [CrossRef]

Santos-Eggimann, B., Cuénoud, P., Spagnoli, J., & Junod, J. (2009). Prevalence of frailty in middle-aged and older community-dwelling Europeans living in 10 countries. *Journal of Gerontology series A, 64*, 675–681.

Saraiva, M. D., Suzuki, G. S., Lin, S. M., de Andrade, D. C., Jacob-Filho, W., & Suemoto, C. K. (2018). Persistent pain is a risk factor for frailty: A systematic review and meta-analysis from prospective longitudinal studies. *Age and Ageing, 47*, 785–793.

SHARE-ERIC. (2024). *Survey of health, ageing and retirement in europe (SHARE) wave 8: COVID-19 Survey 1*. Release version: 9.0.0. SHARE-ERIC. Data set. [CrossRef]

Sim, J., Bartlam, B., & Bernard, M. (2011). The CASP-19 as a measure of quality of life in old age: Evaluation of its use in a retirement community. *Quality of Life Research, 20*, 997–1004. [CrossRef]

Smith, T. O., Dainty, J. R., Williamson, E., & Martin, K. R. (2019). Association between musculoskeletal pain with social isolation and loneliness: Analysis of the English longitudinal study of ageing. *British Journal of Pain, 13*, 82–90. [CrossRef] [PubMed]

Song, X., & Lee, S. (2012). *Basic and advanced bayesian structural equation modeling: With applications in the medical and behavioral sciences.* John Wiley. [CrossRef]

Towers, A., Yeung, P., Stevenson, B., Stephens, C., & Alpass, F. (2015). Quality of life in indigenous and non-indigenous older adults: Assessing the CASP-12 factor structure and identifying a brief CASP-3. *Quality of Life Research*, *24*, 193–203. [CrossRef] [PubMed]

Turner, B. (1995). Aging and identity. Some reflectionson the somatization of the self. In M. Featherstone, & A. Wernick (Eds.), *Images of aging* (pp. 245–260). Routledge.

UN-Population. (2020). *World population ageing highlights.* October 2020. Available online: https://www.un.org/development/desa/pd/ (accessed on 22 May 2022).

Vestjens, L., Cramm, J. M., & Nieboer, A. P. (2018). The influence of quality of primary care on productive interactions among community-living frail older persons and their general practitioners and practice nurses. *International Journal of Integrated Care*, *18*(s2), 107. [CrossRef]

Wang, S., Zhao, M., Shi, Y., Zhang, M., Ying, J., Li, H., Li, Y., Xing, Z., Zhang, H., & Sun, J. (2021). Associations of frailty, loneliness and the quality of life of empty nesters: A cross-sectional study in rural areas. *International Journal of Nursing Practice*, *25*, e12947. [CrossRef]

Wood, B. M., Nicholas, M. K., Blyth, F., Asghari, A., & Gibson, S. (2010). Assessing pain in older people with persistent pain: The NRS is valid but only provides part of the picture. *The Journal of Pain*, *11*(12), 1259–1266. [CrossRef]

Woolford, S. J., Sohan, O., Dennison, E. M., Cooper, C., & Patel, H. P. (2020). Approaches to the diagnosis and prevention of frailty. *Aging Clinical and Experimental Research*, *32*(9), 1629–1637. [CrossRef]

World Health Organization. (2024). *Ageing and health.* Available online: https://www.who.int/news-room/fact-sheets/detail/ageing-and-health (accessed on 22 May 2022).

Wu, S. Y., Hsu, L. L., Hsu, C. C., Hsieh, T. J., Su, S. C., Peng, Y. W., Guo, T., Kang, Y., & Pan, W. H. (2018). Dietary education with customised dishware and food supplements can reduce frailty and improve mental well-being in elderly people: A single-blind randomized controlled study. *Asia Pacific Journal of Clinical Nutrition*, *7*, 1018–1030. [CrossRef]

Yu, R., Tong, C., Ho, F., & Woo, J. (2020). Effects of a multicomponent frailty prevention program in prefrail community-dwelling older persons: A randomized controlled trial. *Journal of the American Medical Directors Association*, *21*(2), 294.e1–294.e10. [CrossRef]

Zapata-Lamana, R., Poblete-Valderrama, F., Ledezma-Dames, A., Pavón-León, P., Leiva, A. M., Fuentes-Alvarez, M. T., Cigarroa, I., & Parra-Rizo, M. A. (2022). Health, functional ability, and environmental quality as predictors of life satisfaction in physically active older adults. *Social Sciences*, *11*(6), 265. [CrossRef]

European Journal of
Investigation in Health, Psychology and Education

MDPI

Article

Meaning in Life Among Aged People: A Qualitative Study of an Institutionalized Elderly Sample

Lăcrămioara Cojocaru, Camelia Soponaru, Daniela Muntele-Hendreș and Ciprian Ceobanu *

Faculty of Psichology and Educational Sciences, Alexandru Ioan Cuza University, 700554 Iaşi, Romania; lacramioara.cojocaru@uaic.ro (L.C.); camelia.soponaru@uaic.ro (C.S.); hendres@uaic.ro (D.M.-H.)
* Correspondence: ciprian@uaic.ro

Abstract: As individuals grow older, they experience notable shifts in their health conditions, social positions, and personal identity. Studies show that finding meaning in life correlates with healthier lifestyle choices and enhanced overall well-being. This sense of meaning functions as a protective factor against life's challenges, strengthening resilience during later years. The research utilized thematic analysis within a qualitative methodology to investigate the subjective sources of meaning among elderly people living in Romanian institutional settings. The analysis revealed several interconnected themes. Religiosity and spirituality emerged as a fundamental anchor, with participants often mentioning God, Divinity, and Higher Power in their narratives. They typically conceptualized life as a sacred gift and emphasized the importance of religious practices such as prayer and church attendance as essential to their sense of purpose. The intergenerational transmission of values also proved significant, with elderly individuals finding meaning in passing down moral and spiritual principles to younger family members, viewing this as their enduring legacy. Interpersonal connections played a crucial role as well, with quality relationships with family and friends fostering a sense of belonging, while broken relationships or isolation negatively impacted well-being. Daily life objectives, including short-term goals like maintaining routines or anticipating family visits, along with preserving functional independence, provided structure and immediate purpose for many participants. The research distinguished between religiosity and spirituality as related but separate concepts: while formal religious rituals offered community-based meaning, those less engaged with organized religion discovered transcendence through personal spiritual experiences such as connecting with nature. This study highlights cultural specificities, particularly how Orthodox Christian traditions shape existential narratives among Romanian elderly, and proposes practical interventions for retirement facilities to incorporate activities focused on spiritual engagement, relationship building, and opportunities for elders to share their wisdom with younger generations.

Keywords: old adults; qualitative research; religiosity/spirituality; intergenerational values transmission; interpersonal relationships

1. Introduction

Older adults derive meaning from various components, including purpose, moral worth, self-worth, control, coherence, excitement, and connectedness. These elements are crucial in shaping life narratives and providing a framework for understanding life experiences in older age (Derkx et al., 2020). Meaning in life refers to the significance and purpose individuals attribute to their existence. It encompasses the beliefs, values, and goals that give life direction and coherence. Research has shown that having a sense of meaning is associated with various positive outcomes, including better mental and physical health, enhanced well-being, and improved coping mechanisms in the face of stressors (Schnell, 2009, 2020).

The influence of these outcomes on the meaning in life was found to be significant. When referring to health and well-being, studies indicate that individuals who perceive their lives as meaningful tend to engage in healthier behaviors and experience better overall health (Bratt & Fagerström, 2023). Meaningfulness has been linked to lower levels of stress and better recovery from illness (Steptoe & Fancourt, 2019) and was found to be a protective factor against cognitive decline (Kim et al., 2019). Meaning acts as a moderator in the relationship between stressors and distress. Individuals with a strong sense of meaning are better equipped to handle life's challenges, experiencing less severe suffering during difficult times (Mäkikangas & Kinnunen, 2003).

The individual's need to search for meaning in life is a phenomenon known and highlighted in the literature within humanistic-existentialist approaches as found in the works of authors such as Frankl, Maslow, and Antonovsky.

The search for meaning is the primary motivation in one's life and not a 'secondary rationalization' of instinctual drives, as Viktor Frankl (2000) wrote in his fundamental book *Man's Search for Meaning*. This task of finding meaning in life does not diminish with age, and in fact, its pursuit can become more pronounced as life goes by. Among older populations, the concept of meaning of life can be interpreted from different theoretical perspectives.

Among these, Antonovsky's theory on the sense of coherence might be considered a cornerstone in understanding how individuals find meaning in life, particularly in the context of health and well-being (Eriksson & Lindström, 2005). Meaningfulness is a multidimensional construct that is applicable across different cultures and life stages, providing a framework for understanding how individuals find meaning and manage stress in their lives. The integration of meaningfulness into health models highlights its importance in both psychological and physical health outcomes (Eriksson & Mittelmark, 2017). Although considerable research has explored sources of meaning in life among older adults internationally, much of this work has been conducted in Western contexts, with relatively little attention paid to Eastern European cultural settings. Romania—with its distinct socio-historical evolution, religious traditions, and social structures—offers a unique context for investigating how older adults construct meaning in life.

2. Theoretical Background

Meaning in life is often understood as a multidimensional construct (Schnell, 2009, 2020; Schnell & Becker, 2006), which means it encompasses various components or dimensions that contribute to an individual's overall sense of meaning. This complexity reflects the diverse ways in which people find significance in their lives. The key features typically associated with the construct of meaning in life are as follows:

Purpose in life is defined by having core goals, aims, and a sense of direction. It involves setting and pursuing meaningful goals that align with one's values and aspirations (Martela & Steger, 2016). A strong sense of purpose is associated with numerous adaptive benefits, including improved mood, motivation, and goal achievement. It also enhances cognitive function and supports better cognitive aging outcomes (Sutin, 2023). Individuals with a clear sense of purpose are more likely to set and achieve goals, which in turn reinforce their sense of meaning and direction in life (Owen et al., 2022).

Significance denotes the belief that one's life possesses inherent value and contributes meaningfully within a broader social or existential context. It encompasses a sense of personal worth and the perception that one's existence holds relevance both for oneself and for others. Meaning in life often arises from activities that are grounded in love for objectively valuable objects, rather than from a mere interest in meaningfulness itself. However, what constitutes a "worthy" object is subjective and cannot be determined from a completely neutral standpoint (Wolf, 2014). Research suggests that meaning in life includes feelings of coherence, purpose, and external value, such as significance or mattering. Internal value, or one's perceived internal worth, is also considered a fundamental component of meaning in life (Li et al., 2020).

Coherence, in the context of life experiences, refers to the ability to perceive life as comprehensible, manageable, and meaningful. These components influence how individuals perceive their quality of life over time. Comprehensibility affects the importance of present and past events, while manageability relates to the control over life events. Studies have shown that individuals exposed to organized patterns report higher levels of meaning compared to those exposed to random patterns (Heintzelman et al., 2013). Other research suggests that life experiences such as consistency, load balance, migration, and integration experiences play a role in influencing life's sense of coherence (Slootjes et al., 2017). In this respect, individuals with a strong sense of coherence are better equipped to integrate their experiences into a meaningful narrative, which is linked to improved psychological well-being and quality of life. While coherence is a component of meaning in life, existential mattering (feeling significant) is a stronger precursor to judgments of life meaning. This suggests that feeling significant may be more crucial than coherence or purpose alone (Costin & Vignoles, 2020).

The belonging dimension of meaning in life emphasizes the importance of social connections and relationships, which can significantly enhance one's sense of meaning. Different studies have found a strong positive correlation between the sense of belonging and the perceived meaningfulness of life, across various methodologies, including correlational, longitudinal, and experimental studies (Zhang et al., 2018; Lambert et al., 2013). Threats to belongingness can reduce the importance of social relationships as a source of meaning in life, but individuals may compensate by seeking autonomy (Zhang et al., 2018). Another significant observation is related to the bidirectional relationship between social connectedness and meaning in life (O'Rourke & Sidani, 2017). Among different types of connectedness, collective connectedness is particularly associated with meaning in life (Stavrova & Luhmann, 2016). This bidirectional relationship highlights the importance of fostering social connections to enhance one's sense of meaning in life.

Transcendence involves experiences that extend beyond the self, such as spirituality, connection to nature, and activities that evoke awe and wonder. This concept is explored through various lenses, including gero-transcendence, self-transcendence, and collective transcendence. Transcendence is considered a crucial aspect of successful aging, providing a framework for interventions that enhance life satisfaction and well-being among older adults (McCarthy & Bockweg, 2013).

While religiosity and spirituality are often intertwined, research suggests they serve distinct psychological functions. Among older adults with low institutional religiosity, spirituality (e.g., connection to nature, cosmic transcendence) may compensate for the absence of structured religious frameworks by providing alternative avenues for meaning-making. This pattern is particularly pronounced in adults over 75, who may prioritize personal spiritual experiences over dogma as they confront mortality. The apparent contradiction—that spirituality matters more for the less religious—reflects a broader existential adaptation: when traditional religiosity wanes, transcendent beliefs persist as a resilient source of coherence (Braam et al., 2006). Other studies indicate that people perceive meaning in life more through self-transcendence (benefits to society) than self-enhancement (benefits to the self). This contrasts with happiness judgments, where self-enhancement plays a more significant role (Huang & Yang, 2022). The concept of self-transcendence, as described by Viktor Frankl, is seen as essential for well-being, emphasizing a shift from materialistic pursuits to spiritual fulfillment. This approach is linked to better mental health and is particularly beneficial for those facing chronic illness or end-of-life situations (Wong, 2016).

Self-transcendence is also explained by Tatjana Schnell (2012), as vertical—through explicit religiosity and spirituality—and horizontal—through self-knowledge, social commitment, as well as health, generativity, and union with nature. This means that religious practices and spiritual beliefs are important sources of meaning for the elderly, as well as personal growth, relatedness, and generativity as a part of social commitment.

All the key factors depicted above indicate that meaning in life among elderly people is influenced in various ways. Research consistently shows that these factors significantly contribute to older people's mental health and overall well-being. Among these, closely linked to the old person's meaning in life are their levels of religiosity and spirituality and the quality of their relationships.

Understanding meaning in life as a multidimensional construct allows for a more nuanced approach to research and interventions aimed at enhancing well-being. It recognizes that individuals may derive meaning from different sources and that these sources can interact in complex ways to shape their overall sense of purpose and significance in life.

3. Methods

3.1. Research Question

It is obvious that sources of meaning in life differ with age. For young adults, the main sources of meaning in life are considered to be relationships, especially family connections (Debats, 1999), personal and professional goals (Bhattacharya, 2011), and parental influence; young adults with supportive parental backgrounds tend to have a stronger sense of meaning in life (Kealy et al., 2020).

In middle-aged adults, the meaning in life is influenced by various sources and factors, which are essential to their psychological well-being and life satisfaction. Key sources of meaning include relationships and health (Karwetzky et al., 2021; Debats, 1999), spirituality and intrinsic religious orientation (Hee & Nam, 2018), as well as personal growth (Fave et al., 2013; Dolberg & Ayalon, 2018). Also, factors such as social support, self-esteem, and stress play significant roles (Hee & Nam, 2018; Chang & Sohn, 2017).

Older adults often find meaning in life through various sources, which significantly impact their well-being, health, and quality of life. For older people, family and close relationships are consistently highlighted as primary sources of meaning (Hupkens et al., 2018; Zhou et al., 2019). Many older adults find meaning through spirituality and religious practices (Jonsén et al., 2015). Engaging in unselfish activities that promote personal growth and contributing to future generations (Sørensen et al., 2021), as well as maintaining good health, having a sense of life, and security are crucial sources of meaning in life for older adults (Hoeyberghs et al., 2019; Zhou et al., 2023). Finally, some older adults find meaning in their connection to nature and their role as a link between generations, which involves passing on traditions and values (Jonsén et al., 2015).

Starting from all these premises, our research question is: What are the main sources of meaning in life for elderly adults, and what are the main features of meaning in life within the research group?

3.2. Methodology

This study employed a qualitative–exploratory research design, guided by a phenomenological approach, aiming to explore the subjective sources of meaning in life among institutionalized elderly individuals. Because of the small number of participants, the results cannot be generalized to a larger population. Qualitative research seeks to understand social phenomena by capturing participants' perspectives and interpreting them within their relational and cultural contexts (Rossman & Rallis, 2016; Bradbury-Jones et al., 2017).

The research began in January 2024 and involved the development of a semi-structured interview guide, constructed based on the main orientations identified in the existing literature. The guide included open-ended questions exploring existential meanings, interpersonal relationships, spirituality, and intergenerational value transmission, as well as several dichotomous and demographic questions. The study protocol was reviewed and approved by the Research Ethics Committee of the affiliated academic institution. The study included 25 institutionalized residents (11 women and 14 men), aged between 65 and 93 years. The participants were aged as follows: 65–74 years—9, 75–84 years—7, 85–93 years—9. Educational backgrounds varied: the majority had completed secondary education (high school or lower), while a smaller number had attended higher education institutions. Marital status was also diverse: several were widowed or divorced, while others remained married. Participants had a range of former occupations, including skilled trades (e.g., foreman, electrician), education, law enforcement, agriculture, and domestic work. This demographic diversity provided a rich context for exploring subjective sources of meaning in later life. Each interview lasted approximately 60 min and was audio-recorded with the participant's permission. The recordings were securely stored on encrypted drives. Interviews were conducted by L.C. and C.S., both trained psychologists, under the coordination of L.C. Inclusion criteria were: institutionalization, age 65+, cognitive ability to sustain dialogue, and informed consent. Those with significant cognitive impairment were excluded. Audio recordings were transcribed via Transkriptor© v.1 and manually verified for accuracy by the research team (L.C., C.S., D.M.H., and C.C.) prior to thematic analysis.

Following data collection, the interviews were transcribed verbatim using Transkriptor© v.1 software and manually corrected for accuracy. Translation from Romanian to English for analytic and reporting purposes was conducted by two independent bilingual researchers. A third bilingual reviewer verified the translations to ensure semantic and contextual fidelity. For data analysis, we employed thematic analysis as described by Braun and Clarke (2006), following a rigorous six-phase process: familiarization with data, initial coding, theme searching, theme reviewing, theme defining and naming, and report production. Initially, NVivo 14© software was used for preliminary coding; however, due to the limitations of semantic recognition in Romanian, manual thematic coding was subsequently undertaken.

L.C. and C.S. independently coded a subset of transcripts, then discussed initial codes with D.M.H. and C.C. to refine the thematic structure. Themes were derived inductively, reflecting patterns across the dataset, and involved triangulation between two independent researchers to enhance analytic credibility. Five major patterns emerged from the data: (1) principles of life, (2) spirituality, (3) religiosity, (4) subjective well-being, and (5) meaning of life through objectives. The thematic analysis enabled us to capture both shared and divergent experiences, linked to participants' demographic profiles and personal life histories. In summary, the methodological design was carefully structured to ensure methodological rigor, transparency, and adherence to COREQ guidelines (Appendix A), allowing an in-depth exploration of the subjective meaning in life among elderly individuals in an institutional setting.

4. Results

Four codes were identified following the analysis of the interviews carried out with the participants (institutionalized elderly), which allowed for the integration of similar themes under one "umbrella" (Figure 1). The "sources of meaning for the elderly" codebook encompasses the following general themes:

- Religious and spiritual faith and practices describe the elderly's convictions about life as a "gift" from God, in the form of an individual destiny, offered by Divinity. These are accompanied by religious practices that anchor faith in a behavioral manner, both at the individual and community levels.
- Intergenerational heritage transmission describes the fact that elderly people consider the spiritual legacy they leave behind to be very important; the legacy is described in terms of moral values and includes, in addition to religious values, secular values, carried out through parental and institutional education (school or workplace). Again, religious practices appear as a sub-theme, representing a traditional value that should be preserved and transmitted to the younger generation, as a complementary source of meaning.
- The quality of relationships is described as positive or negative, and it is linked to the present moment or to previous life experiences, regarding family or friends. The quality of the family relationships influences the tendency toward self-isolation, accompanied by the feeling of loneliness.
- Life objectives describe daily routines and short-term plans (1–3 months, up to a year) and include recreational activities, intentions to visit children who live and work abroad, and tourist visits.

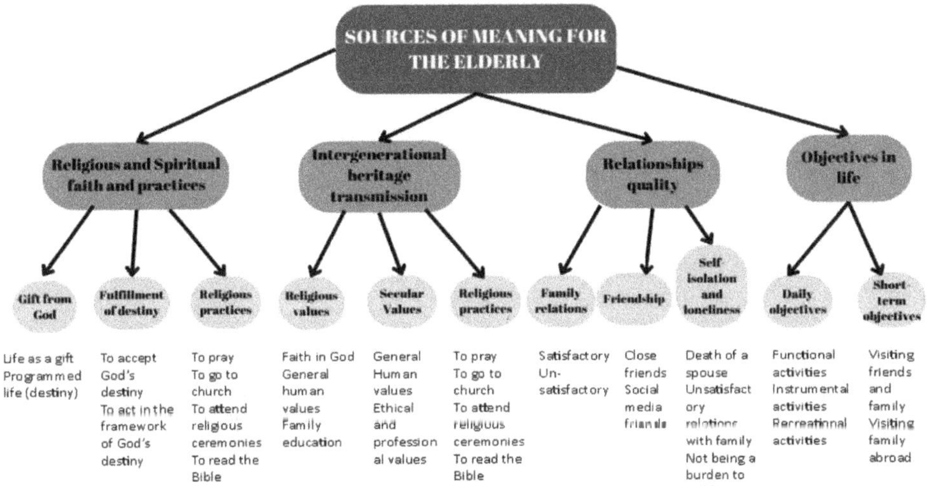

Figure 1. The theme structure: "sources of meaning for the elderly".

With the exception of the intergenerational heritage transmission theme and the unsatisfactory relationships within the family context, to which they refer in the past tense, the remaining themes are derived from their present experiences and convictions, formulated in the present tense.

To provide a clearer picture of the relative significance of these themes within the study group, we summarized the number of statements for each theme in the study group (Figure 2). These proportions suggest the prominence of transcendental and relational dimensions in constructing meaning in life among the participants.

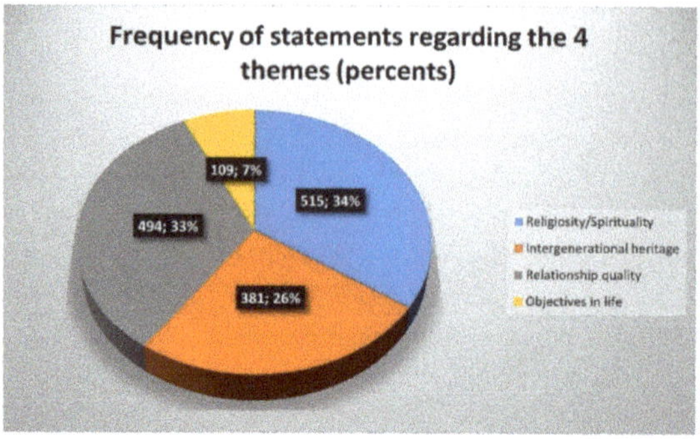

Figure 2. Frequency of statements regarding the four themes.

4.1. Religiosity and Spirituality as Foundations for Meaning in Life

Religiosity and spirituality emerged as the primary frameworks through which participants structured and interpreted their existence, offering coherence, purpose, and resilience in the face of life's challenges. In general, spirituality and religiosity, while often interconnected (Agniete et al., 2021), refer to different concepts. While spirituality was described as an individual search for existential connection and personal transcendence, religiosity represented adherence to communal beliefs and rituals. However, for the participants, these two dimensions were deeply intertwined, jointly shaping their understanding of life's meaning. Faith was recurrently articulated as the source of existential significance, grounding participants in a larger, transcendent order: "I believe in God; faith is very important, without faith there is no meaning in life." (I67, female, late 60s).

Such statements illustrate that for these individuals, faith is not merely an abstract belief but the very medium through which life acquires meaning, providing assurance that existence itself is part of a divine design.

The concept of vertical transcendence (Tatjana Schnell, 2012)—striving toward connection with a higher power—was deeply embedded in participants' narratives. Ritual practices (prayer, worship, fasting) were not perceived solely as obligations, but as acts of reaffirmation of their connection to a meaningful, sacred order: "In the morning, we worship God… it keeps me grounded and thankful every day." (I65, male, mid 80s). Through these actions, participants actively anchored their daily experiences within a spiritual framework, thereby reinforcing the perceived meaningfulness of their lives.

Destiny and divine will were also key components of meaning-making. Participants conceptualized life events—both positive and negative—as parts of a divinely orchestrated plan, which they were called to accept and fulfill: "It is destiny up to a certain point." (I82, female, early 70s); "Both good and bad come from God, and we must respect Him." (I65, male, mid 80s).

Acceptance of destiny thus emerged as an existential orientation that infused suffering and uncertainty with meaning, transforming adversity into opportunities for reaffirming faith and moral growth.

Importantly, the internalization of religious values shaped participants' moral decision-making, reinforcing life's coherence and sense of purpose: "When I do something, I think if it's right or wrong—it's doing God's will." (I62, female, late 60s).

Through aligning personal choices with divine principles, participants embedded moral worth into their daily lives, thus actively constructing meaning in accordance with a higher ethical framework. Adversity—such as illness or family hardships—often prompted a deepened reengagement with faith. Participants described experiences where suffering became a catalyst for reaffirming or transforming their relationship with God: "My son got sick and from that moment I stopped swearing." (I66, male, early 70s); "[Now] I immediately come to terms with the idea that this is the way it was meant to be." (I66, male, early 70s).

This process illustrates how faith was dynamically reconstructed across the lifespan, adapting to existential crises and providing tools for emotional regulation and acceptance. Moreover, meaning was not only found in transcendent beliefs but also in concrete life achievements interpreted through a religious lens—procreation, ethical family life, community contribution, and personal integrity: "I brought up a child." (I62, female, late 60s); "Spouses must love and understand each other and raise their children calmly." (I78, female, mid 80s); "You must think about what you are doing." (I81, male, mid 80s).

Through these domains, participants expressed a profound sense that everyday actions were spiritually significant, contributing cumulatively to the meaningfulness of their existence.

Engagement in religious practices—attending church, praying, maintaining sacred objects—was seen as a continuous act of reaffirmation and anchoring of meaning, especially in older age: "In my house, you will find a cross consecrated by the priest and everything." (I77, female, early 80s); "Go to church, take communion." (I67, female, late 60s).

However, some participants also demonstrated a reflective and individualized stance toward religious observances, suggesting a nuanced, critical engagement with traditional practices: "No one can force me to worship Saint Parascheva only on the feast day. I can visit anytime." (I70, male, early 80s).

This flexibility highlights that spiritual meaning-making was not static but evolved with personal experiences, convictions, and critical reflection, emphasizing participants' agency in shaping their religious lives.

In summary, religiosity and spirituality in later life served as multi-layered frameworks of meaning-making, combining belief, practice, moral action, and existential acceptance into a dynamic, resilient structure that sustained participants' sense of purpose, coherence, and fulfillment.

4.2. Intergenerational Heritage Transmission

Intergenerational heritage transmission plays a crucial role in shaping the meaning of life for older adults. This process involves the exchange of values, traditions, and knowledge between generations, which can significantly impact the well-being and life satisfaction of older individuals. Intergenerational interactions have been shown to positively affect older adults' physical and mental health. These interactions can reduce feelings of loneliness and stress, provide a greater sense of purpose, and enhance life satisfaction. They also foster appreciation for generational differences and strengthen social connections, which can improve mental and physical health and reduce the risk of depression (Zhong et al., 2020; Krzeczkowska et al., 2021).

The values received from elders are often reflected in the values that individuals pass on to their descendants, suggesting a significant familial influence (Albanese et al., 2014).

It has been observed that there are two main bodies of principles and values that are transmitted from the older generation to the younger ones: (i) *religious beliefs* that are considered to be parts of the individual and social identity and (ii) *secular principles and values* that serve as sources for meaning in life. The axiological orientation has become an important part of defining meaning in life for this age group. As mentioned earlier, these values have served as both sources of meaning in life and as axiological objects that have been transmitted to the younger generation.

The early years of a child's life are pivotal for religious education, with family members, particularly older adults, playing a significant role in this process. Older adults frequently become key figures in nurturing children's spirituality, providing support and guidance in religious education activities (Allana et al., 2017).

The involvement of grandparents in religious education is seen as enabling and supportive, helping to embed spirituality in young children and fostering a conducive environment for faith development.

The transmission of religious values (which are closely related to religious covenants) is another element that can be noted in the context of this analysis: "And I think another principle (that can be transmitted) is the relationship with divinity." (I66, male, early 70s); "The values that come through (the philosophy of religious life) religion, religion doesn't teach us anything wrong." (I84, male, early 80s).

The transmission of religious values within families is a pivotal process, with grandparents playing a significant role as educators and role models. Despite the challenges posed by time constraints and cultural pluralism, effective strategies, such as family involvement and integrated educational approaches, have been shown to enhance the transmission of religious and moral values to the next generation. Addressing these challenges is imperative for maintaining the impact of family education on children's spiritual and moral development: "Reaching the stage where I had to realize that there is divinity, telling my granddaughters to develop (faith)." (I67, female, late 60s); "I never had an in-depth discussion with my daughter or my son about the church, about God, about the spirit. That would be part of the spiritual heritage." (I70, male, early 80s); "Because I have two children left. Let them also follow, let them believe in the good Lord as we believe." (I73, female, late 60s); "A spiritual inheritance is a spiritual education. Love of parents, faith, love of friends, of children, of family." (I83, male, mid 80s).

Religion significantly influences human values. The transmission of these values occurs through familial and societal structures, impacting individual and collective behaviors: "The greatest values are trust, kindness, sincerity, love. [...] This code of moral values comes through religion." (I82, female, early 70s).

Grandparents provide both emotional and material support, which is crucial for the transmission of family legacies, including secular values such as education, solidarity, and order (Schuler & De Souza Brito Dias, 2019). Their influence is shaped by family dynamics, cultural contexts, and the quality of their relationships with grandchildren: "Friendship and honesty are the guiding principles of my life." (I74, male, early 70s); "Respect for people. Respect for laws for customs, for unwritten laws." (I84, male, early 80s); "Something that people leave behind that is not material. For example, (life) lessons." (I87, male, early 80s); "Spiritual heritage (depends) on the family. It is about the transmitted values through family education." (I82, female, early 70s); "A way of behavior, the ABC of good behavior." (I81, male, mid 80s).

General human values were also listed as meaning-making for the older people in the study group. They often rely on basic values such as dignity, honesty, and respect for tradition and values. These values provide a sense of continuity and integrity: "Let something be seen behind us, that something of value remains." (I64, female, mid 80s); "Justice is a principle that has guided me throughout my life." (I72, male, early 70s); "I am an honest person. I am guided by truth." (I73, female, late 60s); "In general, I was a man of moderation. Being good, being kind, doing my duty." (I86, male, mid 80s); "To be correct, a man of my word." (I126, male, early 90s); "Love and respect for parents, love for country, and love of humankind." (I81, male, mid 80s); "My guiding principles in life are punctuality and discipline." (I75, male, mid 80s); "...fairness, perseverance" (I67, female, late 60s).

The values related to ethical and professional issues, which have previously and continue to provide meaning to the lives of older adults: "I would put first work ethic. Honesty, humanity. To have as much knowledge as possible, so self-development." (I66, male, early 70s); "My profession, my work, honest and loyal to your friends, to everybody." (I71, female, late 70s).

Older adults often experience increased religiosity as they age, which can influence their role in religious transmission. Their religious biographies, shaped by personal and societal changes, contribute to a flexible and open approach to religious discussions within families, facilitating successful transmission across generations (Spannari et al., 2021). The religious intensity and practices of parents, including older adults, have a lasting impact on their children's religiosity. This influence is often mediated by early and midlife religious experiences, creating a momentum that carries into old age (Silverstein et al., 2022). Although religious practices are mentioned as creators of meaning, it should be noted that they represent a double source of meaning, both as a moral duty and as an anchor for fixing, preserving and transmitting faith and religious heritage: "In the morning, we worship God." (I65, male, mid 80s); "I pray to God . . . give them (my boy and girl) good health." (I70, male, early 80s).

4.3. The Quality of Relationships

The self-assessment component of the interview, which was designed to evaluate the current state of well-being among the elderly, offered valuable insights into the quality of family relationships and the presence of significant others in their lives. These relationships appear to be a source of meaning and a life objective, both of which are closely tied to religious belief and practice. Regular interactions with family, friends, and religious communities enhance the sense of belonging and contentment, contributing to a meaningful life (De Oliveira & De Oliva Menezes, 2018). The quality of social relationships, including support from religious congregations, is linked to better life satisfaction and quality of life in the elderly (Gallardo-Peralta, 2017). Older adults rely on family and friends for emotional, instrumental, and financial support. Those with strong ties to both groups are generally more socially and psychologically well adjusted (Adams & Blieszner, 1995). Social engagement (in-person interactions and group engagements), including interactions with family and friends, helps satisfy the need to belong and reduces feelings of loneliness (Tomstad et al., 2024). It is noticeable that the quality of relationships, particularly with friends, is a stronger predictor of life satisfaction than the frequency of contact. Friendships often provide more positive and meaningful interactions compared to family relationships (Larson et al., 1986; O'Connor, 1995). Interactions with friends are associated with increased positive affect and life satisfaction and decreased negative impact, while family interactions can increase both positive and negative affect, highlighting the complex dynamics of family relationships (Huxhold et al., 2014; Ng et al., 2020).

"(The meaning of life is given by relationships, only if human) makes himself useful to the community, to other people." (I84, male, early 80s). It has been suggested that socializing can be a source of meaning: "I have very good relationships, relationships with friends and family... yes, relationships give meaning to life." (I66, male, early 70s).

Engaging in social activities and leveraging technology to maintain connections can further support these relational aspects (Saarelainen et al., 2020). These relationships provide emotional support, reduce feelings of isolation, and enhance the overall quality of life: "My mom lived with my dad until they were 73 years old. When he died, after 3 years, she withdrew completely." (I62, female, late 60s); "(It's important) to have your grandchildren visiting." (I74, male, early 70s); "Relationships give meaning" (I83, male, mid 80s).

Family relationships significantly influence the meaning of life and well-being in older adults. The quality of relationships enhances quality of life and raises the well-being of the elderly person (Saarelainen et al., 2020). Positive relationships enhance life satisfaction and mental health, while negative interactions can detract from these outcomes. Addressing both positive and negative aspects of these relationships is crucial for supporting older adults in finding meaning and improving their quality of life: "If there would be no meaning in people working together, there would be no (quality) life, there would be no meaning in life they wouldn't be able to create things." (I67, female, late 60s).

Satisfactory family relationships increase life satisfaction: "You also have to match yourself with the person you're in a relationship with, so that you can talk about the same fear. And you can create a thing." (I63, female, early 70s).

While the interviews were conducted in the present tense, the elderly preferred to answer certain topics in the past tense. In order to maintain discretion and motivation to participate, we did not delve deeper into the interview but instead focused on extracting the themes from the life story that the elderly felt comfortable sharing: "It was very good how I programmed (life) him (my husband) and how I lived with him for so many years and had (together) three children, three boys, how I brought them up, I also did (work) in the house and worked, and I sent (the children) to school." (I79, female, mid 80s); "I understand that a fulfilled life means a fulfilled life for others in the family." (I80, male, mid 70s).

Unsatisfactory family relationships can significantly undermine the sense of meaning in life for older adults, primarily through increased depression and reduced quality of life. These effects are compounded by relational gaps and negative interactions, highlighting the importance of fostering positive family dynamics to support the well-being of older adults: "The only thing I would like is to have a good relationship with my daughter-in-law (she won't let me visit my son and grandchildren)." (I62, female, late 60s); "Deep relationships (give meaning to life)... my wife wouldn't let me talk to my maiden until I was 18. I have tried, I have tried to get close to someone, but everything is on the surface, we just see each other." (I72, male, early 70s); "It makes me sad, the relationship with my wife. I don't hate her... she says it's all my fault." (I86, male, mid 80s); "I haven't been in touch with my boys. They are in France. They only came to Romania to pay their taxes and for other things, often they didn't even come to see me. They don't even know I'm in the foster house." (I74, male, early 70s).

Engaging in activities with peers and maintaining friendships can bring joy and a sense of connectedness, which are vital for meaning in life (Saarelainen et al., 2020). Both subjective (perceived) and objective (actual) social supports are linked to higher life satisfaction and health in older adults (Fiori et al., 2007). The quality of relationships with friends is determined by the quality of connection and the emotional distance between individuals: "Yes, relationships give meaning to life. To help them, (friends) to give them advice." (I80, male, mid 70s); "If you're friends with someone, you have to be a good friend, not a false one." I64, female, mid 80s).

Older adults who maintain friendships tend to be more socially and psychologically well adjusted, benefiting from the emotional and instrumental support that these relationships provide (Adams & Blieszner, 1995). While larger networks can enhance life satisfaction, the quality and composition of these networks, particularly the presence of friends, play a crucial role in the well-being of older adults. Older adults prefer small groups of friends due to the immediate emotional benefits, opportunities for meaningful social engagement, and the supportive nature of these relationships: "[...] to make a small group, three or four people. I have made this group here [...]. And we meet every day a quarter of an hour before breakfast, before lunch, another quarter of an hour." (I70, male, early 80s).

Older adults can significantly benefit from social media friendships by enhancing social connections and reducing loneliness. The overall effectiveness of social media as a tool for improving well-being in older adults depends on individual circumstances and the nature of their online interactions: "I don't get bored, (at home). I have friends on WhatsApp, Messenger." (I86, male, mid 80s); "I was alone, ... now I have (friends) if you believe me, on Facebook, a hundred of friends I have. And they all call me. There's a community here." (I74, male, early 70s).

Solitude in older adults can be both beneficial and detrimental, depending on whether it is voluntary or not, and it also depends on the quality of their social relationships. While solitude can enhance positive affect and provide personal time, it can also lead to loneliness and depression if not balanced with meaningful social interactions and valuable relationships (Ong et al., 2015).

Self-isolation and loneliness are significant for older adults, with implications for their physical and mental health. Addressing self-isolation and loneliness in older adults requires a multifaceted approach that considers individual, cultural, and contextual factors. These issues are prevalent among the aging population, particularly in the context of increasing life expectancy and societal changes: "You end up retreating, . . . like a turtle in its shell, and you sit and you think. . . maybe where I went wrong, maybe I did something wrong, right?" (I62, female, late 60s); "Most of the time I feel isolated. I mean not isolated, because no one isolates me, but. . . it's hard not to have anyone close." (I64, female, mid 80s); "Loneliness is very hard." (I65, male, mid 80s); "My wife died June 16 last year. The truth is that it was very hard and still is to me. I live alone in my room, I have nobody close to me." (I70, male, early 80s).

The death of a spouse in elderly adults leads to increased depression, anxiety, and cognitive decline, with social isolation being a significant risk (Hung et al., 2020). Interventions focusing on emotional support and social engagement can aid in mitigating these impacts: "After my husband died, I felt so lonely. I chose to stay alone, and after a while, after a year, I found out about this [retirement] home, and I thought it would be better to be somewhere, not to disturb my daughter." (I63, female, early 70s).

Unsatisfactory social relationships can have significant negative impacts on the well-being of older adults. These impacts manifest in various aspects of mental and physical health, as well as overall life satisfaction (Santini et al., 2015). While older adults may develop resilience to some negative interactions, the overall impact of poor relationship quality remains significant, particularly for mental health: "Most of the (time) I stay isolated. . . no one isolates me, but. . . it's hard to have someone close to you." (I64, female, mid 80s); "You get criticized that it's too much, . . . so, you end up retreating, just like a turtle in its shell and you [start] thinking [yourself] I did something wrong?" (I62, female, late 60s); "Relationships make sense. If you don't relate to people, you're lonely. You drift away. Loneliness kills." (I81, male, mid 80s).

The importance of not being a burden for older adults is multifaceted, involving cultural, emotional, and practical dimensions. Older adults' concerns about being a burden are shaped by their cultural background and emotional relationships with their children (Cahill et al., 2009). The concept of not wanting to be a burden was found to be significant among older adults, particularly in the context of their relationships with their children: "The children decided to put me in the nursing home." (I70, male, early 80s); "I am here because my children relocated abroad, and I didn't want to be a burden for the children." (I71, female, late 70s).

4.4. Life Objectives

It is important to recognize the value of short-term and long-term objectives for older adults. These objectives can provide structure, enhance quality of life, and support successful aging. Short-term objectives, such as engaging in enjoyable activities and physical exercise, can provide immediate benefits and motivation for older adults (Devereux-Fitzgerald et al., 2016). Long-term objectives focus on maintaining health and cognitive function, supported by effective self-management and communication strategies (Lawless et al., 2021). Both types of objectives are essential for enhancing the quality of life and supporting successful aging in older adults.

By focusing on health (Travers et al., 2021), socialization and independence (Pfund et al., 2021), older adults may be able to maintain a sense of purpose and engagement, which are key to defining meaning in life. It has been suggested that there are several types of goals that are common to older adults: (i) goals related to purpose and engagement (Howard & Louvar, 2017); (ii) goals related to autonomy, health, relationships, and emotional comfort which are integral to older adults' quality of life (Van Leeuwen et al., 2019); (iii) for older adults with long-term conditions, self-care and self-management objectives are essential (Lawless et al., 2021). In the current research, we identified two categories of objectives: daily objectives and short-term objectives

The following daily objectives (day-to-day functioning, religious practices, entertainment, purpose, and engagement) have been proposed by the members of the research group: "here (in the nursing home, my wife and I) have a schedule that I aim to be as exact as possible; after we get up in the morning and have breakfast, we go to the city center on foot, then at the church. We had lunch at noon, then we went to the art exhibitions." (I66, male, early 70s); "In the morning, we worship God." (I65, male, mid 80s).

Functional activities are essential for older adults as they promote physical health, enhance psychological well-being, and improve quality of life (Owen et al., 2022). These activities help maintain independence, manage chronic conditions, and reduce the risk of falls, making them a vital component of care for the elderly: "We go out to eat, come back, rest and that's about it." (I64, female, mid 80s); "In the morning, to do my chores, to have my clothes clean." (I87, male, early 80s).

Instrumental activities of daily living are vital for the independence and well-being of older adults, influencing their health, social engagement, and overall quality of life. Effective interventions and an active lifestyle can enhance instrumental activities of daily living performance, while psychosocial factors and technological advancements also play significant roles in their lives: "I still go, and I still help my daughter on holidays, when she's busy." (I63, female, early 70s); "I have in my room, TV, laptop, I talk on WhatsApp and Messenger." (I86, male, mid 80s).

Recreational activities play a vital role in promoting health, happiness, and social connectedness among older adults (Ryu & Heo, 2018). By providing opportunities for physical activity, social interaction, and purposeful engagement, these activities contribute significantly to the well-being and quality of life in aging populations: "I read a book, go to the club, play a Rummy, do tailoring." (I62, female, late 60s); "Out for a walk." (I67, female, late 60s); "I'd like to go to the seaside, to Slănic Moldova (mountain resort), where I've been (when I was younger)." (I87, male, early 80s).

Traveling in later life offers older adults a pathway to spiritual and emotional enrichment, social connection, and personal development. By addressing the challenges and barriers they face, we can support their journeys toward finding meaning and satisfaction in life (Moal-Ulvoas, 2017). Traveling is a common goal among older adults, often linked with finding a calling and mastering new skills. This pursuit not only provides enjoyment but also contributes to a sense of achievement and personal growth: "... in the summer, for example, I planned to go to Denmark, to my sons." (I71, female, late 70s); "...to go and see Florence (where my son lives)." (I84, male, early 80s).

Considering their age, the elderly mentioned that they do not imagine and do not have long-term plans: "I like to live the moment, day by day, because you don't know how far (life goes)." (I62, female, late 60s), or they have plans within a maximum time horizon of one year: "I have always had the plan to go somewhere, to go in summer, spring... I would like to go to Sovata... there is the swimming pool." (I75, male, mid 80s); "... let's go on a trip with our coach from here (from the nursing home)." (I85, female, mid 80s).

5. Discussions and Conclusions

The majority of the themes identified in the present research appear to corroborate findings from previous studies (e.g., North & Fiske, 2015), suggesting shared characteristics among elderly individuals that may transcend geographical and cultural boundaries.

However, our investigation group exhibited distinctive orientations, notably a more individualized and critical approach to religious practice, rather than strict adherence to institutionalized rituals, as well as a pronounced focus on moral transmission and personal legacy as primary sources of meaning. These particularities likely reflect the socio-cultural context and historical experiences specific to the studied region, shaping unique meaning-making pathways among the elderly participants.

For a considerable number of old individuals, religiosity is defined as the extent of religious belief and practice in an individual's life, and it has been historically regarded as a fundamental source of meaning. Its role as a cornerstone of meaning can be analyzed as a link to transcendence, as it often provides individuals with a connection to something greater than themselves, whether it is God, a divine principle, or the cosmic order.

In the group of older adults who were the focus of the study, the qualitative analysis yielded four sources of meaning, as outlined below: (i) religiosity/spirituality, (ii) the relations with others, (iii) the moral principles that govern life, and (iv) specific life goals.

The analysis of the frequency of statements pertaining to "God", "Divinity", "Universe", and "Higher force" has identified religiosity/spirituality as a primary source of meaning, one that is more or less connected to the other sources of meaning that emerged from this study. This phenomenon can be attributed to two factors. First, the frequency with which this theme emerged in the interviews exceeded that of other themes. Second, this theme was a recurring topic that manifested across the entire discourse of the interviewed individuals, irrespective of the subject under discussion. There are several directions and conclusions that can be identified as elements of novelty brought by the current research.

One noticeable conclusion is the way religiosity is seen in various forms:

- as a matter of religious conviction;
- as a matter of religious practice;
- as content in the process of intergenerational transmission;
- as a value in itself;
- as a grid for reinterpreting reality;
- as a filter for selecting choices/decisions;
- as a foundational element in the grounding of the meaning of life.

As evidenced in previous research (Abeyta & Routledge, 2018; AbdAleati et al., 2016), religiosity manifests in various forms, and it has been demonstrated to exert influence on mental health, life satisfaction, and social relationships.

We have to underline that the interpretation of religiosity and spirituality by older people is unique in its own right. Important ideas that are part of the mainstream of religion, such as the punitive or rewarding character of life after death and the influence of destiny by divinity, take particular forms in this context (e.g., the non-acceptance of the existence of life after death, implacable destiny are not sources of meaning for older adults). These forms are transferred to the current life (fulfilled or unfulfilled life, the meaning of suffering, etc.), observations confirmed by previous research (Zimmer et al., 2016).

Another significant observation, which is in line with previous studies (Chamberlain & Zika, 1988), is that a substantial number of the values expressed by the subjects in the study seem to be influenced by previous religious traditions and practices. This assertion is supported by the fact that religious practices and beliefs offer a sense of purpose and direction, thereby providing psychological support. Another observation is that the presence of a community that shares similar religious beliefs and intentions has the potential to foster a sense of social cohesion, thereby offering additional psychological comfort. Finally, another observation is linked to the notion of predetermined destiny, influenced by a divine entity, that provides elderly people with a sense of purpose and induces the idea that it is a contribution to a larger plan. This plan can pertain to the evolution of society as a whole or to a divine plan that is believed to promote unanimity.

The second source of meaning in life identified by the research group, which refers to interpersonal relationships, has the potential to endow the lives of elderly individuals with significance and foster well-being. Some believe that as people age, the importance of relationships may increase, enhancing their sense of coherence and continuity in life (Schnell, 2009). It has been observed that elderly individuals appear to be aware of the significant role that relationships may play in providing meaning and well-being (Adams & Blieszner, 1995).

In these circumstances, while relationships with friends are typically regarded as a positive source of emotional meaning (O'Connor, 1995), we can observe that family relationships are considered both positive and negative emotional sources. It has been acknowledged in the literature that family relationships can have a positive impact on the elderly. However, the impact of dysfunctional family relationships on the elderly has received less attention in research. Within the frame of the current research, one can observe that this phenomenon has the capacity to modify the behavioral profile of the elderly regarding their own family.

In the research group, it was observed that in cases where the relationship is deemed dysfunctional, the elderly person may endeavor to adapt to the family dynamics, which can prove to be a substantial source of stress. Older adults' perceptions of their roles within the family are considered to be a multilayered topic that involves understanding their contributions, the dynamics of family relationships, and social attitudes toward aging.

When the elderly person perceives their relationship with their family as a source of burden for their children, they opt for self-isolation, withdrawing from their family within the nursing home. A significant number of elderly individuals have chosen to relocate to a nursing facility due to their children's international migration.

The third significant source of meaning that was identified in the current research refers to the moral principles, which encompass attitudes and instruments of behavioral regulation. It can be postulated that religion, as stated above, serves as the predominant source of moral values and behavioral principles. In this paradigm, the responsibility for educating younger generations and for the transmission of life principles by elders is viewed as occurring within the broader context of religious belief systems.

Within this theme that emerged from the interviews, we found the notion of *intergenerational transmission of fundamental values and principles* that govern human existence as a whole. It is largely accepted that intergenerational transmission of values is a complex process influenced by familial, cultural, and social factors (Schönpflug, 2001). It plays a crucial role in cultural continuity and the socialization of future generations, and in this context, several broad categories were identified; the respondents believe that these should be transmitted to younger generations as an expression of life experience. The identified categories encompass: *faith as such* (religious values and principles), *general human values* (which may align with those proposed by religion), and *professional values* (which appear to be independent of religious faith).

Based on the current research, *the process of intergenerational transmission of values and principles* can be regarded as a generator of meaning in itself. One of the most important conclusions from our study is that the elderly population perceives this transmission as a moral obligation, intrinsically linked to their life stage and their status as elders within the family structure, particularly with regard to their grandchildren. Within the paradigm of intergenerational transmission, religious practices assume the role of both an instrument and a means, contributing to the perpetuation of religious and spiritual faith. In this context, the religious practices function as an external source of meaning, serving, on one hand, as a tool for educating the young and, on the other hand, as a resource to fortify the internal source of meaning embodied by religion.

The life objectives of the elderly population constitute another substantial source of meaning in life (Hupkens et al., 2018). These objectives are oriented toward daily activities related to functionality and autonomy (Pirhonen & Pietilä, 2015). However, some goals, particularly those of a recreational nature, are associated with family or friends and are designed for a period of time ranging from several months to a maximum of one year.

In contrast to other age demographics, we observed that when we queried the members of the research group about their long-term aspirations, they frequently asserted the absence of long-term goals. We explained this phenomenon in two ways. Firstly, it can be attributed to the awareness of advanced age and impending death. Secondly, it can be explained by the uncertainties related to their fragile physical state. A significant number of elderly individuals have been observed to articulate objectives that are oriented toward the present moment and the pursuit of enjoyment in life. This phenomenon, characterized by the deliberate savoring of life's pleasures (Smith & Hollinger-Smith, 2015), is particularly notable within the context of this specific age demographic.

Apart from the four main sources of meaning that were identified within the research group, some particular topics appear to present certain contradictions. One of these topics is the discourse surrounding older adults' matter of "life after death". It is interesting to note that, despite the strong religious beliefs expressed by the study participants, their views on life after death vary greatly. Although religious perceptions propose and encourage behaviors and attitudes from a rewarding or punitive perspective in the afterlife, it was expected that individuals with a strong religious belief would find motivation for certain behaviors and attitudes, having by default a source of meaning in the idea of life after death. However, the opinions regarding life after death do not necessarily seem to relate to religious beliefs. Also, a large number of respondents stated that they do not believe in life after death, despite their strong religious belief: "I believe in God. I don't believe in life after death." (I71, female, late 70s); "I can't say that it (life after death) exists." (I64, female, mid 80s); "It could be (life after death)." (I65, male, mid 80s); "It exists (life after death). I think hell is on earth here." (I62, female, late 60s); "It's a continuation of present life." (I63, female, early 70s); "I don't believe in life after death (as the orthodox religion describes it). "I believe in reincarnation." (I66, male, early 70s).

Another marginal topic was found in a negligible proportion of the participants self-identified as atheists, attributing human existence to Darwinist evolutionism: "Fear of (life after) death has not affected my decisions in life, as long as I live here, I do what I think is right, not to affect others, to be good, with family and friends." (I63, female, early 70s). This assertion is supported by the observation that "life choices and actions in life are not influenced by the idea of death, but rather by the idea of life" (I66, male, early 70s). In this context of analysis, the concept of life after death does not inherently signify a source of meaning.

In the end, we can state that the existence of all these sources of meaning does not guarantee a state of well-being or a high quality of life. However, it appears to provide the necessary intentional coherence, acceptance of reality, and access to coping mechanisms, whose adaptive nature depends on the rigidity of thinking of old people. Further research is necessary to fully elucidate the implications of this phenomenon.

While this study provides valuable insights into the sources of meaning for institutionalized elderly adults, future research should expand the sample to include non-institutionalized and culturally diverse populations to improve generalizability. Additionally, a mixed-methods approach (combining qualitative depth with quantitative validation) could further verify thematic patterns. Exploring the interplay between religiosity, intergenerational transmission, and social relationships may reveal deeper mechanisms by which older adults construct meaning. Such investigations could inform more tailored interventions to enhance well-being in aging populations.

Although broadly consistent with international findings, the results of this study highlight culturally specific orientations among Romanian institutionalized elderly individuals, including a critical and personalized approach to religious practice and a pronounced emphasis on intergenerational moral legacy. These findings underline the necessity of considering cultural and socio-historical contexts when interpreting meaning-making processes in older adulthood.

This study highlights key areas that could guide interventions aimed at enhancing meaning in life among institutionalized elderly residents. Encouraging opportunities for spiritual engagement, promoting intergenerational value transmission, fostering social connectedness, and supporting personal goal-setting could strengthen residents' sense of purpose and fulfillment. By addressing these dimensions, retirement homes may significantly improve the psychological well-being and overall quality of life of their residents.

Author Contributions: All four authors contributed equally to all phases of the article's development. All authors have read and agreed to the published version of the manuscript.

Funding: This research received no external funding.

Institutional Review Board Statement: The study was conducted in accordance with the Declaration of Helsinki, and approved by the Institutional Ethics Committee of Faculty of Psychology and Education Sciences, "Alexandru Ioan Cuza" University from Iasi, Romania, nr.1381/09.29.23 for studies involving humans.

Informed Consent Statement: Informed consent was obtained from all subjects involved in the study.

Data Availability Statement: All data related to this article are available upon request (in the Romanian language).

Conflicts of Interest: The authors declare no conflicts of interest.

Appendix A. COREQ Checklist

The following table summarizes the reporting of the applicable items from the COREQ 32-item checklist for this study.

Domain 1: Research team and reflexivity

Item	Description in the Study
Research team	Interviews were conducted by two doctoral students and a coordinating professor.
Education and occupation	All researchers had higher education in psychology, and prior experience in qualitative research.
Relationship with participants	No prior relationship with participants; recruitment was voluntary after study objectives were explained.
Personal relevance and reflexivity	Researchers used reflexivity techniques to minimize personal bias.

Domain 2: Study design	
Item	**Description in the Study**
Setting	Interviews were conducted at "Saint Pious Parascheva" nursing home, in private dedicated spaces.
Participants	25 individuals aged between 67 and 93 years; inclusion criterion: institutionalized residents.
Recruitment	Voluntary recruitment after presenting study objectives.
Interview guide	Semi-structured, based on specialist literature; informally pre-tested.
Data collection	Audio-recorded interviews with explicit consent; approx. 60 min each.
Data saturation	Thematic saturation reached after 20 interviews; remaining interviews confirmed findings.
Domain 3: Analysis and findings	
Item	**Description in the Study**
Transcription	Full transcription with Transkriptor© software; manually validated by researchers.
Software used	NVivo© used for initial coding; manual processing later due to language limitations.
Method of analysis	Inductive thematic analysis; coding triangulation between researchers.
Validity and rigor	Continuous reflexivity; consensus on main themes.
Confidentiality	Anonymization through coded identifiers; secured storage of audio and text data.

References

AbdAleati, N. S., Mohd Zaharim, N., & Mydin, Y. O. (2016). Religiousness and mental health: Systematic review study. *Journal of Religion and Health*, *55*, 1929–1937. [CrossRef] [PubMed]

Abeyta, A. A., & Routledge, C. (2018). The need for meaning and religiosity: An individual differences approach to assessing existential needs and the relation with religious commitment, beliefs, and experiences. *Personality and Individual Differences*, *123*, 6–13. [CrossRef]

Adams, R., & Blieszner, R. (1995). Aging well with friends and family. *American Behavioral Scientist*, *39*, 209–224. [CrossRef]

Agniete, A., Cepuliene, A., Pucinskaite, B., Spangelyte, K., Skruibis, P., & Gailiene, D. (2021). Spirituality and Religiosity during Suicide Bereavement: A Qualitative Systematic Review. *Religions*, *12*, 766. [CrossRef]

Albanese, G., Blasio, G., & Sestito, P. (2014). My parents taught Me. Evidence on the family transmission of values. *Journal of Population Economics*, *29*, 571–592. [CrossRef]

Allana, A., Tennant, G., & Petrucka, P. (2017). Embedding spirituality in young children: An inter-generational challenge. *International Journal of Children's Spirituality*, *22*, 239–259. [CrossRef]

Bhattacharya, A. (2011). Meaning in life: A qualitative inquiry into the life of young adults. *Psychological Studies*, *56*, 280–288. [CrossRef]

Braam, A., Bramsen, I., Van Tilburg, T., Van Der Ploeg, H., & Deeg, D. (2006). Cosmic transcendence and framework of meaning in life: Patterns among older adults in the Netherlands. *The Journals of Gerontology, Series B, Psychological Sciences and Social Sciences*, *61*(3), S121–S128. [CrossRef]

Bradbury-Jones, C., Breckenridge, J., Clark, M., Herber, O., Wagstaff, C., & Taylor, J. (2017). The state of qualitative research in health and social science literature: A focused mapping review and synthesis. *International Journal of Social Research Methodology*, *20*(6), 627–645. [CrossRef]

Bratt, A. S., & Fagerström, C. (2023). Perceptions of general attitudes towards older adults in society: Is there a link between perceived life satisfaction, self-compassion, and health-related quality of life? *International Journal of Environmental Research and Public Health*, *20*(4), 3011. [CrossRef]

Braun, V., & Clarke, V. (2006). Using thematic analysis in psychology. *Qualitative Research in Psychology*, *3*(2), 77–101. [CrossRef]

Cahill, E., Lewis, L., Barg, F., & Bogner, H. (2009). "You don't want to burden them": Older Adults' Views on Family Involvement in Care. *Journal of Family Nursing*, *15*, 295–317. [CrossRef] [PubMed]

Chamberlain, K., & Zika, S. (1988). Religiosity, life meaning and wellbeing: Some relationships in a sample of women. *Journal for the Scientific Study of Religion, 27*, 411–420. [CrossRef]

Chang, H., & Sohn, J. (2017). Factors related to meaning of life in middle adults. *Asia-Pacific Journal of Multimedia Services Convergent with Art, Humanities, and Sociology, 7*, 609–621. [CrossRef]

Costin, V., & Vignoles, V. (2020). Meaning is about mattering: Evaluating coherence, purpose, and existential mattering as precursors of meaning in life judgments. *Journal of Personality and Social Psychology, 118*(4), 864–884. [CrossRef]

Debats, D. (1999). Sources of meaning: An investigation of significant commitments in life. *Journal of Humanistic Psychology, 39*, 30–57. [CrossRef]

De Oliveira, A., & De Oliva Menezes, T. (2018). The meaning of religion/religiosity for the elderly. *Revista Brasileira de Enfermagem, 71*(Suppl. S2), 770–776. [CrossRef]

Derkx, P., Bos, P., Laceulle, H., & Machielse, A. (2020). Meaning in life and the experience of older people. *International Journal of Ageing and Later Life, 14*(1), 37–66. [CrossRef]

Devereux-Fitzgerald, A., Powell, R., Dewhurst, A., & French, D. (2016). The acceptability of physical activity interventions to older adults: A systematic review and meta-synthesis. *Social science & medicine, 158*, 14–23. [CrossRef]

Dolberg, P., & Ayalon, L. (2018). Subjective meanings and identification with middle age. *The International Journal of Aging and Human Development, 87*, 52–76. [CrossRef]

Eriksson, M., & Lindström, B. (2005). Validity of Antonovsky's sense of coherence scale: A systematic review. *Journal of Epidemiology and Community Health, 59*, 460–466. [CrossRef] [PubMed]

Eriksson, M., & Mittelmark, M. (2017). The sense of coherence and its measurement. In M. Eriksson, M. B. Mittelmark, S. Sagy, M. Eriksson, G. F. Bauer, J. M. Pelikan, B. Lindström, & G. A. Espnes (Eds.), *The handbook of salutogenesis* (pp. 97–106). Springer Open. [CrossRef]

Fave, A., Brdar, I., Wissing, M., & Vella-Brodrick, D. (2013). Sources and motives for personal meaning in adulthood. *The Journal of Positive Psychology, 8*, 517–529. [CrossRef]

Fiori, K., Smith, J., & Antonucci, T. (2007). Social network types among older adults: A multidimensional approach. *The Journals of Gerontology. Series B, Psychological Sciences and Social Sciences, 62*, 322–330. [CrossRef]

Frankl, V. (2000). *Man's search for meaning*. Beacon Press.

Gallardo-Peralta, L. (2017). The relationship between religiosity/spirituality, social support, and quality of life among elderly Chilean people. *International Social Work, 60*, 1498–1511. [CrossRef]

Hee, J., & Nam, Y. (2018). The factors influencing the meaning in life in middle-aged adult. *Journal of the Korea Academia Industrial Cooperation Society, 19*, 432–440. [CrossRef]

Heintzelman, S., Trent, J., & King, L. (2013). Encounters with objective coherence and the experience of meaning in life. *Psychological Science, 24*, 991–998. [CrossRef]

Hoeyberghs, L., Verté, E., Verté, D., Schols, J., & Witte, N. (2019). The importance of sources of meaning in life of community dwelling psychologically frail older people. *Working with Older People, 23*(2), 65–76. [CrossRef]

Howard, E., & Louvar, K. (2017). Examining life goals of community-dwelling, low-income older adults. *Research in Gerontological Nursing, 10*, 205–214. [CrossRef]

Huang, M., & Yang, F. (2022). Self-transcendence or self-enhancement: People's perceptions of meaning and happiness in relation to the self. *Journal of Experimental Psychology: General, 152*(2), 590–610. [CrossRef]

Hung, Y., Chen, Y., Lee, M., & Yeh, C. (2020). Effect of spousal loss on depression in older adults: Impacts of time passing, living arrangement, and spouse's health status before death. *International Journal of Environmental Research and Public Health, 18*, 13032. [CrossRef]

Hupkens, S., Machielse, A., Goumans, M., & Derkx, P. (2018). Meaning in life of older persons: An integrative literature review. *Nursing Ethics, 25*, 973–991. [CrossRef] [PubMed]

Huxhold, O., Miche, M., & Schüz, B. (2014). Benefits of having friends in older ages: Differential effects of informal social activities on well-being in middle-aged and older adults. *The Journals of Gerontology, Series B, Psychological Sciences and Social Sciences, 69*(3), 366–375. [CrossRef] [PubMed]

Jonsén, E., Norberg, A., & Lundman, B. (2015). Sense of meaning in life among the oldest old people living in a rural area in northern Sweden. *International Journal of Older People Nursing, 10*(3), 221–229. [CrossRef]

Karwetzky, C., Werdecker, L., & Esch, T. (2021). What matters most in life? A german cohort study on the sources of meaning and their neurobiological foundations in four age groups. *Frontiers in Psychology, 12*, 777751. [CrossRef]

Kealy, D., Ben-David, S., & Cox, D. (2020). Early parental support and meaning in life among young adults: The mediating roles of optimism and identity. *Current Psychology, 41*, 3865–3872. [CrossRef]

Kim, G., Shin, S., Scicolone, M., & Parmelee, P. (2019). Purpose in life protects against cognitive decline among older adults. *Innovation in Aging, 3*, S650–S651. [CrossRef]

Krzeczkowska, A., Spalding, D., McGeown, W., Gow, A., Carlson, M., & Nicholls, L. (2021). A systematic review of the impacts of intergenerational engagement on older adults' cognitive, social, and health outcomes. *Ageing Research Reviews, 71*, 101400. [CrossRef]

Lambert, N., Stillman, T., Hicks, J., Kamble, S., Baumeister, R., & Fincham, F. (2013). To belong is to matter. *Personality and Social Psychology Bulletin, 39*, 1418–1427. [CrossRef]

Larson, R., Mannell, R., & Zuzanek, J. (1986). Daily well-being of older adults with friends and family. *Psychology and Aging, 1*(2), 117–126. [CrossRef]

Lawless, M., Tieu, M., Feo, R., & Kitson, A. (2021). Theories of self-care and self-management of long-term conditions by community-dwelling older adults: A systematic review and meta-ethnography. *Social Science & Medicine, 287*, 114393. [CrossRef]

Li, Z., Liu, Y., Peng, K., Hicks, J., & Gou, X. (2020). Developing a quadripartite existential meaning scale and exploring the internal structure of meaning in life. *Journal of Happiness Studies, 22*, 887–905. [CrossRef]

Martela, F., & Steger, M. (2016). The three meanings of meaning in life: Distinguishing coherence, purpose, and significance. *The Journal of Positive Psychology, 11*, 531–545. [CrossRef]

Mäkikangas, A., & Kinnunen, U. (2003). Psychosocial work stressors and well-being: Self-esteem and optimism as moderators in a one-year longitudinal sample. *Personality and Individual Differences, 35*, 537–557. [CrossRef]

McCarthy, V., & Bockweg, A. (2013). The role of transcendence in a holistic view of successful aging. *Journal of Holistic Nursing, 31*, 84–92. [CrossRef]

Moal-Ulvoas, G. (2017). Positive emotions and spirituality in older travelers. *Annals of Tourism Research, 66*, 151–158. [CrossRef]

Ng, Y., Huo, M., Gleason, M., Neff, L., Charles, S., & Fingerman, K. (2020). Friendships in old age: Daily encounters and emotional well-being. *The Journals of Gerontology, Series B, Psychological Sciences and Social Sciences, 76*(3), 551–562. [CrossRef]

North, M. S., & Fiske, S. T. (2015). Modern attitudes toward older adults in the aging world: A cross-cultural meta-analysis. *Psychological Bulletin, 141*(5), 993. [CrossRef]

O'Connor, B. (1995). Family and friend relationships among older and younger adults: Interaction motivation, mood, and quality. *The International Journal of Aging and Human Development, 40*, 9–29. [CrossRef]

Ong, A., Uchino, B., & Wethington, E. (2015). Loneliness and health in older adults: A mini-review and synthesis. *Gerontology, 62*, 443–449. [CrossRef]

O'Rourke, H. M., & Sidani, S. (2017). Definition, determinants, and outcomes of social connectedness for older adults: A scoping review. *Journal of Gerontological Nursing, 43*(7), 43–52. [CrossRef]

Owen, R., Berry, K., & Brown, L. J. (2022). Enhancing older adults' well-being and quality of life through purposeful activity: A systematic review of intervention studies. *The Gerontologist, 62*(6), e317–e327. [CrossRef] [PubMed]

Pfund, G., Allemand, M., & Hofer, M. (2021). Daily social interactions as a route to purposeful days in older adulthood. *Innovation in Aging, 5*, 212–213. [CrossRef]

Pirhonen, J., & Pietilä, I. (2015). Patient, resident, or person: Recognition and the continuity of self in long-term care for older people. *Journal of Aging Studies, 35*, 95–103. [CrossRef]

Rossman, G. B., & Rallis, S. F. (2016). *An introduction to qualitative research: Learning in the field*. Sage Publications.

Ryu, J., & Heo, J. (2018). Relationships between leisure activity types and well-being in older adults. *Leisure Studies, 37*(3), 331–342. [CrossRef]

Saarelainen, S., Mäki-Petäjä-Leinonen, A., & Pöyhiä, R. (2020). Relational aspects of meaning in life among older people—A group-interview gerontechnology study. *Ageing and Society, 42*, 1035–1053. [CrossRef]

Santini, Z. I., Koyanagi, A., Tyrovolas, S., Mason, C., & Haro, J. M. (2015). The association between social relationships and depression: A systematic review. *Journal of Affective Disorders, 175*, 53–65. [CrossRef]

Schnell, T. (2009). The sources of meaning and meaning in life questionnaire (SoMe): Relations to demographics and well-being. *The Journal of Positive Psychology, 4*(6), 483–499. [CrossRef]

Schnell, T. (2012). Spirituality with and without religion—Differential relationships with personality. *Archive for the Psychology of Religion, 34*(1), 33–61. [CrossRef]

Schnell, T. (2020). *The psychology of meaning in life*. Routledge.

Schnell, T., & Becker, P. (2006). Personality and meaning in life. *Personality and Individual Differences, 41*(1), 117–129. [CrossRef]

Schönpflug, U. (2001). Intergenerational transmission of values: The role of transmission belts. *Journal of Cross-Cultural Psychology, 32*(2), 174–185. [CrossRef]

Schuler, E., & De Souza Brito Dias, C. (2019). The great and the grand: The roles of great-randparents and grandparents in multigenerational families. *Innovation in Aging, 3*, S283–S284. [CrossRef]

Silverstein, M., Yoon, J., Harris, R., & Hwang, W. (2022). Tracing the religious life course: Inter-and intragenerational sources of later life religiosity in baby boomers. *Innovation in Aging, 6*, 57. [CrossRef]

Slootjes, J., Keuzenkamp, S., & Saharso, S. (2017). The mechanisms behind the formation of a strong Sense of Coherence (SOC): The role of migration and integration. *Scandinavian Journal of Psychology, 58*(6), 571–580. [CrossRef] [PubMed]

Smith, J. L., & Hollinger-Smith, L. (2015). Savoring, resilience, and psychological well-being in older adults. *Aging & Mental Health, 19*(3), 192–200. [CrossRef]

Sørensen, T., Hestad, K., & Grov, E. (2021). Relationships of sources of meaning and resilience with meaningfulness and satisfaction with life: A population-based study of norwegians in late adulthood. *Frontiers in Psychology*, *12*, 685125. [CrossRef]

Spannari, J., Tervo-Niemela, K., & Kallatsa, L. (2021). Transformations and transmission—A contextual look at religious biographies of older adults. *Innovation in Aging*, *5*, 930. [CrossRef]

Stavrova, O., & Luhmann, M. (2016). Social connectedness as a source and consequence of meaning in life. *The Journal of Positive Psychology*, *11*, 470–479. [CrossRef]

Steptoe, A., & Fancourt, D. (2019). Leading a meaningful life at older ages and its relationship with social engagement, prosperity, health, biology, and time use. *Proceedings of the National Academy of Sciences of the United States of America*, *116*, 1207–1212. [CrossRef]

Sutin, A. (2023). New directions in research on the dynamics of purpose in life and cognitive aging. *Innovation in Aging*, *7*, 308. [CrossRef]

Tomstad, S., Sundsli, K., Sævareid, H., & Söderhamn, U. (2024). Social contact and belonging among older people receiving home care nursing. *Journal of Multidisciplinary Healthcare*, *17*, 1189–1198. [CrossRef]

Travers, J., Hirschman, K., & Naylor, M. (2021). Older adults' goals and expectations when using long-term services and supports. *Journal of Applied Gerontology*, *41*, 709–717. [CrossRef]

Van Leeuwen, K., Van Loon, M., Van Nes, F., Bosmans, J., De Vet, H., Ket, J., Widdershoven, G., & Ostelo, R. (2019). What does quality of life mean to older adults? A thematic synthesis. *PLoS ONE*, *14*, e0213263. [CrossRef] [PubMed]

Wolf, S. (2014). Meaning in life: Meeting the challenges. *Foundations of Science*, *21*, 279–282. [CrossRef]

Wong, P. (2016). Meaning-seeking, self-transcendence, and well-being. In A. Batthyány (Ed.), *Logotherapy and existential analysis proceedings of the viktor frankl institute vienna* (Vol. 1, pp. 311–321). Springer. [CrossRef]

Zhang, H., Sang, Z., Chan, D., & Schlegel, R. (2018). Threats to belongingness and meaning in life: A test of the compensation among sources of meaning. *Motivation and Emotion*, *43*, 242–254. [CrossRef]

Zhong, S., Lee, C., Foster, M., & Bian, J. (2020). Intergenerational communities: A systematic literature review of intergenerational interactions and older adults' health-related outcomes. *Social Science & Medicine*, *264*, 113374. [CrossRef]

Zhou, J., Li, T., Liao, M., & Gao, Y. (2019). Qualitative research on the sources of meaning in life in community elderly people. *The Journal of Practical Nursing*, *35*, 2840–2844. [CrossRef]

Zhou, J., Zhang, Y., Ren, Q., Li, T., Lin, G., Liao, M., Chen, S., Tong, P., & Gao, Y. (2023). Mediating effects of meaning in life on the relationship between family care, depression, and quality of life in Chinese older adults. *Frontiers in Public Health*, *11*, 1079593. [CrossRef]

Zimmer, Z., Jagger, C., Chiu, C. T., Ofstedal, M. B., Rojo, F., & Saito, Y. (2016). Spirituality, religiosity, aging and health in global perspective: A review. *SSM-Population Health*, *2*, 373–381. [CrossRef]

European Journal of
Investigation in Health, Psychology and Education

MDPI

Article

Innovative Health Promotion Strategies: A 6-Month Longitudinal Study on Computerized Cognitive Training for Older Adults with Minor Neurocognitive Disorders

Anna Tsiakiri [1,*], Spyridon Plakias [2], Pinelopi Vlotinou [3], Paraskevi Athanasouli [1], Aikaterini Terzoudi [1], Sotiria Kyriazidou [1], Aspasia Serdari [4], Georgia Karakitsiou [5,6], Kalliopi Megari [6], Nikolaos Aggelousis [7], Konstantinos Vadikolias [1] and Foteini Christidi [1]

1 Department of Neurology, Democritus University of Thrace, 68100 Alexandroupolis, Greece; athanasoulip@gmail.com (P.A.); terzoudi@med.duth.gr (A.T.); sokyriaz@med.duth.gr (S.K.); kvadikol@med.duth.gr (K.V.); christidi.f.a@gmail.com (F.C.)
2 Department of Physical Education and Sport Science, University of Thessaly, 42100 Trikala, Greece; spyros_plakias@yahoo.gr
3 Department of Occupational Therapy, University of West Attica, 12243 Athens, Greece; pvlotinou@uniwa.gr
4 Department of Child and Adolescent, Democritus University of Thrace, 68100 Alexandroupolis, Greece; aserntar@med.duth.gr
5 Department of Psychiatry, Medical School, Democritus University of Thrace, 68100 Alexandroupolis, Greece; gkarakit@med.duth.gr
6 School of Social Sciences and Humanities, Department of Psychology, University of Western Macedonia, 53100 Florina, Greece; kmegari@psy.auth.gr
7 Department of Physical Education and Sport Science, Democritus University of Thrace, 69100 Komotini, Greece; nagelous@phyed.duth.gr
* Correspondence: atsiakir@med.duth.gr

Abstract: Minor neurocognitive disorders (NCDs) represent a transitional phase between normal cognitive aging and dementia, highlighting the importance of early interventions. This study assessed the efficacy of a structured 6-month computerized cognitive training (CCT) program in stabilizing cognitive decline among older adults with minor NCDs. One hundred participants were randomly assigned to an intervention group or a non-intervention group. The intervention group underwent weekly, personalized CCT sessions using the MeMo program, which targeted memory, attention, and adaptability. Cognitive performance was measured at baseline and after six months using the Cambridge Cognitive Examination (CAMCOG). Statistical analysis showed significant cognitive decline in the non intervention group in orientation ($p = 0.032$), language expression ($p = 0.008$), praxis ($p = 0.008$), and memory ($p = 0.01$). In contrast, the intervention group showed no significant changes, except for a minor decline in perception ($p = 0.003$). These results suggest that CCT may help delay cognitive deterioration in minor NCDs. However, while cognitive decline was stabilized, no significant improvement was observed. Further research is recommended to investigate the long-term benefits and the transferability of cognitive gains. The findings support the use of CCT as a non-pharmacological health promotion strategy for enhancing cognitive resilience in aging populations. The novelty of this research lies in its focus on adaptive CCT as a non-pharmacological intervention, highlighting the potential role of neuroplasticity in delaying cognitive decline and offering new insights into personalized cognitive health strategies for aging populations.

Keywords: minor neurocognitive disorders; computerized cognitive training; cognitive decline; health promotion; neuroplasticity; aging

1. Introduction

Minor neurocognitive disorders (minor NCDs), historically known as Mild Cognitive Impairment (MCI), represent a transitional stage between normal aging and dementia, characterized by noticeable but not disabling cognitive decline. Over the years, various terms have been used to describe mild cognitive deterioration, including "benign senescent forgetfulness" (Kral, 1958) and "age-associated memory impairment" (Crook & Larrabee, 1988). However, Petersen and colleagues proposed the widely accepted term MCI, which remains a benchmark in clinical and research contexts (Petersen et al., 1999). The introduction of the DSM-5 in 2013 marked another important development, broadening the concept under the category of neurocognitive disorders (NCDs), which includes both mild and major types (Simpson, 2014). Early identification of minor NCDs is essential for promoting healthy aging, as timely interventions may delay or prevent progression to severe NCDs. Epidemiological data indicate that minor NCD prevalence increases with age, affecting approximately 15.8% of individuals over 60 and 28.6% over 80 (Petersen et al., 2018). While some cases of minor NCDs revert to normal cognitive levels, others progress to dementia, with depression and genetic factors (e.g., the APOE ε4 allele) playing critical roles in determining outcomes. Thus, early detection can enhance clinical decision-making and support preventive health strategies (Liu et al., 2013; Petersen et al., 2014).

Neuroplasticity refers to the brain's ability to reorganize and form new neural connections throughout life and plays a crucial role in maintaining cognitive function during aging (Smith, 2013). While aging is generally associated with a decline in neuroplastic potential, research highlights that the brain retains a significant capacity for adaptive changes even in later life stages (Bruel-Jungerman et al., 2007; Swaab, 1991). Factors such as cognitive stimulation, physical activity, and social engagement have been shown to enhance synaptic plasticity, promote neurogenesis, and improve overall brain resilience (Stern, 2002; Stern & Barulli, 2019). Moreover, interventions aimed at boosting neuroplasticity, including structured cognitive training and lifestyle modifications, have been linked to improved outcomes in individuals with minor NCDs (Scarmeas et al., 2003). Having an understanding of neuroplasticity during aging offers a promising path for the development of preventive strategies to slow cognitive decline and delay the onset of neurodegenerative diseases such as Alzheimer's disease (AD) (Alexopoulos, 2005; Kolb et al., 2017; Sachs-Ericsson & Blazer, 2015). Therefore, promoting neuroplasticity through lifelong learning and a healthy lifestyle is considered essential for healthy brain aging.

Extensive research highlights the potential benefits of cognitive interventions for older adults with minor NCDs. A meta-analysis by Li et al. showed that while no pharmacological treatment provides long-term benefits, cognitive training improves both cognitive performance and self-assessment (Li et al., 2011). Finn and McDonald observed enhanced performance through computer-based training, noting that participants retained the ability to transfer skills across domains (Finn & McDonald, 2011). Similarly, Fiatarone Singh and colleagues found that combining physical exercise with cognitive training significantly improved cognitive function over 18 months (Fiatarone Singh et al., 2014). Barban and colleagues demonstrated superior outcomes from cognitive training combined with positive memory recall therapy in minor NCDs and healthy older adults across four European countries (Barban et al., 2016). Further, Hill and colleagues highlighted the advantages of computer-based interventions, including low cost, adaptability, and scalability (Hill et al., 2017). Recent studies emphasize that combined interventions, including exercise and cognitive training, are among the most effective strategies for cognitive improvement in minor NCDs (Xu et al., 2021).

Computerized cognitive training (CCT) involves the use of specially designed computerized programs, often referred to as "serious games" delivered via computers, tablets, or smart TVs. Zyda defines "serious games" as interactive digital competitions, developed with an educational goal alongside entertainment, aiming to improve skills or impart knowledge (Zyda, 2005). These games combine narrative, artistic design, and software engineering with a pedagogical dimension, emphasizing that while education is critical, entertainment should take precedence to ensure engagement. Several studies have explored the effectiveness of these programs on cognitive functions in older adults with minor NCDs (Barnes et al., 2009; Chae & Lee, 2023; Delbroek et al., 2017; Hagovská et al., 2017; Han et al., 2014; Hyer et al., 2016; Rozzini et al., 2007; Unverzagt et al., 2007). Improved cognitive functions have been reported following NPT software-based training, specifically in areas such as memory (short-term, long-term, verbal, and visual), attention (both spread and divided), perception (including perceptual recognition and identification), verbal fluency, and psychomotor learning (Cipriani et al., 2006). Similarly, Talassi et al. (Talassi et al., 2007) and Rozzini et al. (Rozzini et al., 2007) found enhanced cognitive and emotional outcomes from combined interventions, including behavioral therapy and pharmacological treatments. Barnes et al. highlighted improvements in visual memory and language skills (Barnes et al., 2009), while Herrera et al. observed positive effects on episodic recall and recognition after 12 weeks of training (Herrera et al., 2012). González-Palau and colleagues demonstrated that the "Long Lasting Memories" (LLM) program improved general cognitive function and reduced depressive symptoms over a 12-week period (González-Palau et al., 2014). Moreover, research on virtual reality-based programs has shown promising results. Thapa and colleagues and Maeng and colleagues observed cognitive improvements and enhanced visuospatial skills in participants undergoing VR-based training (Maeng et al., 2021; Thapa et al., 2020). Recent systematic reviews and meta-analyses (Bahar-Fuchs et al., 2017; Ge et al., 2018) have confirmed that CCT leads to improvements in both cognitive and emotional functioning.

Building on the extensive literature review, it becomes evident that CCT offers significant potential for promoting cognitive resilience in older adults with mild neurocognitive disorders (NCDs). However, important gaps persist regarding its long-term efficacy and the most effective implementation protocols. While existing research has predominantly focused on short-term cognitive improvements, sustained benefits and the transferability of these gains to untrained cognitive domains or everyday functional tasks remain underexplored. Therefore, the present study aims to assess the effectiveness of a structured CCT program, specifically designed to improve cognitive function and/or delay progression to severe cognitive impairment in this vulnerable population. By focusing on adaptive, computer-based interventions, this research seeks to contribute valuable insights into health promotion strategies tailored to aging individuals.

2. Materials and Methods

2.1. Subjects

All participants were regularly monitored by the interdisciplinary team of the Dementia Outpatient Clinic at the Department of Neurology, University General Hospital of Alexandroupolis, were recruited from the broader region of Thrace, and represented a diverse sample in terms of age, educational background, and reported duration of cognitive decline. All participants were initially interviewed to collect demographic data and detailed medical history, including any previous diagnoses, as well as information regarding cardiovascular, metabolic, and neurological disorders, and past or current emotional or psychiatric conditions. Following the interview, each participant underwent a thorough clinical evaluation, which included a neurological examination, cognitive assessment, brain imaging, and specialized biochemical and hematological testing. The inclusion criteria were the following: age over 50 years old; subjective cognitive decline or cognitive decline reported by an informant (e.g., spouse, adult child, or primary caregiver) who had regular contact with the participant and who could provide reliable observations of cognitive changes lasting at least six months prior to study enrollment; cognitive impairment verified through formal cognitive testing, preserved functional capacity in daily life activities; Greek as the native language; and adequate sensory and motor functions to ensure reliable participation in psychometric assessments and cognitive training sessions. Sensory and motor abilities were evaluated during the initial clinical examination, including basic vision and hearing screening (with corrective aids if necessary) and a brief neurological assessment to verify fine and gross motor skills, ensuring participants could effectively interact with the touchscreen device used in cognitive training. Cognitive impairment was verified through formal cognitive testing, including the Montreal Cognitive Assessment (MoCA) (Nasreddine et al., 2005; Tsiakiri et al., 2021) and the Cambridge Cognitive Examination (CAMCOG) (Roth et al., 1986; Tsolaki et al., 2000), in accordance with DSM-5 criteria. The diagnostic process also involved a comprehensive clinical evaluation that included medical history, neurological examination, neuroimaging, and laboratory tests to rule out secondary causes of cognitive impairment. Subjective cognitive complaints were validated through both self-reports and informant reports provided by close family members or caregivers with regular contact with the participant. To differentiate between normal cognitive aging and minor NCD, we applied neuropsychological criteria based on age- and education-adjusted normative data, considering scores 1 to 1.5 standard deviations below the mean as indicative of cognitive decline. Potential confounding factors, such as comorbid medical conditions, were systematically evaluated and considered in the diagnostic process. The exclusion criteria were the following: prior diagnosis of dementia, other neurological disease; other major psychiatric disorder (such as psychosis, major depressive disorder, bipolar disorder, etc.), major cardiovascular diseases; current pharmacological treatment with cholinesterase inhibitors, antipsychotic medications, anticholinergic drugs, benzodiazepines, or neuroleptics.

After completing the screening process, 100 individuals met the diagnostic criteria for minor NCD, as defined in the DSM-5 (Simpson, 2014), as well as the inclusion/exclusion criteria of this study, and were further allocated into the two groups of this study (i.e., an intervention group and a non-intervention group). All participants provided written informed consent prior to their inclusion in this study. Ethical approval was obtained from the Scientific Board of the University General Hospital of Alexandroupolis (ΔΣ1/Θ68/06-04-2020). The data were analyzed anonymously.

2.2. *Materials*

2.2.1. Clinical Assessment

Participants' clinical assessment and follow-up at the Dementia Outpatient Clinic were carried out by a multidisciplinary team, which consisted of experienced medical professionals, nursing staff, and experts from various other fields. All relevant information was systematically documented in an electronic medical record, including demographic details, provisional diagnoses, findings from clinical and laboratory testing, vascular risk factors, and data regarding the onset and progression of the disease.

2.2.2. Neuropsychological Assessment

The primary tool used in this evaluation was the Cambridge Cognitive Examination (CAMCOG), a subscale of the Cambridge Mental Disorders of the Elderly Examination (CAMDEX), first introduced by Roth and colleagues (Roth et al., 1986; Tsolaki et al., 2000). CAMCOG is widely regarded as a reliable instrument for detecting cognitive deficits and assessing patients with minor NCDs. It provides a total score ranging from 0 to 107, based on responses to 60 individual items, and covers nine distinct cognitive domains: orientation, language comprehension, language expression, attention, praxis, calculation, abstraction, memory, and perception. The administration of the CAMCOG typically requires 30 to 40 min, but may take longer depending on the severity of the participant's cognitive deficits. This tool has been recommended for the detection of mild NCDs and is considered effective in differentiating between normal aging and pathological cognitive decline (Aprahamian et al., 2011; Conde-Sala et al., 2012). In accordance with the study design, the assessments were conducted at two key points: initially upon the participants' enrollment in the study (T0), and exactly six months later (T1), for both the intervention and non-intervention groups. This ensured consistency in the assessment timeline across groups, with the intervention group completing their cognitive training and the non-intervention group undergoing routine clinical follow-up during this same period.

2.2.3. Computerized Cognitive Training (CTT) Program

In this study, the Memory Motivation (MeMo) program served as a primary tool for cognitive training (Memory Motivation, n.d.; P. Robert et al., 2020). The MeMo is an online application developed to support individuals with cognitive disorders, healthcare professionals engaged in the prevention of cognitive decline and stimulation, and anyone seeking to enhance their memory and attention. Designed by a team of healthcare experts from the Institut Claude Pompidou, Association IA, CoBTeK lab, and Université Côte d'Azur in Nice, France, the MeMo program was translated into Greek for the purpose of the present study (Department of Neurology, University General Hospital of Alexandroupolis, Democritus University of Thrace), following authorization from its creators. MeMo offers a variety of recreational activities and exercises specifically designed to strengthen and train cognitive functions. The program focuses on three core areas: memory, adaptability, and attention. Each exercise is tailored to target a specific cognitive skill, allowing for personalized training based on the individual's identified deficits. The training activities in MeMo are divided into two main sections. The first section focuses on memory, offering three distinct exercises: "Recognition", aimed at improving visual memory; "MeMo Quiz", designed to train working memory; and "Faces", which helps users practice memory recall. The second section emphasizes mental flexibility and attention, featuring three additional exercises: "Arrows", which targets processing speed, inhibitory control, and cognitive flexibility; "Complex Cards", which is geared toward enhancing working memory; and "Square Jumps", aimed at training response prediction and inhibitory control. Each exercise includes graded difficulty levels and tracks users' personal scores and progress over time. When a user achieves the highest score in a specific level, they are automatically promoted to the next level. The adaptive nature of the MeMo program lies in its dynamic adjustment of exercise difficulty. While the content of the exercises is standardized, the program automatically advances participants to more challenging levels when tasks are successfully completed. Conversely, if a participant struggles, the program retains them at the current level, allowing for continued practice until mastery is achieved. This adaptive mechanism ensures that each individual engages with tasks that correspond to their cognitive performance, promoting effective and personalized cognitive stimulation. After creating an account, users can monitor their performance and progress, while therapists can also track the long-term development of their patients. The MeMo application is freely accessible at the following link, http://www.memory-motivation.org/home-4/, and is available in four different languages: English, French, Italian, and Greek. It has been primarily utilized in studies conducted by its developers to evaluate its effectiveness in cognitive training for older adults with minor neurocognitive disorders. Although external studies are currently limited, the available research highlights its potential as a valuable non-pharmacological intervention.

2.3. Procedure

All participants were randomly assigned to one of two groups: the intervention group, consisting of participants who completed the cognitive intervention program, and The non-intervention group, which comprised individuals who continued with their standard clinical follow-up, which included routine medical monitoring, health consultations, and general advice provided by the Dementia Outpatient Clinic. However, they did not receive any structured cognitive training or specific cognitive stimulation during the study period.

For the intervention group, each individual cognitive training session consisted of activities from the MeMo program. Sessions were scheduled to last 45 min each. Sessions were held once a week over a period of six consecutive months. All interventions were tailored to individual needs, and appropriate electronic equipment was available for delivering the CCT programs. The program sessions were conducted in a dedicated space provided by the Department of Neurology, located within the urban area of the city. This environment was carefully selected to ensure minimal distractions and was equipped with adequate lighting to create an optimal setting for cognitive training. A laptop with a touchscreen was primarily used, as it was observed that using a computer mouse reduced performance in time-sensitive tasks, while tablets were deemed inadequate due to their smaller screens.

Before starting the program, participants attended two introductory sessions to become familiar with the computer equipment and software. Participation in the program was entirely voluntary, and individuals were free to withdraw at any time if they wished. The recruitment of the 50 participants was carried out in staggered phases to ensure that the program could be delivered consistently by a single researcher, who conducted all sessions to maintain uniformity and reduce the likelihood of participant dropout.

2.4. Statistical Analysis

Comparisons between the intervention and non-intervention groups at baseline demographic and clinical characteristics were made using an independent *t*-test (age), a Mann–Whitney U test (education, MoCA), and chi-square (sex distribution). Generalized linear mixed models (GLMMs) were applied to examine the effect of the interaction TIME*intervention on nine dependent variables of CAMCOG (orientation, language comprehension, language expression, attention, praxis, calculation, abstraction, memory, perception). A negative binomial distribution was chosen in all cases based on the Akaike Information Criterion (AIC) and Bayesian Information Criterion (BIC). The significance level was set at $p = 0.05$, adjusted for multiple comparisons with Bonferroni correction. IBM SPSS Statistics software (Version 29, IBM SPSS Inc., Chicago, IL, USA) was used for statistical analyses.

3. Results

The final sample consisted of 100 participants of both sexes. The demographic characteristics and MoCA scores of the participants at baseline are presented in Table 1. The groups did not differ in age ($p = 0.172$), sex distribution ($p = 0.260$), education ($p = 0.057$), or MoCA score ($p = 0.068$).

Table 2 presents descriptive statistics comparing two groups (i.e., non-intervention and intervention) at two time points, t0 (baseline) and t1 (follow-up), across various cognitive domains as measured by CAMCOG. Each cognitive domain was assessed at both time points. The results are reported separately for the groups, and the data format includes the mean value followed by the SD.

Table 3 presents the results of pairwise comparisons for the CAMCOG target variables measured at two time points (t0 vs. t1) for the two groups (the intervention and non-intervention group). Post hoc analysis revealed significant differences between the two time points (t0 vs. t1) for the non-intervention group in several CAMCOG variables, but not for the intervention group. Specifically, the non-intervention group showed significantly worse performance at t1 in orientation (p = 0.032), language expression (p = 0.008), praxis (p = 0.008), and memory (p = 0.01). Furthermore, there were significant differences for both intervention and non-intervention groups in CAMCOG-perception (intervention group: p = 0.003; non-intervention group, p = 0.03), with both groups showing worse performance at t1.

Table 1. Demographic characteristics and MoCA scores of groups at baseline (t0).

	Total Sample	Non-Intervention Group	Intervention Group	p-Value
Age (yrs)	69.92 ± 7.45	68.90 ± 8.35	70.94 ± 6.35	0.172
Sex (M/F)	27/73	16/34	11/39	0.260
Education (yrs)	9.48 ± 4.96	8.48 ± 5.32	10.48 ± 4.39	0.057
MoCA	24.72 ± 2.07	24.40 ± 2.15	25.04 ± 1.96	0.068

Notes. yrs = years; M/F = male/female; MoCA = Montreal Cognitive Assessment.

Table 2. Descriptive statistics (mean ± SD) of CAMCOG scores across intervention and non-intervention groups at baseline (t0) and follow-up (t1).

	Baseline (t0) Groups		Follow-Up (t1) Groups	
	Non-Intervention	Intervention	Non-Intervention	Intervention
Orientation	9.96 ± 0.20	9.94 ± 0.31	9.78 ± 0.58	9.92 ± 0.40
Language comprehension	6.38 ± 0.75	6.44 ± 0.76	6.24 ± 0.74	6.50 ± 0.68
Language expression	23.82 ± 2.72	24.22 ± 2.35	23.00 ± 2.93	24.10 ± 2.64
Attention	6.40 ± 1.03	6.68 ± 0.65	6.46 ± 0.73	6.62 ± 0.67
Praxis	26.42 ± 2.32	26.76 ± 2.02	25.68 ± 2.80	26.48 ± 2.10
Calculation	2.02 ± 0.14	2.00 ± 0.00	2.02 ± 0.14	2.00 ± 0.00
Abstraction	5.30 ± 1.66	5.52 ± 1.52	5.42 ± 1.68	5.52 ± 1.50
Memory	26.16 ± 3.55	25.86 ± 3.60	25.42 ± 3.99	25.46 ± 3.94
Perception	8.80 ± 1.92	9.14 ± 1.05	8.54 ± 1.93	8.76 ± 1.22

Notes. SD = standard deviation; CAMCOG = Cambridge Cognitive Examination.

Table 3. Pairwise comparisons of CAMCOG target variables across time points (t0 vs. t1) for the two groups (non-intervention, intervention).

CAMCOG Target Variables	Groups	Contrast Estimate (SE)	Statistics (t, df, p_{adj})
Orientation	Non-intervention	0.180 (0.083)	t (196) = 2.159; $\mathbf{p_{adj}}$ **= 0.032**
	Intervention	0.020 (0.045)	t (196) = 0.448; p_{adj} = 0.655
Language comprehension	Non-intervention	0.139 (0.080)	t (196) = 1.749; p_{adj} = 0.082
	Intervention	−0.060 (0.071)	t (196) = −0.838; p_{adj} = 0.403
Language expression	Non-intervention	0.816 (0.304)	t (196) = 2.683; $\mathbf{p_{adj}}$ **= 0.008**
	Intervention	0.120 (0.228)	t (196) = 0.524; p_{adj} = 0.601
Attention	Non-intervention	−0.060 (0.130)	t (196) = −0.458; p_{adj} = 0.647
	Intervention	0.060 (0.059)	t (196) = 1.010; p_{adj} = 0.314
Praxis	Non-intervention	0.738 (0.273)	t (196) = 2.701; $\mathbf{p_{adj}}$ **= 0.008**
	Intervention	0.279 (0.179)	t (196) = 1.565; p_{adj} = 0.119

Table 3. *Cont.*

CAMCOG Target Variables	Groups	Contrast Estimate (SE)	Statistics (t, df, p_{adj})
Calculation	Non-intervention	0.000 (0.000)	n/a
	Intervention	−0.000 (0.000)	n/a
Abstraction	Non-intervention	−0.115 (0.153)	t (196) = −0.754; p_{adj} = 0.452
	Intervention	−0.000 (0.117)	t (196) = −0.000; p_{adj} = 1.000
Memory	Non-intervention	0.734 (0.283)	t (196) = 2.592; $\mathbf{p_{adj}}$ **= 0.010**
	Intervention	0.397 (0.440)	t (196) = 0.902; p_{adj} = 0.368
Perception	Non-intervention	0.256 (0.117)	t (196) = 2.180; $\mathbf{p_{adj}}$ **= 0.030**
	Intervention	0.378 (0.125)	t (196) = 3.012; $\mathbf{p_{adj}}$ **= 0.003**

Notes. CAMCOG = Cambridge Cognitive Examination; SE = standard error; p_{adj} = Bonferroni adjusted *p*-value. Bold *p*-values represent significant differences between t0 and t1, after Bonferroni correction for multiple comparisons.

The CAMCOG variables with statistically significant differences are graphically represented in Figure 1a, Figure 1b, Figure 1c, Figure 1d, and Figure 1e, respectively.

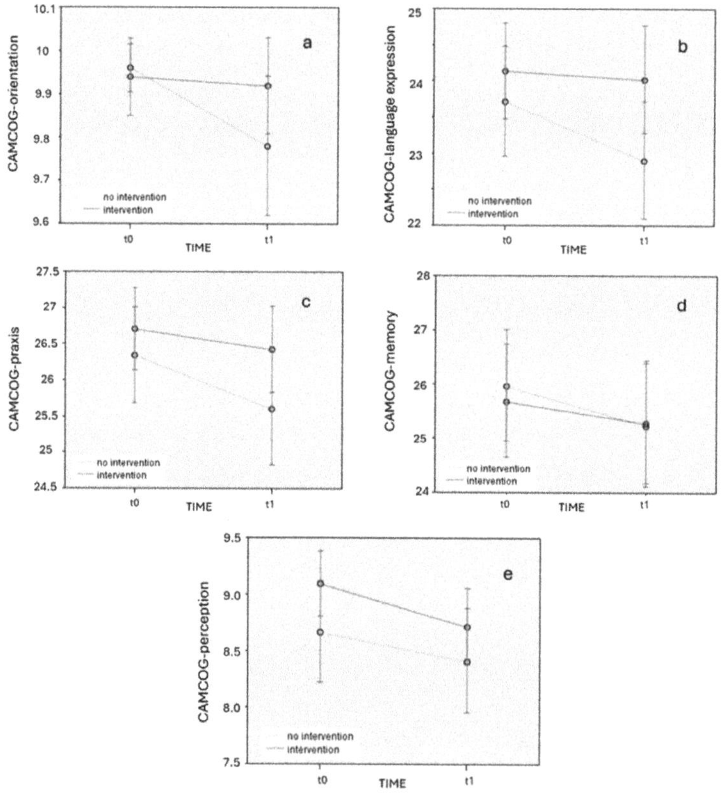

Figure 1. (**a**). Changes in target CAMCOG variable of orientation over time (t0 and t1) for intervention and non-intervention groups. (**b**). Changes in target CAMCOG variable of language expression over time (t0 and t1) for intervention and non-intervention groups. (**c**). Changes in target CAMCOG variable of praxis over time (t0 and t1) for intervention and non-intervention groups. (**d**). Changes in target CAMCOG variable of memory over time (t0 and t1) for intervention and non-intervention groups. (**e**). Changes in target CAMCOG variable of perception over time (t0 and t1) for intervention and non-intervention groups.

4. Discussion

The present study highlights a critical distinction between the cognitive trajectories of participants receiving a 6-month intervention and those without any structured cognitive support. Specifically, our study suggests that a CCT program provided through a 6-month period may stabilize cognitive decline in individuals with minor NCD; while significant cognitive decline was observed across multiple domains in the non-intervention group, the intervention group mainly demonstrated a pattern of no changes over time.

4.1. CCT and Underlying Mechanisms in Cognitive Decline

One of the key findings of the present study is that overall cognitive functioning in the intervention group did not show any significant decline (except for CAMCOG-perception), a result that supports the hypothesis regarding the efficacy of the proposed personalized CCT intervention. Although no significant improvement was identified, the absence of significant decline in most cognitive domains indicates that the CCT intervention may have played a protective role against progressive cognitive deterioration. In contrast to the intervention group, the non-intervention group showed statistically significant declines in various cognitive domains. Orientation exhibited a notable reduction, reflecting diminished spatial and temporal awareness over time in the absence of external cognitive engagement. Language expression also showed a marked decline, highlighting progressive deterioration in verbal fluency and communication abilities. Similarly, praxis was negatively affected, indicating a worsening capacity to perform learned motor sequences, potentially linked to reduced coordination and planning functions. Memory performance declined as well, aligning with the expected trajectory of cognitive aging in the absence of active cognitive stimulation. Additionally, sensory perception demonstrated a significant decrease, underscoring the natural progression of cognitive impairment over time.

Our findings are in line with the existing literature suggesting that cognitive training can be a promising approach for slowing cognitive decline (Butler et al., 2018) and/or improving cognitive performance and behavioral symptoms (Ge et al., 2018; Hill et al., 2017), as well as neuropsychiatric symptoms (Liang et al., 2018). Similar trends were reported in a previous study, where the most notable changes were observed in language and memory (Barnes et al., 2009). Additionally, two other studies documented improvement tendencies in memory, although these were not supported by statistically significant results in neuropsychological tests (Rapp et al., 2002; Troyer et al., 2008). This observation aligns with previous findings, suggesting that older adults with minor NCDs can benefit from cognitive interventions across multiple cognitive and non-cognitive domains (Hughes et al., 2014).

The sustainability of cognitive improvement over time has been questioned in previous studies and cannot be answered in the present study, where only short-term effects were examined. The SMART study highlighted that cognitive training preserved memory performance, but only during the intervention period, suggesting that the benefits of cognitive interventions are contingent on continuous practice across multiple cognitive domains (Fiatarone Singh et al., 2014). Similarly, short-term improvement in cognition has been found in subjects with mild cognitive deficits following the implementation of a computer-assisted cognitive rehabilitation program (Mansbach et al., 2017). However, a systematic review of 32 studies emphasizes both short- and long-term benefits of cognitive interventions (Hong et al., 2015). Of note, CCT has been proposed as a technique with potential long-term benefits for cognitive health (Bahar-Fuchs et al., 2017; Lampit et al., 2014; Shah et al., 2017; Tsiakiri, 2022). It has been suggested that computer-based interventions are more effective for cognitive training, while structured instructional interventions are superior in fostering self-assessment skills (Li et al., 2011). CCT has also been effective for the improvement of emotional well-being. A previously published sub-study by Tsiakiri and colleagues reported similar results, showing enhancements in emotional status (Tsiakiri et al., 2024c). Furthermore, not only CCT, but also other digital activities, such as brain-training games, have been shown to enhance overall cognitive functioning (Gooding et al., 2016).

The absence of significant improvement in memory performance in the intervention group is a noteworthy finding, particularly since memory is a core domain targeted in cognitive training for individuals with NCDs. Several factors may account for this outcome. While the MeMo program includes exercises designed to stimulate memory-related processes, such as working memory and recall tasks, it is possible that the program's structure did not provide sufficient intensity or task specificity to elicit measurable gains in memory. The adaptive design of the program focuses primarily on performance-based progression, which may favor improvements in cognitive flexibility and attention rather than engaging the deeper encoding and consolidation processes necessary for enhancing memory. Additionally, the memory tasks within the MeMo program may have been more focused on short-term and working memory rather than on episodic memory, which tends to be more vulnerable in individuals with minor NCDs. This focus could partially explain the discrepancy between our findings and those of previous studies that reported significant memory improvements following cognitive interventions specifically tailored to episodic memory, such as those incorporating spaced retrieval or associative learning techniques.

To enhance memory-related outcomes, future iterations of the program could benefit from modifications aimed at increasing task complexity with a greater emphasis on long-term memory processes. Incorporating strategy-based training approaches, such as mnemonic devices and visualization techniques, may also strengthen memory performance. Furthermore, increasing the overall training intensity and frequency, along with repeated exposure to memory-specific tasks, could contribute to more pronounced cognitive gains. Combining computerized cognitive training with real-life memory exercises or dual-task paradigms may further support the transfer of cognitive improvements to everyday memory functions.

In our study, the absence of significant cognitive decline in the intervention group, compared to the significant cognitive deterioration in several domains in the non-intervention group, support the potential of CCT in delaying progression to dementia. Although not specifically examined in the current study, the beneficial effects of cognitive training interventions are believed to result from neuroplastic changes at the synaptic level. For instance, training in sensory and motor functions has the potential to alter synaptic connections in these regions, as well as in the prefrontal cortex (Hu et al., 2021). It can also increase levels of neurotrophic factors in the brain, enhancing resistance to neural damage (Verghese et al., 2003). In addition, cognitive–neuroimaging studies support neuroplastic alterations in several brain regions following cognitive training sessions, including functional changes in the hippocampus in subjects with MCI (Rosen et al., 2011). The hippocampus is a key area for memory functions (Bartsch & Wulff, 2015), while hippocampal and medial temporal atrophy have been identified as key predictors of cognitive decline (van de Pol et al., 2007). Another study combining cognitive and neuroimaging measures in MCI subjects with and without a 7-month combined cognitive/physical training revealed significant cognitive decline in a non-intervention group and significant cognitive improvement in an intervention group, followed by a neural efficiency decline in a non-intervention group (Maffei et al., 2017). Similarly, Klados and colleagues found that cognitive training combined with physical exercise can reorganize the functional connectivity of the beta band in individuals with NCDs (Klados et al., 2016). Therefore, not only is physical exercise effective for cognitive enhancement (Pamboris et al., 2024; Vlotinou et al., 2023), but combined physical and cognitive exercises maximize the benefits for brain health by pairing physical activity and cognitive effort (Styliadis et al., 2015). The references to neuroplastic changes are grounded in findings from prior research on the effects of cognitive training in older adults, which suggest that cognitive stimulation may promote neural adaptability and support hippocampal function. However, these neurobiological mechanisms remain speculative within the context of our results. Future studies incorporating neuroimaging or biological markers would be necessary to validate such interpretations and provide direct evidence of underlying neural changes associated with CCT.

Of note, cognitive training may be more effective for patients in very early stages of cognitive impairment, with the optimal window of intervention being when individuals report subjective cognitive decline. Previous studies have shown that the early stages of Alzheimer's disease benefit more from cognitive training (Clare et al., 2003). In contrast, reversing cognitive decline in the later stages of dementia is challenging, as deficits become severe. However, restoring residual cognitive and emotional functioning remains possible (Sakamoto et al., 2013), as the hippocampus in NCDs may retain sufficient neuroplasticity to benefit from cognitive training (Rosen et al., 2011). Therefore, considering that many subjects with minor NCDs progress to have major NCDs (Tsiakiri et al., 2024a), cognitive training interventions may have an added value by enhancing neuroplasticity and thus delaying cognitive decline in both healthy aging and NCD populations (González-Palau et al., 2014).

Although this study revealed statistically significant effects of computerized cognitive training (CCT) in preventing cognitive decline, it is important to consider whether these findings reflect clinically meaningful improvements in cognitive function. Statistical significance indicates that the observed changes are unlikely due to chance; however, this does not necessarily imply that the magnitude of change has a tangible impact on individuals' daily functioning. The effect sizes observed in our study suggest modest improvements, particularly in domains such as memory, language, and praxis, which are crucial for maintaining functional independence in older adults. While these improvements may not represent dramatic shifts in neuropsychological test scores, even small gains in cognitive performance can be meaningful in real-world contexts, such as enhancing the ability to manage daily tasks, maintain social engagement, and reduce the risk of further cognitive deterioration. Moreover, the cumulative effect of cognitive stability over time, as observed in the intervention group, could delay progression to more severe cognitive impairment. Future research should incorporate functional outcome measures, such as activities of daily living (ADLs) and quality of life assessments, to better capture the clinical relevance of cognitive changes observed in CCT interventions.

4.2. Clinical Considerations and Training Effectiveness

Cognitive Training and Transfer Effects: Although the applied CCT mainly offers activities related to memory, adaptability, and attention, we found significant post-intervention differences in memory, but also in orientation, language expression, praxis, and perception. This highlights a key question in cognitive intervention research, i.e., whether improvement in a specific cognitive domain can be transferred to other untrained domains, thereby enhancing the brain's neuroplasticity. Despite reports on limited such generalization across cognitive domains (Mansbach et al., 2017), previous studies have demonstrated that healthy older adults can benefit from cognitive training in both near-transfer tasks (similar to the trained tasks) and far-transfer tasks (dissimilar to the trained tasks) (Karbach & Kray, 2009; Willis et al., 2006). A previous meta-analysis also found significant improvement in functional abilities among individuals with minor NCDs following cognitive training, suggesting a transfer effect of cognitive training (Li et al., 2011), which can also benefit subjects' quality of life (Hagovská et al., 2017). Of note, in other clinical groups, such as stroke, training in processing speed in particular has shown promise in improving working memory and daily functioning by maintaining two key neural networks involved in cognitive regulation: the central executive network and the default mode network (Tsiakiri et al., 2024b). The potential for transfer effects from training of one cognitive function to untrained cognitive functions holds significant clinical relevance. Two interpretations have been proposed to explain this phenomenon (Lin et al., 2016). The first posits that individuals with minor NCDs, having lower baseline cognitive abilities, possess greater room for improvement across both trained and untrained domains. The second highlights the benefits of enriched training protocols that incorporate a combination of multiple tasks.

In this study, a total of 24 sessions per participant, with a weekly frequency of one session lasting 45 min, offered over a period of 6 months, has not been clearly established in the literature as sufficient for long-term outcomes. The largest cognitive gains are thought to occur through repeated practice of a skill over an extended period, even when learned later in life. Intensive training or practice of a novel skill can alter neural structures and functions within a relatively short time frame of 1 week to 3 months (Rabipour & Raz, 2012). In another study, researchers concluded that brief sessions under 30 min may be ineffective, possibly because synaptic plasticity is more likely to occur after 30 to 60 min of stimulation (Lampit et al., 2014). On the other hand, conducting training more than three times per week might reduce the effectiveness of computer-based cognitive programs. These findings raise the possibility of an optimal "dose" of training, beyond which factors such as cognitive fatigue may diminish the benefits of the intervention. In fact, the "dose effect" of cognitive intervention is a key area of research, aimed at determining whether the effectiveness of an intervention correlates with the duration of cognitive training or the number of training sessions (Basak et al., 2008; Miller et al., 2013; Sood et al., 2019). To date, there is no strong evidence that longer sessions or a greater number of total sessions are positively associated with improved outcomes in individuals with minor NCDs. In fact, some studies with higher session counts and longer total durations reported smaller effect sizes (Li et al., 2011). Regarding the appropriate intervention duration, evidence suggests that the number of sessions may not directly influence intervention outcomes. Furthermore, a large-scale study indicated a negligible correlation between the number of training sessions and observed transfer benefits (Owen et al., 2010).

The schedule of the present study was designed to balance cognitive stimulation with feasibility, ensuring high adherence among older adults with minor neurocognitive disorders. However, the literature presents mixed findings regarding the optimal 'dose' of cognitive training for maximizing cognitive benefits. In fact, higher session counts and longer intervention durations do not consistently correlate with improved cognitive outcomes, with some studies reporting smaller effect sizes under more intensive protocols. Given these discrepancies, our protocol represents a moderate-intensity approach aimed at providing sufficient cognitive stimulation while maintaining long-term engagement and minimizing the risk of fatigue. Future research should focus on systematically evaluating different training frequencies, session durations, and intervention lengths to determine the most effective combination for enhancing cognitive outcomes, particularly in populations with minor NCDs.

While our study demonstrated that the intervention group maintained cognitive function over the study period, no significant cognitive improvements were observed, which contrasts with prior research reporting cognitive gains following computerized cognitive training (CCT). Several factors may account for this discrepancy. Firstly, the duration of the intervention may have influenced the outcomes. Although the six-month training period aligns with other CCT studies, it is possible that a longer intervention might be required to produce measurable cognitive gains, particularly in populations with existing cognitive impairments. Training frequency could also be a contributing factor; variations in adherence or engagement levels may have limited the cumulative cognitive stimulation necessary to drive significant improvements. Additionally, sample characteristics may have played a role. Our study focused on older adults with minor neurocognitive disorders (NCDs), a group that may have reduced neuroplasticity compared to cognitively healthy individuals, potentially limiting their capacity for cognitive gains. In contrast, studies reporting significant improvements often include younger or healthier populations with greater cognitive reserve. Finally, it is worth considering that the primary benefit of CCT in populations with minor NCD may lie in the preservation of cognitive function rather than marked improvement. Preventing decline in such vulnerable groups can be clinically meaningful, even in the absence of measurable cognitive enhancement. Future research should explore the impact of longer interventions, increased training intensity, and tailored programs to maximize cognitive outcomes.

A key limitation of this study is the lack of follow-up assessments beyond the 6-month intervention period, which limits our ability to determine the long-term sustainability of the observed cognitive benefits. While the intervention group maintained cognitive function during the study period, it remains unclear whether these effects persist over time or if cognitive decline resumes once the training is discontinued. Cognitive training interventions may produce temporary gains that diminish without continued practice, as suggested by some longitudinal studies. Conversely, sustained cognitive benefits have been reported in studies with extended follow-up periods, highlighting the potential role of booster sessions or ongoing cognitive engagement in maintaining improvements. Future research should incorporate longitudinal follow-up assessments to evaluate the durability of cognitive training effects, ideally over periods of 12 months or longer. Such studies could provide insights into the optimal frequency and duration of interventions required to achieve and maintain long-term cognitive health, particularly in populations at risk for neurocognitive decline.

The results of the present study are consistent with the existing literature on the efficacy of computerized cognitive training (CCT) in older adults with cognitive impairments. Prior studies, such as those by Smith (2013) and Lampit et al. (2014), have demonstrated that CCT interventions can lead to significant improvements in cognitive domains, including memory, attention, and executive functions. These studies emphasized the role of adaptive training protocols, where task difficulty dynamically adjusts based on the participant's performance, thereby enhancing cognitive engagement, and promoting neuroplasticity. In line with these findings, our study employed an adaptive CCT approach through the MeMo platform, which not only adjusts the complexity of cognitive tasks in real-time, but also allows for remote, unsupervised implementation, offering greater flexibility compared to traditional, clinic-based interventions.

4.3. Delivery Mode in Cognitive Training

Another important aspect of the present study is the therapeutic framework in which the intervention program was delivered. It consisted exclusively of individualized, face-to-face sessions, with a personalized approach for each participant. These components have been shown to enhance the effectiveness of similar interventions (Belleville et al., 2006; Hwang et al., 2012), although some research also supports the superiority of group-based interventions (Lampit et al., 2014; Verhaeghen et al., 1992). Direct supervision by the researcher ensured adherence to the therapeutic protocol, provided encouragement for completing demanding tasks, assisted in resolving technical issues, and promoted social interaction, all of which may further contribute to the overall efficacy of such interventions.

4.4. Motivation in Cognitive Training

A crucial element reported in cognitive training studies is the role of motivation (Ben-Sadoun et al., 2016; Manera et al., 2015) in encouraging participation in cognitive training programs (Ben-Sadoun et al., 2018). Motivation is considered a central component of intervention theory for older adults with cognitive impairment (Savulich et al., 2017; Valentijn et al., 2005). Within the motivational framework of this program, two primary mechanisms—perceived benefit and support—were shown to influence the degree to which older adults with cognitive dysfunction are motivated to engage in exercise-based interventions. The MeMo program has been designed to enhance intrinsic motivation for continued engagement through several key features (P. Robert et al., 2020). First, the game interface is specifically tailored to older adults with cognitive dysfunction, incorporating a simplified graphical user interface, straightforward instructions with regular reminders, and clear gameplay rules, making it highly accessible to participants. Additionally, the difficulty level of the exercises is dynamically adjusted to participants' performance, providing an error-free learning environment, and keeping them in a "challenge zone" to maintain engagement. Finally, the program is implemented on a touchscreen device to reduce barriers associated with unfamiliar technological interfaces, such as a mouse and keyboard, which older adults often find difficult to use (P. H. Robert et al., 2014).

4.5. Strengths and Limitations of the Study

This study presents strengths that enhance the reliability and validity of its findings. The rigorous inclusion criteria were based on DSM-5 standards for minor NCD, and the comprehensive assessments ensured accurate participant selection and minimized diagnostic bias. Additionally, the personalized CCT intervention, delivered through the MeMo application and supervised individually, promoted high engagement and adherence, resulting in minimal participant dropout. However, certain limitations must be acknowledged. The relatively small sample size and the six-month duration of the intervention may have restricted this study's ability to detect long-term cognitive changes. Additionally, the lack of long-term follow-up makes it difficult to determine whether the observed absence of cognitive changes in the intervention group is sustainable over time. One potential limitation of this study is the absence of an active control condition for the non-intervention group. While the intervention group received structured cognitive training, the non-intervention group continued with standard clinical follow-up without any cognitive stimulation. This difference in engagement levels may introduce bias, as participants receiving active cognitive stimulation could benefit not only from the training itself, but also from increased mental activity and social interaction. Future studies should consider including an active control group engaged in non-cognitive activities (e.g., social or recreational activities) to better isolate the specific effects of computerized cognitive training. Another limitation of this study is that one of the inclusion criteria was applied by non-specialized informants, such as family members, which may somehow detract from the reliability of the sample. Furthermore, a notable limitation of this study is the geographic and cultural homogeneity of the sample, as participants were recruited exclusively from a specific region in Greece. This may limit the generalizability of the findings to broader populations with different cultural, educational, and socio-economic backgrounds. Cognitive training outcomes can be influenced by cultural factors, such as cognitive reserve, lifestyle habits, and educational systems, which may affect both baseline cognitive performance and responsiveness to interventions. Future research should aim to replicate these findings in more diverse, multicultural cohorts to enhance the external validity and applicability of computerized cognitive training (CCT) programs across different settings.

5. Conclusions

This longitudinal study evaluated the efficacy of a structured 6-month CCT program for older adults with minor mNCDs as part of a broader health promotion strategy. Our findings indicate that such personalized, computerized interventions can play a pivotal role in delaying cognitive decline, particularly in domains vulnerable to age-related decline, such as orientation, memory, language, and praxis. CCT aligns with health promotion principles by offering an accessible, non-pharmacological approach to enhancing mental well-being and preventing further cognitive deterioration in aging populations. Further research with larger cohorts, longer follow-up periods, and diverse populations is necessary to confirm the long-term benefits of this intervention. Additionally, integrating multimodal strategies, including physical activity and social engagement, may amplify the positive outcomes of cognitive training by addressing multiple determinants of health. These findings highlight the potential of personalized digital tools to serve as effective, scalable components of health promotion programs aimed at supporting cognitive health among older adults.

Author Contributions: Conceptualization, A.T. (Anna Tsiakiri) and F.C.; methodology, S.P. and P.V.; software, S.P.; validation, A.T. (Aikaterini Terzoudi), P.A. and A.S.; formal analysis, S.P. and G.K.; investigation, A.T. (Anna Tsiakiri); resources, K.V. and N.A.; data curation, A.T. (Anna Tsiakiri) and S.P.; writing—original draft preparation, K.M., P.A. and S.K.; writing—review and editing, K.V. and F.C.; visualization, A.T. (Anna Tsiakiri) and S.P.; supervision, K.V. and N.A.; project administration, A.T. (Anna Tsiakiri); funding acquisition, A.T. (Anna Tsiakiri). All authors have read and agreed to the published version of the manuscript.

Funding: This research received no external funding.

Institutional Review Board Statement: This study was conducted in accordance with the Declaration of Helsinki and approved by the Scientific Board of the University General Hospital of Alexandroupolis (ΔΣ1/Θ68/06-04-2020).

Informed Consent Statement: Informed consent was obtained from all subjects involved in this tudy.

Data Availability Statement: The data are available upon request.

Conflicts of Interest: The authors declare no conflicts of interest.

References

Alexopoulos, G. S. (2005). Depression in the elderly. *The Lancet (London, England)*, *365*(9475), 1961–1970. [CrossRef]

Aprahamian, I., Diniz, B. S., Izbicki, R., Radanovic, M., Nunes, P. V., & Forlenza, O. V. (2011). Optimizing the CAMCOG test in the screening for mild cognitive impairment and incipient dementia: Saving time with relevant domains. *International Journal of Geriatric Psychiatry*, *26*(4), 403–408. [CrossRef] [PubMed]

Bahar-Fuchs, A., Webb, S., Bartsch, L., Clare, L., Rebok, G., Cherbuin, N., & Anstey, K. J. (2017). Tailored and adaptive computerized cognitive training in older adults at risk for dementia: A randomized controlled trial. *Journal of Alzheimer's Disease: JAD*, *60*(3), 889–911. [CrossRef] [PubMed]

Barban, F., Annicchiarico, R., Pantelopoulos, S., Federici, A., Perri, R., Fadda, L., Carlesimo, G. A., Ricci, C., Giuli, S., Scalici, F., Turchetta, C. S., Adriano, F., Lombardi, M. G., Zaccarelli, C., Cirillo, G., Passuti, S., Mattarelli, P., Lymperopoulou, O., Sakka, P., ... Caltagirone, C. (2016). Protecting cognition from aging and Alzheimer's disease: A computerized cognitive training combined with reminiscence therapy. *International Journal of Geriatric Psychiatry*, *31*(4), 340–348. [CrossRef]

Barnes, D. E., Yaffe, K., Belfor, N., Jagust, W. J., DeCarli, C., Reed, B. R., & Kramer, J. H. (2009). Computer-based cognitive training for mild cognitive impairment: Results from a pilot randomized, controlled trial. *Alzheimer Disease and Associated Disorders*, *23*(3), 205–210. [CrossRef]

Bartsch, T., & Wulff, P. (2015). The hippocampus in aging and disease: From plasticity to vulnerability. *Neuroscience*, *309*, 1–16. [CrossRef]

Basak, C., Boot, W. R., Voss, M. W., & Kramer, A. F. (2008). Can training in a real-time strategy video game attenuate cognitive decline in older adults? *Psychology and Aging*, *23*(4), 765–777. [CrossRef]

Belleville, S., Gilbert, B., Fontaine, F., Gagnon, L., Ménard, E., & Gauthier, S. (2006). Improvement of episodic memory in persons with mild cognitive impairment and healthy older adults: Evidence from a cognitive intervention program. *Dementia and Geriatric Cognitive Disorders*, *22*(5–6), 486–499. [CrossRef]

Ben-Sadoun, G., Manera, V., Alvarez, J., Sacco, G., & Robert, P. (2018). Recommendations for the design of serious games in neurodegenerative diseases. *Frontiers in Aging Neuroscience*, *10*, 13. [CrossRef]

Ben-Sadoun, G., Sacco, G., Manera, V., Bourgeois, J., König, A., Foulon, P., Fosty, B., Bremond, F., d'Arripe-Longueville, F., & Robert, P. (2016). Physical and cognitive stimulation using an exergame in subjects with normal aging, mild and moderate cognitive impairment. *Journal of Alzheimer's Disease: JAD*, *53*(4), 1299–1314. [CrossRef]

Bruel-Jungerman, E., Rampon, C., & Laroche, S. (2007). Adult hippocampal neurogenesis, synaptic plasticity and memory: Facts and hypotheses. *Reviews in the Neurosciences*, *18*(2), 93–114. [CrossRef]

Butler, M., McCreedy, E., Nelson, V. A., Desai, P., Ratner, E., Fink, H. A., Hemmy, L. S., McCarten, J. R., Barclay, T. R., Brasure, M., Davila, H., & Kane, R. L. (2018). Does cognitive training prevent cognitive decline?: A systematic review. *Annals of Internal Medicine*, *168*(1), 63–68. [CrossRef] [PubMed]

Chae, H. J., & Lee, S. H. (2023). Effectiveness of online-based cognitive intervention in community-dwelling older adults with cognitive dysfunction: A systematic review and meta-analysis. *International Journal of Geriatric Psychiatry*, *38*(1), e5853. [CrossRef]

Cipriani, G., Bianchetti, A., & Trabucchi, M. (2006). Outcomes of a computer-based cognitive rehabilitation program on Alzheimer's disease patients compared with those on patients affected by mild cognitive impairment. *Archives of Gerontology and Geriatrics*, *43*(3), 327–335. [CrossRef] [PubMed]

Clare, L., Woods, R. T., Moniz Cook, E. D., Orrell, M., & Spector, A. (2003). Cognitive rehabilitation and cognitive training for early-stage Alzheimer's disease and vascular dementia. *The Cochrane Database of Systematic Reviews*, *4*, CD003260. [CrossRef]

Conde-Sala, J. L., Garre-Olmo, J., Vilalta-Franch, J., Llinàs-Reglà, J., Turró-Garriga, O., Lozano-Gallego, M., Hernández-Ferrándiz, M., Pericot-Nierga, I., & López-Pousa, S. (2012). Predictors of cognitive decline in Alzheimer's disease and mild cognitive impairment using the CAMCOG: A five-year follow-up. *International Psychogeriatrics*, *24*(6), 948–958. [CrossRef] [PubMed]

Crook, T., & Larrabee, G. J. (1988). Age-associated memory impairment: Diagnostic criteria and treatment strategies. *Psychopharmacology Bulletin*, *24*(4), 509–514.

Delbroek, T., Vermeylen, W., & Spildooren, J. (2017). The effect of cognitive-motor dual task training with the biorescue force platform on cognition, balance and dual task performance in institutionalized older adults: A randomized controlled trial. *Journal of Physical Therapy Science*, *29*(7), 1137–1143. [CrossRef]

Fiatarone Singh, M. A., Gates, N., Saigal, N., Wilson, G. C., Meiklejohn, J., Brodaty, H., Wen, W., Singh, N., Baune, B. T., Suo, C., Baker, M. K., Foroughi, N., Wang, Y., Sachdev, P. S., & Valenzuela, M. (2014). The Study of Mental and Resistance Training (SMART) study—Resistance training and/or cognitive training in mild cognitive impairment: A randomized, double-blind, double-sham controlled trial. *Journal of the American Medical Directors Association*, *15*(12), 873–880. [CrossRef]

Finn, M., & McDonald, S. (2011). Computerised cognitive training for older persons with mild cognitive impairment: A pilot study using a randomised controlled trial design. *Brain Impairment*, *12*(3), 187–199. [CrossRef]

Ge, S., Zhu, Z., Wu, B., & McConnell, E. S. (2018). Technology-based cognitive training and rehabilitation interventions for individuals with mild cognitive impairment: A systematic review. *BMC Geriatrics*, *18*(1), 213. [CrossRef] [PubMed]

González-Palau, F., Franco, M., Bamidis, P., Losada, R., Parra, E., Papageorgiou, S. G., & Vivas, A. B. (2014). The effects of a computer-based cognitive and physical training program in a healthy and mildly cognitive impaired aging sample. *Aging & Mental Health*, *18*(7), 838–846. [CrossRef]

Gooding, A. L., Choi, J., Fiszdon, J. M., Wilkins, K., Kirwin, P. D., van Dyck, C. H., Devanand, D., Bell, M. D., & Rivera Mindt, M. (2016). Comparing three methods of computerised cognitive training for older adults with subclinical cognitive decline. *Neuropsychological Rehabilitation*, *26*(5–6), 810–821. [CrossRef]

Hagovská, M., Dzvoník, O., & Olekszyová, Z. (2017). Comparison of two cognitive training programs with effects on functional activities and quality of life. *Research in Gerontological Nursing*, *10*(4), 172–180. [CrossRef]

Han, J. W., Oh, K., Yoo, S., Kim, E., Ahn, K.-H., Son, Y.-J., Kim, T. H., Chi, Y. K., & Kim, K. W. (2014). Development of the ubiquitous spaced retrieval-based memory advancement and rehabilitation training program. *Psychiatry Investigation*, *11*(1), 52–58. [CrossRef] [PubMed]

Herrera, C., Chambon, C., Michel, B. F., Paban, V., & Alescio-Lautier, B. (2012). Positive effects of computer-based cognitive training in adults with mild cognitive impairment. *Neuropsychologia*, *50*(8), 1871–1881. [CrossRef] [PubMed]

Hill, N. T. M., Mowszowski, L., Naismith, S. L., Chadwick, V. L., Valenzuela, M., & Lampit, A. (2017). Computerized cognitive training in older adults with mild cognitive impairment or dementia: A systematic review and meta-analysis. *The American Journal of Psychiatry*, *174*(4), 329–340. [CrossRef] [PubMed]

Hong, Y. J., Jang, E. H., Hwang, J., Roh, J. H., & Lee, J.-H. (2015). The efficacy of cognitive intervention programs for mild cognitive impairment: A systematic review. *Current Alzheimer Research*, *12*(6), 527–542. [CrossRef]

Hu, M., Wu, X., Shu, X., Hu, H., Chen, Q., Peng, L., & Feng, H. (2021). Effects of computerised cognitive training on cognitive impairment: A meta-analysis. *Journal of Neurology, 268*(5), 1680–1688. [CrossRef]

Hughes, T. F., Flatt, J. D., Fu, B., Butters, M. A., Chang, C.-C. H., & Ganguli, M. (2014). Interactive video gaming compared with health education in older adults with mild cognitive impairment: A feasibility study. *International Journal of Geriatric Psychiatry, 29*(9), 890–898. [CrossRef]

Hwang, H. R., Choi, S. H., Yoon, D. H., Yoon, B.-N., Suh, Y. J., Lee, D., Han, I.-T., & Hong, C.-G. (2012). The effect of cognitive training in patients with mild cognitive impairment and early Alzheimer's disease: A preliminary study. *Journal of Clinical Neurology (Seoul, Korea), 8*(3), 190–197. [CrossRef]

Hyer, L., Scott, C., Atkinson, M. M., Mullen, C. M., Lee, A., Johnson, A., & Mckenzie, L. C. (2016). Cognitive training program to improve working memory in older adults with MCI. *Clinical Gerontologist, 39*(5), 410–427. [CrossRef]

Karbach, J., & Kray, J. (2009). How useful is executive control training? Age differences in near and far transfer of task-switching training. *Developmental Science, 12*(6), 978–990. [CrossRef] [PubMed]

Klados, M. A., Styliadis, C., Frantzidis, C. A., Paraskevopoulos, E., & Bamidis, P. D. (2016). Beta-band functional connectivity is reorganized in mild cognitive impairment after combined computerized physical and cognitive training. *Frontiers in Neuroscience, 10*, 55. [CrossRef]

Kolb, B., Harker, A., & Gibb, R. (2017). Principles of plasticity in the developing brain. *Developmental Medicine and Child Neurology, 59*(12), 1218–1223. [CrossRef] [PubMed]

Kral, V. A. (1958). Senescent memory decline and senile amnestic syndrome. *The American Journal of Psychiatry, 115*(4), 361–362. [CrossRef] [PubMed]

Lampit, A., Hallock, H., & Valenzuela, M. (2014). Computerized cognitive training in cognitively healthy older adults: A systematic review and meta-analysis of effect modifiers. *PLoS Medicine, 11*(11), e1001756. [CrossRef]

Li, H., Li, J., Li, N., Li, B., Wang, P., & Zhou, T. (2011). Cognitive intervention for persons with mild cognitive impairment: A meta-analysis. *Ageing Research Reviews, 10*(2), 285–296. [CrossRef]

Liang, J., Xu, Y., Lin, L., Jia, R., Zhang, H., & Hang, L. (2018). Comparison of multiple interventions for older adults with Alzheimer disease or mild cognitive impairment. *Medicine, 97*(20), e10744. [CrossRef]

Lin, F., Heffner, K. L., Ren, P., Tivarus, M. E., Brasch, J., Chen, D.-G., Mapstone, M., Porsteinsson, A. P., & Tadin, D. (2016). Cognitive and neural effects of vision-based speed-of-processing training in older adults with amnestic mild cognitive impairment: A pilot study. *Journal of the American Geriatrics Society, 64*(6), 1293–1298. [CrossRef]

Liu, C.-C., Kanekiyo, T., Xu, H., & Bu, G. (2013). Apolipoprotein E and Alzheimer disease: Risk, mechanisms and therapy. *Nature Reviews Neurology, 9*(2), 106–118. [CrossRef] [PubMed]

Maeng, S., Hong, J. P., Kim, W.-H., Kim, H., Cho, S.-E., Kang, J. M., Na, K.-S., Oh, S.-H., Park, J. W., Bae, J. N., & Cho, S.-J. (2021). Effects of virtual reality-based cognitive training in the elderly with and without mild cognitive impairment. *Psychiatry Investigation, 18*(7), 619–627. [CrossRef] [PubMed]

Maffei, L., Picano, E., Andreassi, M. G., Angelucci, A., Baldacci, F., Baroncelli, L., Begenisic, T., Bellinvia, P. F., Berardi, N., Biagi, L., Bonaccorsi, J., Bonanni, E., Bonuccelli, U., Borghini, A., Braschi, C., Broccardi, M., Bruno, R. M., Caleo, M., Carlesi, C., . . . Train the Brain Consortium. (2017). Randomized trial on the effects of a combined physical/cognitive training in aged MCI subjects: The Train the Brain study. *Scientific Reports, 7*(1), 39471. [CrossRef]

Manera, V., Petit, P.-D., Derreumaux, A., Orvieto, I., Romagnoli, M., Lyttle, G., David, R., & Robert, P. H. (2015). "Kitchen and cooking", a serious game for mild cognitive impairment and Alzheimer's disease: A pilot study. *Frontiers in Aging Neuroscience, 7*, 24. [CrossRef]

Mansbach, W. E., Mace, R. A., & Clark, K. M. (2017). The efficacy of a computer-assisted cognitive rehabilitation program for patients with mild cognitive deficits: A pilot study. *Experimental Aging Research, 43*(1), 94–104. [CrossRef]

Memory Motivation. (n.d.). Retrieved 10 February 2025. Available online: https://www.memory-motivation.org/home-4/ (accessed on 5 May 2020).

Miller, K. J., Dye, R. V., Kim, J., Jennings, J. L., O'Toole, E., Wong, J., & Siddarth, P. (2013). Effect of a computerized brain exercise program on cognitive performance in older adults. *The American Journal of Geriatric Psychiatry: Official Journal of the American Association for Geriatric Psychiatry, 21*(7), 655–663. [CrossRef]

Nasreddine, Z. S., Phillips, N. A., Bédirian, V., Charbonneau, S., Whitehead, V., Collin, I., Cummings, J. L., & Chertkow, H. (2005). The montreal cognitive assessment, MoCA: A brief screening tool for mild cognitive impairment. *Journal of the American Geriatrics Society, 53*(4), 695–699. [CrossRef]

Owen, A. M., Hampshire, A., Grahn, J. A., Stenton, R., Dajani, S., Burns, A. S., Howard, R. J., & Ballard, C. G. (2010). Putting brain training to the test. *Nature, 465*(7299), 775–778. [CrossRef]

Pamboris, G. M., Plakias, S., Tsiakiri, A., Karakitsiou, G., Bebeletsi, P., Vadikolias, K., Aggelousis, N., Tsiptsios, D., & Christidi, F. (2024). Physical therapy in neurorehabilitation with an emphasis on sports: A bibliometric analysis and narrative review. *Sports, 12*(10), 276. [CrossRef]

Petersen, R. C., Caracciolo, B., Brayne, C., Gauthier, S., Jelic, V., & Fratiglioni, L. (2014). Mild cognitive impairment: A concept in evolution. *Journal of Internal Medicine*, *275*(3), 214–228. [CrossRef]

Petersen, R. C., Lopez, O., Armstrong, M. J., Getchius, T. S. D., Ganguli, M., Gloss, D., Gronseth, G. S., Marson, D., Pringsheim, T., Day, G. S., Sager, M., Stevens, J., & Rae-Grant, A. (2018). Practice guideline update summary: Mild cognitive impairment: Report of the guideline development, dissemination, and implementation subcommittee of the american academy of neurology. *Neurology*, *90*(3), 126–135. [CrossRef] [PubMed]

Petersen, R. C., Smith, G. E., Waring, S. C., Ivnik, R. J., Tangalos, E. G., & Kokmen, E. (1999). Mild cognitive impairment: Clinical characterization and outcome. *Archives of Neurology*, *56*(3), 303–308. [CrossRef] [PubMed]

Rabipour, S., & Raz, A. (2012). Training the brain: Fact and fad in cognitive and behavioral remediation. *Brain and Cognition*, *79*(2), 159–179. [CrossRef]

Rapp, S., Brenes, G., & Marsh, A. P. (2002). Memory enhancement training for older adults with mild cognitive impairment: A preliminary study. *Aging & Mental Health*, *6*(1), 5–11. [CrossRef]

Robert, P., Manera, V., Derreumaux, A., Ferrandez Y Montesino, M., Leone, E., Fabre, R., & Bourgeois, J. (2020). Efficacy of a web app for cognitive training (MeMo) regarding cognitive and behavioral performance in people with neurocognitive disorders: Randomized controlled trial. *Journal of Medical Internet Research*, *22*(3), e17167. [CrossRef]

Robert, P. H., König, A., Amieva, H., Andrieu, S., Bremond, F., Bullock, R., Ceccaldi, M., Dubois, B., Gauthier, S., Kenigsberg, P.-A., Nave, S., Orgogozo, J. M., Piano, J., Benoit, M., Touchon, J., Vellas, B., Yesavage, J., & Manera, V. (2014). Recommendations for the use of serious games in people with Alzheimer's disease, related disorders and frailty. *Frontiers in Aging Neuroscience*, *6*, 54. [CrossRef]

Rosen, A. C., Sugiura, L., Kramer, J. H., Whitfield-Gabrieli, S., & Gabrieli, J. D. (2011). Cognitive training changes hippocampal function in mild cognitive impairment: A pilot study. *Journal of Alzheimer's Disease: JAD*, *26*(Suppl. S3), 349–357. [CrossRef]

Roth, M., Tym, E., Mountjoy, C. Q., Huppert, F. A., Hendrie, H., Verma, S., & Goddard, R. (1986). CAMDEX. A standardised instrument for the diagnosis of mental disorder in the elderly with special reference to the early detection of dementia. *The British Journal of Psychiatry: The Journal of Mental Science*, *149*, 698–709. [CrossRef]

Rozzini, L., Costardi, D., Chilovi, B. V., Franzoni, S., Trabucchi, M., & Padovani, A. (2007). Efficacy of cognitive rehabilitation in patients with mild cognitive impairment treated with cholinesterase inhibitors. *International Journal of Geriatric Psychiatry*, *22*(4), 356–360. [CrossRef]

Sachs-Ericsson, N., & Blazer, D. G. (2015). The new DSM-5 diagnosis of mild neurocognitive disorder and its relation to research in mild cognitive impairment. *Aging & Mental Health*, *19*(1), 2–12. [CrossRef]

Sakamoto, M., Ando, H., & Tsutou, A. (2013). Comparing the effects of different individualized music interventions for elderly individuals with severe dementia. *International Psychogeriatrics*, *25*(5), 775–784. [CrossRef] [PubMed]

Savulich, G., Piercy, T., Fox, C., Suckling, J., Rowe, J. B., O'Brien, J. T., & Sahakian, B. J. (2017). Cognitive training using a novel memory game on an ipad in patients with amnestic mild cognitive impairment (aMCI). *International Journal of Neuropsychopharmacology*, *20*(8), 624–633. [CrossRef] [PubMed]

Scarmeas, N., Zarahn, E., Anderson, K. E., Hilton, J., Flynn, J., Van Heertum, R. L., Sackeim, H. A., & Stern, Y. (2003). Cognitive reserve modulates functional brain responses during memory tasks: A PET study in healthy young and elderly subjects. *NeuroImage*, *19*(3), 1215–1227. [PubMed]

Shah, T. M., Weinborn, M., Verdile, G., Sohrabi, H. R., & Martins, R. N. (2017). Enhancing cognitive functioning in healthly older adults: A systematic review of the clinical significance of commercially available computerized cognitive training in preventing cognitive decline. *Neuropsychology Review*, *27*(1), 62–80. [CrossRef]

Simpson, J. R. (2014). DSM-5 and neurocognitive disorders. *The Journal of the American Academy of Psychiatry and the Law*, *42*(2), 159–164.

Smith, G. S. (2013). Aging and neuroplasticity. *Dialogues in Clinical Neuroscience*, *15*(1), 3–5. [CrossRef]

Sood, P., Kletzel, S. L., Krishnan, S., Devos, H., Negm, A., Hoffecker, L., Machtinger, J., Hu, X., & Heyn, P. C. (2019). Nonimmersive brain gaming for older adults with cognitive impairment: A scoping review. *The Gerontologist*, *59*(6), e764–e781. [CrossRef]

Stern, Y. (2002). What is cognitive reserve? Theory and research application of the reserve concept. *Journal of the International Neuropsychological Society: JINS*, *8*(3), 448–460. [CrossRef]

Stern, Y., & Barulli, D. (2019). Cognitive reserve. *Handbook of Clinical Neurology*, *167*, 181–190. [CrossRef]

Styliadis, C., Kartsidis, P., Paraskevopoulos, E., Ioannides, A. A., & Bamidis, P. D. (2015). Neuroplastic effects of combined computerized physical and cognitive training in elderly individuals at risk for dementia: An eLORETA controlled study on resting states. *Neural Plasticity*, *2015*, 172192. [CrossRef]

Swaab, D. F. (1991). Brain aging and Alzheimer's disease, "Wear and tear" versus "Use it or lose it". *Neurobiology of Aging*, *12*(4), 317–324. [CrossRef] [PubMed]

Talassi, E., Guerreschi, M., Feriani, M., Fedi, V., Bianchetti, A., & Trabucchi, M. (2007). Effectiveness of a cognitive rehabilitation program in mild dementia (MD) and mild cognitive impairment (MCI): A case control study. *Archives of Gerontology and Geriatrics*, *44*(Suppl. S1), 391–399. [CrossRef] [PubMed]

Thapa, N., Park, H. J., Yang, J.-G., Son, H., Jang, M., Lee, J., Kang, S. W., Park, K. W., & Park, H. (2020). The effect of a virtual reality-based intervention program on cognition in older adults with mild cognitive impairment: A randomized control trial. *Journal of Clinical Medicine*, *9*(5), 1283. [CrossRef]

Troyer, A. K., Murphy, K. J., Anderson, N. D., Moscovitch, M., & Craik, F. I. M. (2008). Changing everyday memory behaviour in amnestic mild cognitive impairment: A randomised controlled trial. *Neuropsychological Rehabilitation*, *18*(1), 65–88. [CrossRef]

Tsiakiri, A. (2022). Remote learning for adults with mild cognitive impairment in the new landscape of COVID-19 restrictions. *Advances in Social Sciences Research Journal*, *9*, 382–394. [CrossRef]

Tsiakiri, A., Bakirtzis, C., Plakias, S., Vlotinou, P., Vadikolias, K., Terzoudi, A., & Christidi, F. (2024a). Predictive models for the transition from mild neurocognitive disorder to major neurocognitive disorder: Insights from clinical, demographic, and neuropsychological data. *Biomedicines*, *12*(6), 1232. [CrossRef]

Tsiakiri, A., Christidi, F., Tsiptsios, D., Vlotinou, P., Kitmeridou, S., Bebeletsi, P., Kokkotis, C., Serdari, A., Tsamakis, K., Aggelousis, N., & Vadikolias, K. (2024b). Processing speed and attentional shift/mental flexibility in patients with stroke: A comprehensive review on the trail making test in stroke studies. *Neurology International*, *16*(1), 210–225. [CrossRef]

Tsiakiri, A., Ioannidis, P., Vlotinou, P., Kokkotis, C., Megagianni, S., Toumaian, M., Terzoudi, K., Koutzmpi, V., Despoti, A., Megari, K., Liozidou, A., Kyriazidoy, S., Vadikolias, K., & Tsapanou, A. (2024c). The role of a computerized cognitive intervention program on the neuropsychiatric symptoms in mild cognitive impairment. *Aging Medicine and Healthcare*, *15*(3), 122–128. [CrossRef]

Tsiakiri, A., Vadikolias, K., Tripsianis, G., Vlotinou, P., Serdari, A., Terzoudi, A., & Heliopoulos, I. (2021). Influence of social and demographic factors on the montreal cognitive assessment (MoCA) test in rural population of North-Eastern Greece. *Geriatrics*, *6*(2), 43. [CrossRef]

Tsolaki, M., Fountoulakis, K. N., Chantzi, H., & Kazis, A. (2000). The Cambridge Cognitive Examination (CAMCOG): A validation study in outpatients suffering from dementia and non-demented elderly subjects (including Age Associated Cognitive Decline patients) in Greece. *American Journal of Alzheimer's Disease & Other Dementias®*, *15*(5), 269–276. [CrossRef]

Unverzagt, F. W., Kasten, L., Johnson, K. E., Rebok, G. W., Marsiske, M., Koepke, K. M., Elias, J. W., Morris, J. N., Willis, S. L., Ball, K., Rexroth, D. F., Smith, D. M., Wolinsky, F. D., & Tennstedt, S. L. (2007). Effect of memory impairment on training outcomes in ACTIVE. *Journal of the International Neuropsychological Society*, *13*(6), 953–960. [CrossRef] [PubMed]

Valentijn, S. A. M., van Hooren, S. A. H., Bosma, H., Touw, D. M., Jolles, J., van Boxtel, M. P. J., & Ponds, R. W. H. M. (2005). The effect of two types of memory training on subjective and objective memory performance in healthy individuals aged 55 years and older: A randomized controlled trial. *Patient Education and Counseling*, *57*(1), 106–114. [CrossRef]

van de Pol, L. A., Korf, E. S. C., van der Flier, W. M., Brashear, H. R., Fox, N. C., Barkhof, F., & Scheltens, P. (2007). Magnetic resonance imaging predictors of cognition in mild cognitive impairment. *Archives of Neurology*, *64*(7), 1023–1028. [CrossRef]

Verghese, J., Lipton, R. B., Katz, M. J., Hall, C. B., Derby, C. A., Kuslansky, G., Ambrose, A. F., Sliwinski, M., & Buschke, H. (2003). Leisure activities and the risk of dementia in the elderly. *The New England Journal of Medicine*, *348*(25), 2508–2516. [CrossRef]

Verhaeghen, P., Marcoen, A., & Goossens, L. (1992). Improving memory performance in the aged through mnemonic training: A meta-analytic study. *Psychology and Aging*, *7*(2), 242–251. [CrossRef] [PubMed]

Vlotinou, P., Tsiakiri, A., Frantzidis, C. A., Katsouri, I.-G., & Aggelousis, N. (2023). The effect of an interventional movement program on the mechanical gait characteristics of a patient with dementia. *Engineering Proceedings*, *50*(1), 4. [CrossRef]

Willis, S. L., Tennstedt, S. L., Marsiske, M., Ball, K., Elias, J., Koepke, K. M., Morris, J. N., Rebok, G. W., Unverzagt, F. W., Stoddard, A. M., Wright, E., & ACTIVE Study Group. (2006). Long-term effects of cognitive training on everyday functional outcomes in older adults. *JAMA*, *296*(23), 2805–2814. [CrossRef]

Xu, Z., Sun, W., Zhang, D., Chung, V. C.-H., Sit, R. W.-S., & Wong, S. Y.-S. (2021). Comparative effectiveness of interventions for global cognition in patients with mild cognitive impairment: A systematic review and network meta-analysis of randomized controlled trials. *Frontiers in Aging Neuroscience*, *13*, 653340. [CrossRef]

Zyda, M. (2005). From visual simulation to virtual reality to games. *Computer*, *38*(9), 25–32. [CrossRef]

European Journal of
Investigation in Health, Psychology and Education

MDPI

Article

Olfactory Identification as a Biomarker for Cognitive Impairment: Insights from Healthy Aging, Subjective Cognitive Decline, and Mild Cognitive Impairment

Jaime Bouhaben, Alice Helena Delgado-Lima and María Luisa Delgado-Losada *

Experimental Psychology, Cognitive Processes and Speech Therapy Department, Faculty of Psychology, Complutense University of Madrid, 28223 Pozuelo de Alarcón, Spain; jaimebou@ucm.es (J.B.); alicedel@ucm.es (A.H.D.-L.)
* Correspondence: mldelgad@ucm.es

Abstract: Introduction: This study aims to investigate the relationship between olfactory identification (OI) and cognitive impairment by examining OI abilities across various stages of cognitive deterioration. **Methods**: A total of 264 participants were divided into three groups based on cognitive status: cognitively healthy, subjective cognitive, and mild cognitive impairment. All participants were assessed using the Sniffin' Sticks Olfactory Identification test and a comprehensive neuropsychological test battery. **Results**: Our results highlight the main effects of age and cognitive status on OI scores. Regarding cognitive abilities, OI is associated with measures of short-term memory, long-term, working memory, and selective attention. Finally, logistic regression models showed that OI is a significant predictor for discriminating SCD from CH, MCI from CH, and MCI from SCD. **Discussion**: These findings suggest the addition of olfactory identification measures in neuropsychological assessments could improve the early detection of individuals at risk for cognitive impairment.

Keywords: olfaction; neuroplasticity; aging; subjective cognitive decline; cognitive impairment; mild cognitive impairment; olfactory identification; biomarker

1. Introduction

Cognitive impairment in aging is a physiological process linked to age, which, in some cases, can lead to pathology up to dementia. Within this slow and continuous process of deterioration, two transition phases can be distinguished. Subjective cognitive complaints (SCCs) are defined as concerns about the worsening or malfunctioning of some aspect of cognition, regardless of whether the cognitive impairment is detected by standardized objective tests [1]. Then, the second corresponds to mild cognitive impairment (MCI) in which the person presents a cognitive impairment that does not interfere or minimally interferes with the activities of daily living [2].

Population studies with follow-ups from 3 to 20 years report that SCCs may predict MCI and/or dementia, usually in combination with other variables such as being a woman or having a high educational level [3,4] and being a carrier of the APOE e4 gene [5], causing concern in the patient [6–8]. Patients who manifest these cognitive complaints are more likely to progress to MCI and dementia [6–9]. Results from longitudinal studies with clinical samples are more contradictory. On one side, memory complaints do not often predict progression to dementia [10,11]. However, other studies do find an increased risk of progression to dementia in participants with SCC [11]. The presence of SCC supposes a criterion for subjective cognitive decline (SCD) [6,7]. SCD increases the risk of developing pathologies such as MCI and Alzheimer's disease [6,7]. Some studies and meta-analyses point out that patients with SCD or subjective complaints are 1.73–2 times more likely to develop MCI or dementia [12–16].

In SCD, one should perceive a decline in cognitive performance in daily life with respect to a previous stage of subjectively intact cognition. This transition from normality to a stage of cognitive difficulties is not reflected in standardized tests, whose performance remains within a normal range for age and educational level [6,7]. Criteria also state that SCD is unrelated to an acute event and persists over time, so memory complaints must be present within the past 6 months. This is because it is believed that SCD can arise as a result of both preclinical AD and other non-neurodegenerative conditions. Thus, monitoring the course and progression may provide insight into the possible etiology [6–8].

The prevalence of SCD is estimated between 14% and 54% [17]. It is still unclear what factors moderate the progression between complaints and objective cognitive impairment [16]; therefore, the early identification of the progression from SCD to MCI is of great importance for public health [18].

Olfactory identification (OI), the capacity to recognize and name specific odors, is recognized to be impacted by aging [19–22], MCI [23–25], dementia [21,26,27], and more recently, it has been associated with an asymptomatic preclinical stage of AD, SCD [16,28–30].

A single measure of OI dysfunction might predict, not only an increase in cognitive decline up to 15 years later [31–34] but also a higher risk of conversion from normal cognition to MCI [35] and from MCI to AD [32]. Furthermore, olfactory deficits are associated with neurodegenerative findings detectable by neuroimaging [34,36–38].

Deterioration in OI is intimately related to cognitive decline in various pathological conditions and aging. The association between the neuroanatomy of the olfactory system and cognition [32,39,40] is well supported by the literature. This association highlights a close relationship with memory, given the proximity of the hippocampus and olfactory cortex. Additionally, the prefrontal cortex is also a neocortical region involved in olfactory processing, which suggests a relationship between OI performance and executive functioning. Studies with functional neuroimaging support the relevance of these regions in olfactory functioning [41]. Olfactory and cognitive performance share neural correlates affected by physiological aging. Brain structures closely related to the olfactory system show significant early histopathology in MCI and AD, and the brains of AD patients invariably show neuropathology in the entorhinal cortex [42,43]. It is worth highlighting a correlation between psychophysical measures of olfactory function and hippocampal volumetric loss [43,44]. Several studies have emphasized the potential usefulness of an olfactory identification test and hippocampal volume loss for the early detection of AD [45,46].

Olfactory status is reliably associated with cognitive health, and the severity of olfactory dysfunction appears to be associated with the rate of cognitive impairment [27,34,47–49].

The aim of this study is to understand the association between OI and cognitive impairment by analyzing the olfactory identification abilities across different stages of cognitive deterioration (CH, SCD, MCI) and determining if these variations can help categorize individuals accurately while exploring the relationship between OI and cognitive domains (memory, executive functioning, attention, executive functioning, visuospatial skills, and language) in a sample of older adults representing a continuum of performance capability. Thereby, this study contributes to the broader goal of enhancing early diagnostic capabilities in cognitive impairment.

2. Materials and Methods

2.1. Participants

An initial pool of 297 Spanish-speaking older adults volunteered to participate in this study. All the participants were recruited through advertisements in senior centers and health centers in the Community of Madrid (Spain). All the participants were informed about the study guidelines and gave written informed consent to participate in this study.

The general inclusion criteria were (i) age ranging from 55 to 90 years; (ii) no prior diagnosis of dementia; (iii) no records of any neurological alterations, such as stroke, head trauma, or encephalitis; (iv) absence of current otorhinolaryngological issues; and (v) compliance with testing procedures. Once the general inclusion criteria for this study were fulfilled, the participants were assigned to one of three clinical cohorts, based on their cognitive status. These cohorts were cognitively healthy participants (CH), participants with subjective cognitive decline (SCD), and participants with mild cognitive impairment (MCI). A fourth clinical cohort of participants with a serious risk of dementia and/or probable Alzheimer's disease (AD) was identified. However, due to its limited sample size, this cohort was excluded from further analyses. The inclusion criteria for the cognitively healthy (CH) cohort were screening score > 26 (MoCA > 26), normal performance in neuropsychological tests, and no self-reported complaints about their cognitive status. The diagnostic criteria for subjective cognitive decline were screening score > 26 (MoCA > 26), performance in neuropsychological tests within the normal limits, and self-reported complaints about their cognitive status. These complaints were measured with three questions: (Q1) *Do you have memory problems?*; (Q2) *Do you forget where you put things?* and (Q3) *Do you forget the names of family and acquaintances?* Response options for Q1 were *yes* or *no*. This is a frequently asked question in most population studies about SCD [50]. Both Q2 and Q3 have two alternatives: *Rarely* (interpreted as *no*) or *Frequently* (interpreted as *yes*). Those participants who answered *yes* to Q1, Q2, and Q3 were considered to satisfy the self-reported complaints criteria. These SCD criteria were obtained from Jessen et al. (2020) [7]. MCI diagnosis was performed following the criteria in Albert et al. (2013) [51]: (i) evidence of concerns about cognitive changes compared to a previous level, corroborated by an informant; (ii) evidence of worse than expected performance in at least one cognitive domain (−1.5 SD), according with age and educational background; (iii) preservation of functional independence in activities of daily life; and (iv) disagreement with criteria for diagnosis of dementia.

The exclusion criteria from the study were (i) medical history of olfactory alterations, including nasal polyps, rhinitis, rhinosinusitis, or previous otorhinolaryngological surgery; (ii) medication intake which may affect olfactory performance (such as some antibiotics, antiepileptics, antithyroids, benzodiazepines, or antiarrhythmics); (iii) presence or suspicion of psychiatric alterations, such as depressive or psychotic disorders (self-reported by the participant or present in clinical history); and (iv) presence of olfactory deficits or alterations due to COVID-19 infection (self-reported or present in the clinical history).

The final sample, after eligibility criteria, was composed of 264 participants (68.04 ± 7.58 years; 172 women of 67.4 ± 7.27 years and 92 men of 69.2 ± 8.05 years).

2.2. Study Design

The present study follows a cross-sectional non-experimental design, as no manipulation for independent variables nor random allocation was performed and measures were taken once per participant. The assessment procedure was carried out between September 2021 and September 2022. The complete procedure was administered in one visit. In this visit, all participants underwent the neuropsychological test battery described in Section 2.3 and the Olfactory Identification Test (from Sniffin' Sticks Olfactory Test). Supplementary Table S1 displays a summary of the study methods.

This research followed the tenets of the Declaration of Helsinki (Edinburgh, 2013) and was approved by the Ethics Committee from University Hospital San Carlos (Madrid, Spain, internal codes 17/192-E and 18/422-E_BS). This study was adjusted to standards of good clinical practice (art.34 RD 223/2004; community directive 2001/20/CE) and to the protection of personal data and confidentiality (European Data Protection Regulation, and in accordance with the Organic Law 3/2018 on the Protection of Personal Data and Guarantee of Digital Rights).

2.3. Measures and Procedure

The assessment protocol comprised a screening test of general cognitive status, a questionnaire of cognitive complaints, an olfactory evaluation, and a battery of neuropsychological standardized measures to measure these cognitive domains: semantic memory, episodic memory, executive function, working memory, attention, and language.

- *Global cognitive status*: General cognitive performance was tested with the Spanish adaptation of the Montreal *Cognitive Assessment (MoCA)* instrument [52]. MoCA is a widely used screening tool that assesses several cognitive domains: attention, concentration, memory, language, calculation, orientation, and executive functions. Due to its nature as a screening tool, MoCA grants cutoff points for cognitive impairment, which may accurately guide its diagnosis. MoCA's original publication points to 26 as the cutoff point between cognitive impairment and healthy aging [53]. This cutoff point was adopted in the present study to help with the classification of participants with MCI.
- *Olfactory performance*: Olfaction was assessed with the Spanish adaptation of the Identification Smell Test, from the Sniffin' Sticks Olfactory Test. This adaptation was developed and validated by Delgado-Losada et al. (2020, 2021) [54,55]. In the Spanish version of this test, potential bias due to cultural aspects of odor descriptors was addressed. Recognition and subjective intensity scores were obtained for the present study. Both scores are part of Delgado-Losada et al.'s (2021) study [55]. *Recognition score*: This is the original score of the test. It represents whether each odorant is correctly identified through a four-alternative forced-choice method. The odorant is shown to the participant, and they have to identify the target odor between four odor descriptors. Correct answers from the 16 items are added in order to calculate this score. *Subjective intensity score*: This score intends to measure the subjective intensity of an odor. It was designed and validated by Delgado-Losada et al. (2021) [55]. After each trial, participants have to score the subjective intensity of the smell presented with a 1–10 visual analog scale (1 implies a minimal intensity and 10 implies an extraordinary intensity). This score provides an additional value to olfactory identification performance. The total score is calculated as the arithmetic mean of the 1 to 10 intensity given to each item.
- *California Verbal Learning Test-II (CVLT-II)* [56]: CVLT is a neuropsychological instrument that intends to measure short-term and long-term episodic memory through a wordlist task. Participants listen to a list of 16 words, with 1 s intervals, and they are asked to memorize as many as they are able to. Immediately after five trials, participants are asked to recall the target words (immediate recall). After 20 min, they are asked again to recall the words (delayed recall). Two scores were taken, the immediate recall score and the delayed recall score, both related to episodic memory.
- *Digit Span Test* from Wechsler Adult Intelligence Scales-IV (WAIS-IV) [57]: The test consists of two parts: the digit span forward (DSF) and the digit span backward (DSB). In DSF, a number is spoken each second in various sequences, and the individual is expected to repeat the numbers in the same order. In the DSB section, the individual is asked to repeat the sequences of numbers in reverse order. In both sections, the length of the number of sequences gradually increases. There are two trials for each digit span. Two scores were obtained, including the DSF span score, which measures short-term memory, and the DSB span score, which measures working memory.
- *Cancellation Test.* This is a classic cancellation task, adapted from the ELSA study (https://www.elsa-project.ac.uk; accessed on 10 November 2024) (Huppert et al., 2004) [58] and implemented in the ELES project [59], which measures selective attention and processing speed. The task consists of a matrix of random letters distributed in rows and columns. Participants are asked to mark target letters (P and W) as fast as possible in 1 min. The number of correct (target letters correctly marked) and incorrect answers (omission errors) were considered.
- *Rey-Osterrieth Complex Figure Test (RCFT).* This is also an instrument widely administered in clinical neuropsychology to measure visuospatial skills and non-verbal memory [60]. Participants are exposed to a complex figure they have to copy on paper and memorize. After the first copy, they are asked to repeat the figure immediately (immediate recall). Then, after 20 min, participants are asked to draw the figure again (delayed recall). Total scores from immediate recall and delayed recall were obtained.

- *Verbal Fluency Test*: Verbal fluency measures are often included in neuropsychological protocols to assess language and executive functioning in both cognitively healthy and cognitively impaired conditions. According to Lezak et al. (2012) [61], participants have to verbally declare as many words as they are able to, following a certain condition, in 1 min per condition. In this study, two conditions were administered: phonological (generate as many words starting with the letter F as possible in one minute) and semantic (name as many animals as possible in 1 min). The total score per condition was obtained, as intended measures of phonological and semantic verbal fluency, respectively.

Vocabulary Test, from Wechsler Adult Intelligence Scales-IV [57]. This is a test in which participants are asked to explain and define a concept from its word, starting with easy words that get progressively more difficult. It is usually administered to measure verbal comprehension, crystallized intelligence, lexical knowledge, and the ability to retrieve information. The total score was obtained as a measure of premorbid intelligence and cognitive ability.

Trail Making Test. This is a classic neuropsychological task that aims to measure executive functioning. Two parts were administered [62]. TMT-A consists of a piece of paper composed of 25 randomly distributed circles, numbered from 1 to 25. Participants have to connect them with a constant line, in ascending order, as quickly as possible, but maintaining accuracy in order. TMT-A mainly assesses visuospatial processing speed and sustained attention. Similarly, TMT-B also consists of a piece of paper with randomly distributed circles, but in this case, those circles contain numbers from 1 to 13 and letters from A to L. Participants have to connect them in ascending order, intercalating numbers and letters (1-A-2-B-3-C and so on). TMT-B mainly assesses cognitive flexibility and the ability to alter between two sets of stimuli. Two scores were obtained, including the time of resolution (in seconds) of parts A and B.

2.4. Statistical Analyses

The entire statistical analysis plan was carried out with R software, version 4.3.0 [63]. In the first place, a descriptive analysis was conducted. The mean and standard deviation were calculated for each cognitive status group, as well as chi-squared tests for dichotomous variables and F tests for continuous variables. In addition, percentiles 10 and 5 of the Olfactory Identification-Recognition score were used to describe the participants' olfactory performance as normosmic (>10th percentile), mildly impaired (<10th percentile), and severely impaired (<5th percentile) in Figure 1B [54,55].

Next, a two-way between-subject ANOVA model with Type III sum of squares was adjusted for the Olfactory Identification-Recognition score as a dependent variable, with cognitive status (*CH*, *SCD*, and *MCI*), age, and the interaction cognitive status $\times$ age as factors. Age categories were established as [<60, 60), [60, 70) and [70, >70). Post hoc between-group multiple comparisons were conducted under Tukey's HSD test, with adjusted p values due to multiple comparisons.

After that, relationships between cognitive measures and olfactory performance were studied. Linear regression models were computed for each cognitive measure, with age and olfactory identification as predictors. A stepwise method was applied to identify the contribution of the Olfactory Identification-Recognition score for each cognitive variable: a baseline model (model 1) was firstly computed with *age + sex* as predictors. Model 1 was compared to model 2, which also includes olfactory performance. Regarding sex, due to variable coding, positive estimates favor women, whereas negative estimates favor men. Alpha was set at $\alpha = 0.0038$ under Bonferroni correction ($\alpha = 0.05/13$).

Finally, logistic regression models were conducted in order to categorize the participants into their respective cognitive groups (CH vs. SCD, CH vs. MCI, and SCD vs. MCI). This analysis intended to find how the olfactory identification score is able to help to categorize the participants into their respective cognitive status groups, and hence, the potential clinical use of this test. For each comparison (CH vs. SCD, CH vs. MCI, and SCD vs. MCI), two models were calculated, including a baseline model (model 1) that classifies *age* + *sex* as predictors, and its performance was compared to model 2, which was computed with age, sex, and the Olfactory Identification-Recognition score as predictors. This method was taken from Delgado-Lima et al., 2023 [9]. In these models, positive estimates also favor women and negative ones favor men. For this analysis, alpha was set at $\alpha = 0.017$, under Bonferroni correction ($\alpha = 0.05/3$).

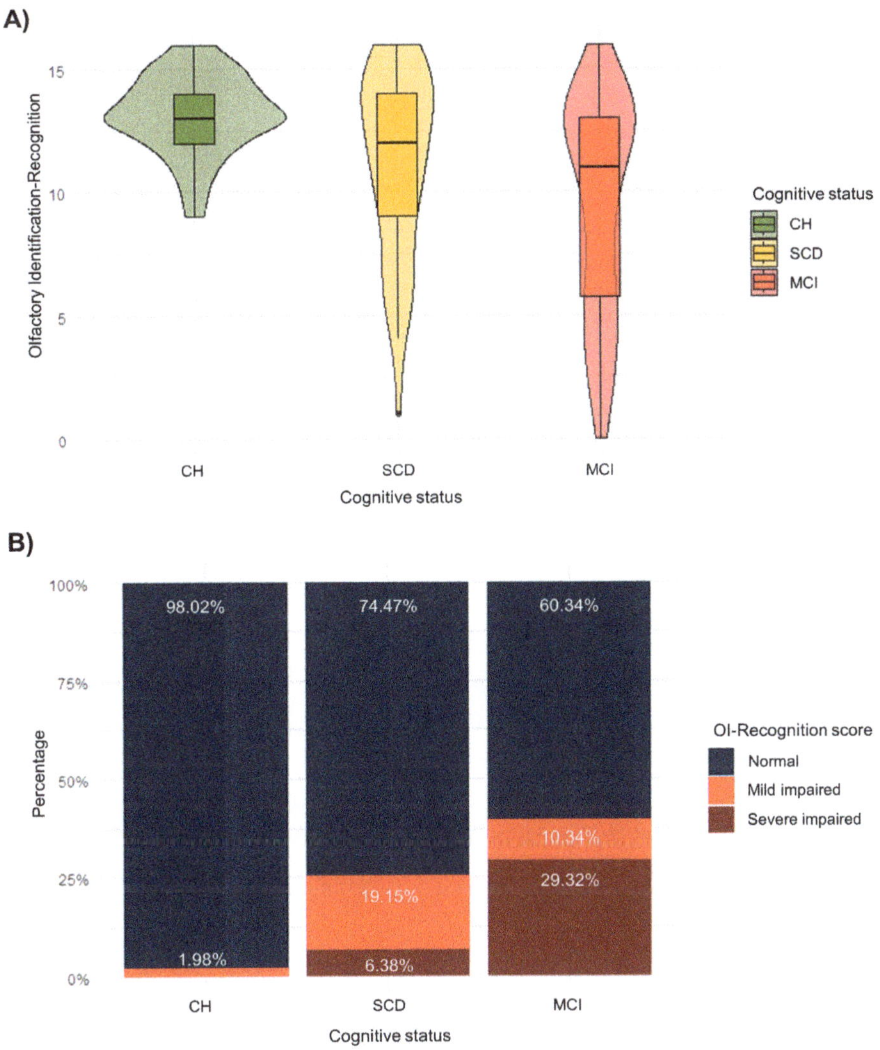

Figure 1. (**A**) Violin and boxplot for each cognitive group. (**B**) Distribution of normal, mild impaired, and severe impaired olfaction per cognitive group.

3. Results

A descriptive analysis of the sample by cognitive status is displayed in Table 1. The effect of *age* is statistically different from 0, due to the mean age in the MCI group being lower. Hence, this effect was considered in subsequent analyses. However, no differences either in sex or frequent alcohol consumption were elucidated. Regarding the Olfactory Identification-Subjective intensity score, there is no evidence of differences between cognitive groups. Consequently, this score was not used in further analyses. Figure 1A shows distributions for each cognitive group with violin plots, whereas Figure 1B reports the percentages of normal, mildly impaired, and severely impaired olfactory identification per cognitive group.

The two-way ANOVA model on the Olfactory Identification-Recognition score shows the main effects of *age* (F = 36.52, df = 2, p < 0.0001) and *cognitive status* (F = 33.65, df = 2, C). There is no evidence to support the *cognitive status* × *age* interaction effect (F = 0.825, df = 3, p = 0.48). The mean graph is shown in Figure 2. Post hoc comparisons on *age* show, on one side, significant differences between [<60, 60) and [70, >70) (dif = 2.151, p = 0.0016) and between [60, 70) and [80, >80) (dif = 2.302, p <= 0.0005). Both differences favor the younger category. On the other side, post hoc comparisons on *cognitive status* report significant differences between the three cohorts, with CH participants scoring higher and MCI participants scoring lower: CH and SCD (dif = 1.801, p = 0.007), SCD and MCI (dif = 1.847, p = 0.005), and CH and MCI (dif = 3.647, p < 0.0001).

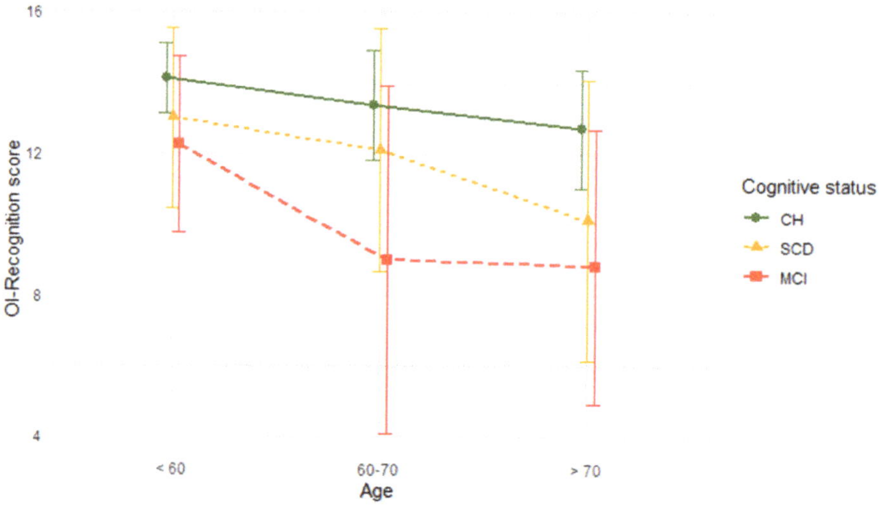

Figure 2. Mean graph of the Olfactory Identification-Recognition score by age and cognitive status.

Linear regression models for each cognitive variable are reported in Table 2. In each case, model 1 predicts cognitive performance with *age*. The stepwise introduction of the Olfactory Identification-Recognition score in model 2 was tested with R^2 and with an F-test comparing both models. These results highlight the effect of olfactory identification performance in measures of short-term memory (CVLT—immediate recall score, b = 0.589, SE = 0.112, p < 0.0001; DSF, b = 0.09, SE = 0.023, p = 0.0001; Rey Complex Figure Test—immediate recall score, b = 0.542, SE = 0.164, p = 0.001), long-term memory (CVLT—delayed recall score, b = 0.254, SE = 0.066, p < 0.0001), semantic memory (semantic verbal fluency—total score, b = 0.391, SE = 0.089, p < 0.0001), working memory (DSI, b = 0.098, SE = 0.025, p = 0.0001), and selective attention (Cancelation—correct answers, b = 0.309, SE = 0.103, p = 0.003). Olfactory identification also relates to cognitive performance in the Vocabulary Test—total score (b = 0.577, SE = 0.248, p = 0.021) and TMT B—seconds (b = −4.258, SE = 1.519, p = 0.005), but these effects are not adjusted for multiple comparisons (p < 0.0038). Hence, these effects should be interpreted carefully. Sex also seems to be a statistically significant predictor of the Vocabulary Test—total score (b = −4.338, SE = 1.525, p = 0.005). The negative association implies that men tend to score higher in this task. However, this effect is not adjusted to corrected p < 0.0038 either, so the interpretation should be careful.

Table 1. Descriptive analysis by cognitive status.

	Cognitively Healthy (CH)	Subjective Cognitive Decline (SCD)	Mild Cognitive Impairment (MCI)			
Sample Size	***101***	***47***	***116***			
	Mean (SD) or Count	**Mean (SD) or Count**	**Mean (SD) or Count**	**F or Chi**	***p***	**Post Hoc [a]**
Sex (women)	62	33	77	1.238	0.538	-
Age	69 (7.98)	69.74 (6.83)	66.52 (7.46)	4.448	0.013 *	CH, SCD > MCI
Frequent alcohol consumption	23	5	17	5.227	0.265	-
Identification-Recognition score	13.18 (1.61)	11.23 (3.74)	9.51 (4.44)	29.89	<0.0001 **	CH > SCD > MCI
Identification-Subjective intensity score	5.61 (1.35)	6.05 (2.03)	6.46 (1.91)	1.487	0.228	-
MoCA	28.96 (1.1)	28.67 (1.12)	23.84 (2.07)	305.5	<0.0001 **	CH, SCD > MCI
CVLT—immediate recall score	31.76 (6.6)	30.51 (5.59)	27.74 (6.99)	9.464	0.0001 **	CH, SCD > MCI
CVLT—delayed recall score	7.94 (3.69)	7.74 (2.58)	6.35 (4.39)	4.732	0.009 **	CH, SCD > MCI
Digits—Direct span	5.44 (1.56)	5.17 (1.23)	5.24 (1.54)	0.743	0.477	-
Digits—Inverse span	4.33 (1.65)	4.09 (1.52)	3.76 (1.34)	3.595	0.029 *	CH, SCD > MCI
Cancelation—correct answers	17.31 (4.27)	15.2 (4.93)	17.06 (4.47)	2.867	0.059	-
Cancelation—omissions	8 (9.2)	14.1 (36.94)	5.25 (6.38)	3.534	0.031 *	MCI > CH, SCD
RCFT—immediate recall score	19.17 (6.81)	17.48 (6.62)	16.96 (9.17)	1.968	0.142	-
RCFT—delayed recall score	20.93 (21.87)	25.13 (38.47)	16.81 (7.72)	1.843	0.161	-
Phonological verbal fluency—total score	14.85 (4.71)	14.21 (3.36)	13.14 (4.5)	3.914	0.021 *	CH, SCD > MCI
Semantic verbal fluency—total score	20.6 (6.52)	17.37 (4.74)	17.88 (5.08)	7.844	0.0005 **	CH > SCD, MCI
Vocabulary Test—total score	48.5 (10.98)	45.61 (11.67)	45.21 (10.23)	2.346	0.098	-
TMT A—seconds	47.93 (20.94)	51.53 (14.73)	50.11 (30.51)	0.376	0.687	-
TMT B—seconds	103.9 (55.67)	120.26 (61)	121.69 (91.85)	1.569	0.211	-

* $p < 0.05$; ** $p < 0.01$. [a] Post hoc comparisons ($p < 0.05$) under FWER correction.

Table 2. Results from multiple linear regression models for cognitive variables.

Cognitive Variables	Predictors	Estimate (b)	Std. Error (SE)	*p*	R^2	F [a]	*p*
CVLT—immediate recall	*Model 1*				0.015	11.067	0.001
	Intercept	7.336	1.057	<0.0001 **			
	Age	−0.033	0.015	0.027 *			
	Sex	0.119	0.241	0.621			
	Model 2				0.059		
	Intercept	5.206	1.216	<0.0001 **			
	Age	−0.023	0.015	0.114			
	Sex	0.043	0.237	0.857			
	Olfactory Identification—Recognition	0.125	0.038	0.001 **			
CVLT—delayed recall	*Model 1*				0.052	14.581	0.0002 **
	Intercept	14.342	2.258	<0.0001 **			
	Age	−0.117	0.032	0.0006 **			
	Sex	0.769	0.512	0.134			
	Model 2				0.104		
	Intercept	10.103	2.461	<0.0001 **			
	Age	−0.092	0.032	0.003 **			
	Sex	0.752	0.498	0.132			
	Olfactory Identification—Recognition	0.253	0.066	0.0001 **			
Digits—Direct span	*Model 1*				0.129	15.646	0.0001 **
	Intercept	10.069	0.778	<0.0001 **			
	Age	−0.067	0.011	<0.0001 **			
	Sex	−0.314	0.185	0.051			
	Model 2				0.177		
	Intercept	8.599	0.849	<0.0001 **			
	Age	−0.059	0.011	<0.0001 **			
	Sex	−0.357	0.231	0.061			
	Olfactory Identification—Recognition	0.09	0.023	0.0001 **			

Table 2. *Cont.*

Cognitive Variables	Predictors	Estimate (b)	Std. Error (SE)	p	R^2	F [a]	p
Digits—Inverse span	*Model 1*					14.581	0.0002 **
	Intercept	7.897	0.864	<0.0001 **	0.068		
	Age	−0.055	0.012	<0.0001 **			
	Sex	−0.191	0.195	0.327			
	Model 2				0.117		
	Intercept	6.247	0.945	<0.0001 **			
	Age	−0.047	0.012	0.0001 **			
	Sex	−0.195	0.189	0.306			
	Olfactory Identification—Recognition	0.097	0.025	0.0001 **			
Cancelation—correct answers	*Model 1*					9.414	0.0024 **
	Intercept	29.214	2.892	<0.0001 **	0.071		
	Age	−0.179	0.041	0.0002 **			
	Sex	−0.365	0.662	0.582			
	Model 2				0.106		
	Intercept	23.817	3.339	<0.0001 **			
	Age	−0.154	0.041	0.0002 **			
	Sex	−0.557	0.652	0.394			
	Olfactory Identification—Recognition	0.309	0.103	0.003 **			
Cancelation—omissions	*Model 1*					2.329	0.128
	Intercept	−5.657	10.775	0.601	0.001		
	Age	0.194	0.153	0.205			
	Sex	0.808	2.465	0.743			
	Model 2				0.004		
	Intercept	−15.815	12.638	0.212			
	Age	0.241	0.255	0.123			
	Sex	0.444	2.469	0.875			
	Olfactory Identification—Recognition	0.598	0.391	0.128			

Table 2. *Cont.*

Cognitive Variables	Predictors	Estimate (b)	Std. Error (SE)	*p*	R^2	F [a]	*p*
RCFT—immediate recall score	*Model 1*					11.977	0.0006 **
	Intercept	30.823	4.675	<0.0001 **	0.027		
	Age	−0.172	0.066	0.009			
	Sex	−1.578	1.06	0.138			
	Model 2				0.074		
	Intercept	20.959	5.379	0.0001			
	Age	−0.126	0.066	0.058			
	Sex	−1.89	1.038	0.071			
	Olfactory Identification—Recognition	0.568	0.164	0.0006 **			
RCFT—delayed recall score	*Model 1*					2.857	0.092
	Intercept	16.423	14.551	0.26	0.001		
	Age	0.093	0.207	0.652			
	Sex	−4.149	3.262	0.205			
	Model 2				0.008		
	Intercept	2.397	16.694	0.886			
	Age	0.149	0.208	0.474			
	Sex	−4.797	3.27	0.144			
	Olfactory Identification—Recognition	0.874	0.518	0.093			
Phonological verbal fluency—total score	*Model 1*					1.399	0.238
	Intercept	13.738	2.634	<0.0001 **	0.001		
	Age	−0.001	0.037	0.973			
	Sex	0.525	0.594	0.378			
	Model 2				0.001		
	Intercept	12.294	2.901	<0.0001 **			
	Age	0.005	0.038	0.899			
	Sex	0.544	0.594	0.361			
	Olfactory Identification—Recognition	0.088	0.076	0.248			

Table 2. *Cont.*

Cognitive Variables	Predictors	Estimate (b)	Std. Error (SE)	p	R^2	F [a]	p
Semantic verbal fluency—total score	*Model 1*					18.737	<0.0001 **
	Intercept	36.276	3.23	<0.0001 **	0.101		
	Age	−0.241	0.046	<0.0001 **			
	Sex	−1.648	0.728	0.025 *			
	Model 2				0.161		
	Intercept	30.038	3.437	<0.0001 **			
	Age	−0.214	0.044	<0.0001 **			
	Sex	−1.534	0.924	0.051			
	Olfactory Identification—Recognition	0.384	0.088	<0.0001 **			
Vocabulary Test—total score	*Model 1*					7.318	0.007 *
	Intercept	47.359	6.745	<0.0001 **			
	Age	0.027	0.096	0.782			
	Sex	−3.82	1.535	0.013 *			
	Model 2				0.049		
	Intercept	35.929	7.874	<0.0001 **			
	Age	0.08	0.097	0.407			
	Sex	−4.338	1.525	0.005 *			
	Olfactory Identification—Recognition	0.577	0.248	0.021 *			
TMT A—seconds	*Model 1*				0.124	2.917	0.089
	Intercept	−26.76	13.314	0.055			
	Age	1.111	0.196	<0.0001 **			
	Sex	1.051	3.15	0.739			
	Model 2				0.128		
	Intercept	−12.237	16.146	0.449			
	Age	1.044	0.199	<0.0001 **			
	Sex	1.575	3.151	0.618			
	Olfactory Identification—Recognition	−0.854	0.5	0.089			

Table 2. *Cont.*

Cognitive Variables	Predictors	Estimate (b)	Std. Error (SE)	p	R^2	F [a]	p
TMT B—seconds	*Model 1*				0.077	8.637	0.004 *
	Intercept	−77.531	42.478	0.069			
	Age	2.709	0.604	<0.0001 **			
	Sex	11.171	9.705	0.251			
	Model 2				0.109		
	Intercept	−1.508	49.116	0.975			
	Age	2.363	0.605	0.0001 **			
	Sex	13.911	9.585	0.148			
	Olfactory Identification—Recognition	−4.473	1.522	0.004 *			

* $p < 0.05$; ** $p < 0.0038$. [a] F test to check if model 2 significantly improves model 1.

Finally, the discrimination power of olfactory identification to differentiate the cognitively healthy participants from the participants with subjective cognitive decline (CH vs. SCD) and the participants with mild cognitive impairment (CH vs. MCI) was tested with logistic regression models. The results are displayed in Tables 3–5. In each table, model 1 is the baseline model, as it shows performance with *age* and *sex* as the unique predictors. Right after model 1, model 2 implies the introduction of the Olfactory Identification-Recognition score for analysis if the model improves. A comparison between model 1 (baseline) and model 2 was performed with ANOVA with the likelihood ratio test.

The results for the CH vs. SCD classification are shown in Table 3. In this first case, model 1 is a null model, with no effect of *age* ($p = 0.572$) or *sex* ($p = 0.186$). However, the addition of the Olfactory Identification-Recognition score significantly improves the logistic model (model 1 vs. model 2, chi = 17.952, df = 1, $p < 0.0001$). Next, the results for the CH vs. MCI comparison are reported in Table 4. Again, model 1 is a null model, with no statistically significant predictor, as the effect of age and sex are not statistically different from 0 ($p = 0.086$ and $p = 0.746$, respectively). Similar to the CH vs. SCD model, the addition of the Olfactory Identification-Recognition score significantly improves the classification power of model 2 (model 1 vs. model 2, chi = 124.06, df = 1, $p < 0.0001$). Plus, with the addition of the OI score, the effect of age is now statistically significant. Nevertheless, there is no evidence to assume the effect of sex. Finally, the results for the CH vs. MCI comparison are displayed in Table 5. The inclusion of the Olfactory Identification-Recognition score in model 2 also improves its classification power (model 1 vs. model 2, chi = 49.782, df = 1, $p < 0.0001$). In model 2, age is also a significant predictor ($p = 0.0009$), whereas sex cannot be considered statistically significant ($p = 0.054$). ROC curves for models with the Olfactory Identification-Recognition score are reported in Figure 3.

Table 3. Logistic regression models (baseline or model 1 and definitive or model 2) of CH vs. SCD.

	Estimate	Error	*p*	Sensitivity	Specificity	AUC
Model 1						
Intercept	2.235	1.759	0.204			
Age	−0.017	0.024	0.702	0.59	-	0.5
Sex	−0.428	0.383	0.263			
Model 2						
Intercept	3.839	2.447	0.117			
Age	−0.014	0.027	0.576	0.76	0.94	0.66
Sex	0.546	0.413	0.186			
Olfactory Identification—Recognition	−0.317	0.083	<0.0001 **			

* $p < 0.05$; ** $p < 0.017$.

Table 4. Logistic regression models (baseline or model 1 and definitive or model 2) of CH vs. MCI.

	Estimate	Error	*p*	Sensitivity	Specificity	AUC
Model 1						
Intercept	2.051	1343.0	0.127			
Age	−0.032	0.019	0.089	0.61	0.6	0.6
Sex	0.098	0.304	0.746			
Model 2						
Intercept	19.822	3.585	<0.0001 **			
Age	−0.128	0.031	<0.0001 **	0.85	0.82	0.83
Sex	0.091	0.447	0.839			
Olfactory Identification—Recognition	−0.967	0.166	<0.0001 **			

* $p < 0.05$; ** $p < 0.017$.

Table 5. Logistic regression models (baseline or model 1 and definitive or model 2) of SCD vs. MCI.

	Estimate	Error	*p*	Sensitivity	Specificity	AUC
Model 1						
Intercept	4.064	1.727	0.019 *			
Age	−0.052	0.025	0.039 *	0.33	0.66	0.5
Sex	−0.321	0.396	0.419			
Model 2						
Intercept	13.883	3.016	<0.0001 **			
Age	−0.109	0.033	0.0009 **			
Sex	−0.949	0.491	0.054	0.71	0.8	0.73
Olfactory Identification—Recognition	−0.479	0.094	<0.0001 **			

* $p < 0.05$; ** $p < 0.017$.

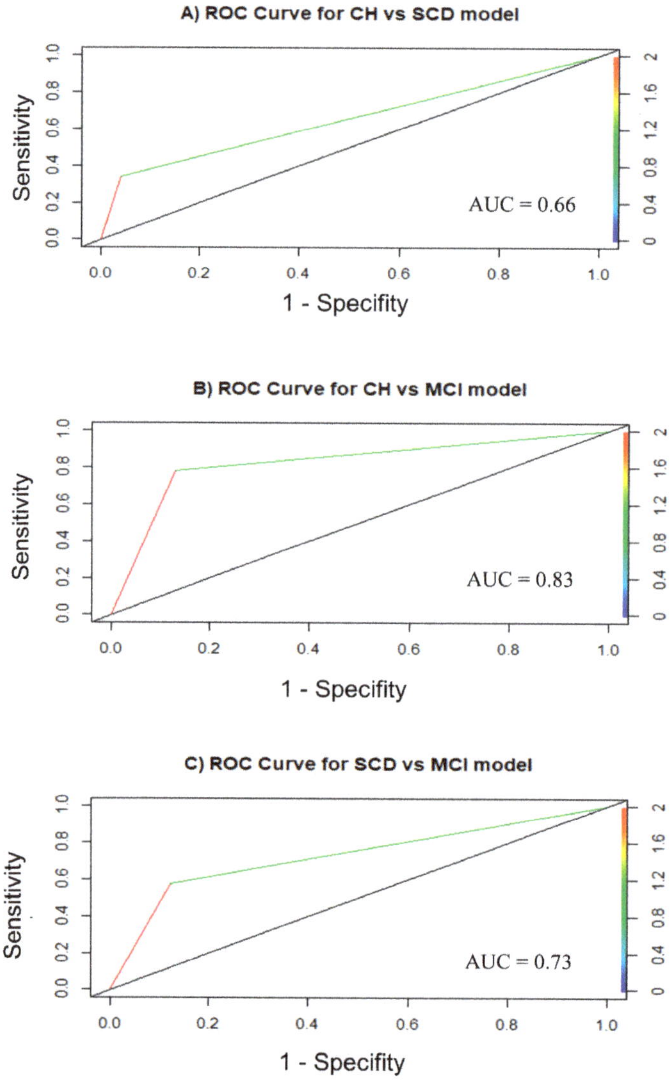

Figure 3. ROC curves for: (**A**) CH vs. SCD, (**B**) CH vs. MCI, and (**C**) SCD vs. MCI.

4. Discussion

In the present study, the association between OI dysfunction and the risk of cognitive impairment (SCD and MCI) was analyzed. OI tests are frequently employed to assess olfactory function in individuals with MCI and dementia [64–66].

We found that OI differed significantly between CH, SCD, and MCI. Across the continuum of cognitive risk, OI decreases in a stepwise manner, as the participants with MCI performed lower than SCD, and SCD performed lower than CH. Our results indicated that 40% of the participants with MCI had OI dysfunction (Figure 1B). Different investigations indicate that sensory impairments, such as OI deficits, may precede cognitive impairment, and several years before symptoms of cognitive impairment manifest in AD, individuals may already exhibit compromised OI abilities [67–69]. The literature is unanimous in its interest in including OI analysis in MCI and SCD groups, whose results are along the same lines as ours, observing a worse performance in OI in the MCI group compared to SCD and in SCD compared to CH [70–72].

Our results are in line with many other authors who have found a pattern of deterioration in OI test performance similar to ours between CH participants and SCD participants [28,29,73]. This trend was also supported by the meta-analysis by Jobin et al. (2021) [48]. Their results noted that individuals with SCD have lower performance on OI tests compared to cognitively healthy (CH) older adults. Moreover, Sohrabi et al. (2009) also found statistically significant differences in OI between CH and SCD cohorts [74]. Therefore, the differences in olfaction between CH and SCD groups seem to be consistent.

In our study, ANOVA analysis on olfactory identification revealed significant main effects for both age and cognitive status. The significant effect of age on olfactory performance is consistent with prior research, indicating that olfactory performance decreases with age. This deterioration is attributed to various factors, including the degeneration of olfactory receptor neurons, changes in the olfactory bulb, and alterations in central processing regions [19,75,76]. This association reflects age-related physiological changes in the central nervous system, which may affect both olfaction and cognitive function [77].

Promising and consistent results about how OI alterations alone predict the progression to AD from its asymptomatic preclinical stage (including MCI and even earlier stages such as SCD) have been reported [78,79]. However, our results suggest that combining cognitive assessments with an olfactory identification measure could improve the early detection of at-risk individuals. Olfactory deficits have been shown to precede cognitive symptoms and correlate with the severity of cognitive impairment. Thus, like other authors, we can point out that the odor identification test scores are influenced by non-olfactory cognitive abilities [39,80,81].

Likewise, when comparing the cognitive status across the three samples, CH scored significantly higher than those with SCD and those with MCI. Similarly, the SCD participants demonstrated better cognitive outcomes compared to the MCI participants. These results align with the existing literature, which consistently shows that cognitive performance declines progressively from CH to SCD and then to MCI [7,15,16,18,82]. Additionally, the SCD participants demonstrated better cognitive outcomes compared to the MCI participants, further supporting the notion that SCD represents an asymptomatic preclinical stage in the continuum of cognitive decline.

When analyzing the results for each cognitive domain and their association with OI, the results indicate that a decrease in OI is associated with lower performance in episodic, semantic, and working memory, executive functions, and attention and processing speed, and there is no relationship with performance in language or visuospatial skills. The relationship between these cognitive domains and odor identification function might suggest overlapping structural and physiological disease processes in regions of the central nervous system related to olfactory factors [83]. Regarding sex differences, there are examples in the literature that support them in OI [76,84,85], so we considered that sex could be a potential covariate within linear and logistic regression models. Our results highlight that sex seems to be a statistically significant predictor for the vocabulary score, under uncorrected p-values. This effect favors men. However, we found no evidence of sex differences predicting any other cognitive score, when combining it with OI. These results regarding sex are in line with our previous studies [54,55].

In episodic memory, our results revealed that OI is related to both verbal episodic memory (measured with CVLT-II immediate and delayed recall scores) and visual episodic memory (measured with RCFT immediate recall score). In relation to semantic memory, OI is associated with the semantic verbal fluency score. There is consensus in indicating that, to a greater extent, in the semantic fluency condition, not in the phonological one, people with progressive cognitive impairment generate significantly fewer words [86,87]. In another meta-analysis by Jobin et al. [88], OI was related to episodic memory and semantic memory, although effect sizes were relatively small. In addition, our findings are in line with several studies in which a relationship was found between semantic memory deficits and lower performance on the OI test [31,70,89,90]. OI relies on prior semantic knowledge, the ability to access that knowledge, and the capacity to link it to linguistic labels, along with organization and information processing strategies. Vocabulary tests are related to this crystalized knowledge [91], so this could explain the results in the vocabulary scores and the potential sex differences found in this score. Difficulties at any level of semantic processing can affect task performance [92]. The entorhinal cortex, which connects with the hippocampus and is essential in the formation and recognition of memories, also plays a very important role in olfactory processing [93,94]. It is now thought that AD likely originates in the entorhinal cortex, a region essential for olfactory processing [28]. Thus, OI could be key in the early detection of AD, as these deficits may appear in individuals with SCD or suspected preclinical AD [73]. Apparent but milder deficits have been observed in at-risk individuals without dementia (i.e., individuals with APOE4 allele genotypes [95] and first-degree relatives of AD patients [96,97]).

In executive functions, our results indicate that OI is related to working memory, verbal fluency, and cognitive flexibility. In working memory, OI dysfunction is associated with lower scores on DSI scores [98]. As noted above, OI is associated with semantic verbal fluency (also an executive function measure). In relation to cognitive flexibility, OI might be related to TMT-B. TMT-B may indicate dysfunction in the dorsolateral prefrontal cortex, so our results suggest that processing in frontal regions is more important than olfactory processing. Our results support Challakere et al. (2022) [99], who found worse performance in TMT-B performance as cognitive impairment progresses. These results may suggest that orbitofrontal processing (an area thought to be relevant in olfactory processing) would be more affected than processing in other frontal regions (i.e., dorsolateral). However, we found no relationship between OI and performance in TMT-A, in disagreement with Uchida et al. (2020) [100].

Lastly, OI was found to be a powerful variable for classifying patients into CH, SCD, and MCI categories. The HC vs. SCD logistic regression model suggests that olfactory identification has a significant role in distinguishing between CH and SCD individuals. Similarly, the CH vs. MCI logistic regression model is also significant in distinguishing MCI from CH when including the OI score, in agreement with our previous findings [19]. Moreover, the present study also evidences that OI is a useful tool for distinguishing patients with MCI from those with just previous SCD. Nevertheless, there is no evidence in any model to assume that sex might be a predictive variable to distinguish CH, SCD, and MCI. Thus, our findings align with and extend those of previous studies. For instance, Wang et al. (2021) [29] found that OI scores were progressively lower from CH to SCD, MCI, and AD. Although OI measures are useful for the early detection of dementia, these are underutilized in clinical examinations. This could indicate a lack of familiarity with these instruments and uncertainty about how they integrate with a traditional neuropsychological assessment. Consequently, our findings may help practitioners by offering a framework for interpreting OI measures.

We consider that a strong point of our study is the application of a broad neuropsychological assessment protocol, which allowed us to deepen the relationship between OI and the different cognitive domains. The combination of the OI test and cognitive tests in various domains can improve the ability to predict future cognitive impairment in older adults without dementia [69]. Nevertheless, the strengths of the present study do not exempt it from some limitations. The main limitation lies in the study design. This is a cross-sectional study, so each cognitive group is composed of different participants. Hence, it is not possible to interpret statistical differences between groups as the development of dementia. Future research should explore the relationship between olfactory identification and cognitive performance using longitudinal data, allowing for conclusions about the progression from SCD to MCI to be made. Our study is also limited by the absence of an educational background variable. Future research should also include educational background as an explanatory variable, due to its association with olfactory identification and cognitive performance [101,102]. Another limitation is the absence of an Alzheimer's cohort. Future investigations with longitudinal data should also include conversion to AD. Finally, an important addition to future studies would be neuroimaging measurement. The combination of olfactory, cognitive, and neuroimaging data would offer a more complete photograph of olfaction as a predictor of dementia. In relation to this, Li et al. (2024) [69], in participants who progressed to cognitive decline within a 5-year span, found a relationship between OI, hippocampal cortical volume, and cognitive decline. Results like this support our hypothesis in further studies.

5. Conclusions

Our results suggest that combining cognitive assessments with olfactory identification tests could enhance the early detection of individuals at risk. Additionally, incorporating olfactory testing into routine assessments for elderly individuals, especially those reporting subjective cognitive complaints, could provide a non-invasive and cost-effective tool for early diagnosis and intervention. Future research should focus on longitudinal studies to confirm the predictive value of olfactory identification deficits in conjunction with cognitive assessments and to explore the underlying mechanisms linking olfactory function and cognitive impairment.

Supplementary Materials: The following supporting information can be downloaded at https://www.mdpi.com/article/10.3390/ejihpe14120196/s1, Table S1: Summary table for the present study's methods.

Author Contributions: Conceptualization, J.B., A.H.D.-L., and M.L.D.-L.; methodology, A.H.D.-L., M.L.D.-L., and J.B.; data collection, A.H.D.-L.; formal analysis, J.B.; investigation, A.H.D.-L., and M.L.D.-L.; writing—original draft preparation, J.B., A.H.D.-L., and M.L.D.-L.; writing—review and editing, J.B., A.H.D.-L., and M.L.D.-L. All authors have read and agreed to the published version of the manuscript.

Funding: This research received no external funding.

Institutional Review Board Statement: Ethics Committee from University Hospital San Carlos Madrid, Spain, internal codes 17/192-E and 18/422-E_BS.

Informed Consent Statement: All participants were informed about the aims of this study and gave written informed consent.

Data Availability Statement: Data at individual level is available upon request.

Acknowledgments: The authors would like to thank all the people who volunteered and participated in this study.

Conflicts of Interest: The authors declare no conflict of interest.

References

1. Mendonça, M.D.; Alves, L.; Bugalho, P. From Subjective Cognitive Complaints to Dementia: Who Is at Risk?: A Systematic Review. *Am. J. Alzheimer's Dis. Other Dement.* **2016**, *31*, 105–114. [CrossRef] [PubMed]
2. Petersen, R.C.; Lopez, O.; Armstrong, M.J.; Getchius, T.S.D.; Ganguli, M.; Gloss, D.; Gronseth, G.S.; Marson, D.; Pringsheim, T.; Day, G.S.; et al. Practice Guideline Update Summary: Mild Cognitive Impairment: Report of the Guideline Development, Dissemination, and Implementation Subcommittee of the American Academy of Neurology. *Neurology* **2017**, *90*, 126–135. [CrossRef] [PubMed]
3. Chary, E.; Amieva, H.; Pérès, K.; Orgogozo, J.; Dartigues, J.; Jacqmin-Gadda, H. Short-versus long-term prediction of dementia among subjects with low and high educational levels. *Alzheimer's Dement.* **2013**, *9*, 562–571. [CrossRef] [PubMed]
4. Van Oijen, M.; de Jong, F.J.; Hofman, A.; Koudstaal, P.J.; Breteler, M.M. Subjective memory complaints, education, and risk of Alzheimer's disease. *Alzheimer's Dement.* **2007**, *3*, 92–97. [CrossRef] [PubMed]
5. Jungwirth, S.; Zehetmayer, S.; Bauer, P.; Weissgram, S.; Tragl, K.H.; Fischer, P. Prediction of Alzheimer's dementia with short neuropsychological instruments. *J. Neural Transm.* **2009**, *116*, 1513–1521. [CrossRef]
6. Jessen, F.; Amariglio, R.E.; van Boxtel, M.; Breteler, M.; Ceccaldi, M.; Chételat, G.; Dubois, B.; Dufouil, C.; Ellis, K.A.; van der Flier, W.M.; et al. A Conceptual Framework for Research on Subjective Cognitive Decline in Preclinical Alzheimer's Disease. *Alzheimer's Dement.* **2014**, *10*, 844–852. [CrossRef]
7. Jessen, F.; Amariglio, R.E.; Buckley, R.F.; van der Flier, W.M.; Han, Y.; Molinuevo, J.L.; Rabin, L.; Rentz, D.M.; Rodriguez-Gomez, O.; Saykin, A.J.; et al. The Characterisation of Subjective Cognitive Decline. *Lancet Neurol.* **2020**, *19*, 271–278. [CrossRef]
8. Molinuevo, J.L.; Rabin, L.A.; Amariglio, R.; Buckley, R.; Dubois, B.; Ellis, K.A.; Ewers, M.; Hampel, H.; Klöppel, S.; Rami, L.; et al. Implementation of subjective cognitive decline criteria in research studies. *Alzheimer's Dement.* **2017**, *13*, 296–311. [CrossRef]
9. Luck, T.; Luppa, M.; Matschinger, H.; Jessen, F.; Angermeyer, M.C.; Riedel-Heller, S.G. Incident subjective memory complaints and the risk of subsequent dementia. *Acta Psychiatr. Scand.* **2015**, *131*, 290–296. [CrossRef]
10. Silva, D.; Guerreiro, M.; Faria, C.; Maroco, J.; Schmand, B.A.; Mendonca, A. Significance of subjective memory complaints in the clinical setting. *J. Geriatr. Psychiatry Neurol.* **2014**, *27*, 259–265. [CrossRef]
11. Gallassi, R.; Oppi, F.; Poda, R.; Scortichini, S.; Maserati, M.S.; Marano, G.; Sambati, L. Are subjective cognitive complaints a risk factor for dementia? *Neurol. Sci.* **2010**, *31*, 327–336. [CrossRef] [PubMed]
12. Reisberg, B.; Shulman, M.B.; Torossian, C.; Leng, L.; Zhu, W. Outcome over seven years of healthy adults with and without subjective cognitive impairment. *Alzheimer's Dement.* **2010**, *6*, 11–24. [CrossRef] [PubMed]
13. van Harten, A.C.; Mielke, M.M.; Swenson-Dravis, D.M.; Hagen, C.E.; Edwards, K.K.; Roberts, R.O.; Petersen, R.C.; Geda, Y.E.; Knopman, D.S.; Petersen, R.C. Subjective cognitive decline and risk of MCI: The Mayo Clinic Study of Aging. *Neurology* **2018**, *91*, e300–e312. [CrossRef] [PubMed]
14. Rabin, L.A.; Smart, C.M.; Amariglio, R.E. Subjective cognitive decline in preclinical Alzheimer's disease. *Annu. Rev. Clin. Psychol.* **2017**, *13*, 369–396. [CrossRef] [PubMed]
15. Mitchell, A.J.; Beaumont, H.; Ferguson, D.; Yadegarfar, M.; Stubbs, B. Risk of Dementia and Mild Cognitive Impairment in Older People with Subjective Memory Complaints: Meta-Analysis. *Acta Psychiatr. Scand.* **2014**, *130*, 439–451. [CrossRef]
16. Pike, K.E.; Cavuoto, M.G.; Li, L.; Wright, B.J.; Kinsella, G.J. Subjective Cognitive Decline: Level of Risk for Future Dementia and Mild Cognitive Impairment, a Meta-Analysis of Longitudinal Studies. *Neuropsychol. Rev.* **2022**, *32*, 703–735. [CrossRef]
17. for Cohort Studies of Memory in an International Consortium (COSMIC); Röhr, S.; Pabst, A.; Riedel-Heller, S.G.; Jessen, F.; Turana, Y.; Handajani, Y.S.; Brayne, C.; Matthews, F.E.; Stephan, B.C.M.; et al. Estimating Prevalence of Subjective Cognitive Decline in and across International Cohort Studies of Aging: A COSMIC Study. *Alzheimer's Res. Ther.* **2020**, *12*, 167. [CrossRef]
18. Jester, D.J.; Vyhnálek, M.; Andel, R.; Marková, H.; Nikolai, T.; Laczó, J.; Matusková, V.; Cechová, K.; Sheardova, K.; Hort, J. Progression from subjective cognitive decline to mild cognitive impairment or dementia: The role of baseline cognitive performance. *J. Alzheime'rs Dis.* **2022**, *86*, 1763–1774. [CrossRef]
19. Delgado-Lima, A.H.; Bouhaben, J.; Martínez-Zujeros, S.; Pallardo-Rodil, B.; Gómez-Pavón, J.; Delgado-Losada, M.L. Could Olfactory Identification Be a Prognostic Factor in Detecting Cognitive Impairment Risk in the Elderly? *GeroScience* **2023**, *45*, 2011–2025. [CrossRef]
20. Adams, D.R.; Kern, D.W.; Wroblewski, K.E.; McClintock, M.K.; Dale, W.; Pinto, J.M. Olfactory Dysfunction Predicts Subsequent Dementia in Older U.S. Adults. *J. Am. Geriatr. Soc.* **2018**, *66*, 140–144. [CrossRef]
21. Devanand, D.P. Olfactory Identification Deficits, Cognitive Decline, and Dementia in Older Adults. *Am. J. Geriatr. Psychiatry* **2016**, *24*, 1151–1157. [CrossRef] [PubMed]
22. Woodward, M.R.; Hafeez, M.U.; Qi, Q.; Riaz, A.; Benedict, R.H.B.; Yan, L.; Szigeti, K.; Pavlik, V.; Massman, P.; Darby, E.; et al. Odorant Item Specific Olfactory Identification Deficit May Differentiate Alzheimer Disease from Aging. *Am. J. Geriatr. Psychiatry* **2018**, *26*, 835–846. [CrossRef] [PubMed]
23. Chen, B.; Espin, M.; Haussmann, R.; Matthes, C.; Donix, M.; Hummel, T.; Haehner, A. The effect of olfactory training on olfaction, cognition, and brain function in patients with mild cognitive impairment. *J. Alzheimer's Dis.* **2022**, *85*, 745–754. [CrossRef] [PubMed]
24. Yoshitake, M.; Maeshima, E.; Maeshima, S.; Osawa, A.; Ito, N.; Ueda, I.; Kamiya, M. Olfactory Identification Ability in Patients with Mild Cognitive Impairment and Alzheimer's Disease. *J. Phys. Ther. Sci.* **2022**, *34*, 710–714. [CrossRef] [PubMed]

25. Roalf, D.R.; Moberg, M.J.; Turetsky, B.I.; Brennan, L.; Kabadi, S.; Wolk, D.A.; Moberg, P.J. A Quantitative Meta-Analysis of Olfactory Dysfunction in Mild Cognitive Impairment. *J. Neurol. Neurosurg. Psychiatry* **2017**, *88*, 226–232. [CrossRef] [PubMed]
26. Velayudhan, L.; Pritchard, M.; Powell, J.F.; Proitsi, P.; Lovestone, S. Smell Identification Function as a Severity and Progression Marker in Alzheimer's Disease. *Int. Psychogeriatr.* **2013**, *25*, 1157–1166. [CrossRef]
27. Tian, Q.; Bilgel, M.; Moghekar, A.R.; Ferrucci, L.; Resnick, S.M. Olfaction, cognitive impairment, and PET biomarkers in community-dwelling older adults. *J. Alzheimer's Dis.* **2022**, *86*, 1275–1285. [CrossRef]
28. Chen, B.; Wang, Q.; Zhong, X.; Mai, N.; Zhang, M.; Zhou, H.; Haehner, A.; Chen, X.; Wu, Z.; Auber, L.A.; et al. Structural and Functional Abnormalities of Olfactory-Related Regions in Subjective Cognitive Decline, Mild Cognitive Impairment, and Alzheimer's Disease. *Int. J. Neuropsychopharmacol.* **2022**, *25*, 361–374. [CrossRef]
29. Wang, Q.; Chen, B.; Zhong, X.; Zhou, H.; Zhang, M.; Mai, N.; Wu, Z.; Huang, X.; Haehner, A.; Chen, X.; et al. Olfactory dysfunction is already present with subjective cognitive decline and deepens with disease severity in the Alzheimer's disease spectrum. *J. Alzheimer's Dis.* **2021**, *79*, 585–595. [CrossRef]
30. Bahar-Fuchs, A.; Moss, S.; Rowe, C.; Savage, G. Awareness of Olfactory Deficits in Healthy Aging, Amnestic Mild Cognitive Impairment and Alzheimer's Disease. *Int. Psychogeriatr.* **2011**, *23*, 1097–1106. [CrossRef]
31. Wilson, R.S.; Arnold, S.E.; Tang, Y.; Bennett, D.A. Odor Identification and Decline in Different Cognitive Domains in Old Age. *Neuroepidemiology* **2006**, *26*, 61–67. [CrossRef] [PubMed]
32. Devanand, D.P.; Lee, S.; Manly, J.; Andrews, H.; Schupf, N.; Doty, R.L.; Stern, Y.; Zahodne, L.B.; Louis, E.D.; Mayeux, R. Olfactory Deficits Predict Cognitive Decline and Alzheimer Dementia in an Urban Community. *Neurology* **2015**, *84*, 182–189. [CrossRef] [PubMed]
33. Roberts, R.O.; Christianson, T.J.H.; Kremers, W.K.; Mielke, M.M.; Machulda, M.M.; Vassilaki, M.; Alhurani, R.E.; Geda, Y.E.; Knopman, D.S.; Petersen, R.C. Association between Olfactory Dysfunction and Amnestic Mild Cognitive Impairment and Alzheimer Disease Dementia. *JAMA Neurol.* **2016**, *73*, 93. [CrossRef] [PubMed]
34. Dintica, C.S.; Marseglia, A.; Rizzuto, D.; Wang, R.; Seubert, J.; Arfanakis, K.; Bennett, D.A.; Xu, W. Impaired Olfaction Is Associated with Cognitive Decline and Neurodegeneration in the Brain. *Neurology* **2019**, *92*, e700–e709. [CrossRef] [PubMed]
35. Wilson, R.S.; Schneider, J.A.; Arnold, S.E.; Tang, Y.; Boyle, P.A.; Bennett, D.A. Olfactory Identification and Incidence of Mild Cognitive Impairment in Older Age. *Arch. Gen. Psychiatry* **2007**, *64*, 802. [CrossRef]
36. Segura, B.; Baggio, H.C.; Solana, E.; Palacios, E.M.; Vendrell, P.; Bargalló, N.; Junqué, C. Neuroanatomical Correlates of Olfactory Loss in Normal Aged Subjects. *Behav. Brain Res.* **2013**, *246*, 148–153. [CrossRef]
37. Hagemeier, J.; Woodward, M.R.; Rafique, U.A.; Amrutkar, C.V.; Bergsland, N.; Dwyer, M.G.; Benedict, R.; Zivadinov, R.; Szigeti, K. Odor Identification Deficit in Mild Cognitive Impairment and Alzheimer's Disease Is Associated with Hippocampal and Deep Gray Matter Atrophy. *Psychiatry Res. Neuroimaging* **2016**, *255*, 87–93. [CrossRef]
38. Lu, J.; Testa, N.; Jordan, R.; Elyan, R.; Kanekar, S.; Wang, J.; Eslinger, P.; Yang, Q.X.; Zhang, B.; Karunanayaka, P.R. Functional Connectivity between the Resting-State Olfactory Network and the Hippocampus in Alzheimer's Disease. *Brain Sci.* **2019**, *9*, 338. [CrossRef]
39. Schubert, C.R.; Carmichael, L.L.; Murphy, C.; Klein, B.E.K.; Klein, R.; Cruickshanks, K.J. Olfaction and the 5-year Incidence of Cognitive Impairment in an Epidemiological Study of Older Adults. *J. Am. Geriatr. Soc.* **2008**, *56*, 1517–1521. [CrossRef]
40. Yaffe, K.; Freimer, D.; Chen, H.; Asao, K.; Rosso, A.; Rubin, S.; Tranah, G.; Cummings, S.; Simonsick, E. Olfaction and Risk of Dementia in a Biracial Cohort of Older Adults. *Neurology* **2017**, *88*, 456–462. [CrossRef]
41. Dade, L.A.; Zatorre, R.J.; Jones-Gotman, M. Olfactory Learning: Convergent Findings from Lesion and Brain Imaging Studies in Humans. *Brain* **2002**, *125*, 86–101. [CrossRef] [PubMed]
42. Devanand, D.P.; Michaels-Marston, K.S.; Liu, X.; Pelton, G.H.; Padilla, M.; Marder, K.; Bell, K.; Stern, Y.; Mayeux, R. Olfactory Deficits in Patients with Mild Cognitive Impairment Predict Alzheimer's Disease at Follow-Up. *Am. J. Psychiatry* **2000**, *157*, 1399–1405. [CrossRef] [PubMed]
43. Al-Otaibi, M.; Lessard-Beaudoin, M.; Castellano, C.-A.; Gris, D.; Cunnane, S.C.; Graham, R.K. Volumetric MRI Demonstrates Atrophy of the Olfactory Cortex in AD. *Curr. Alzheimer Res.* **2021**, *17*, 904–915. [CrossRef] [PubMed]
44. Prandini, M.N.; Nonato, M.B.; Lois, B.J.V. The importance of Hippocampal Volume Reduction in People with Alzheimer's Disease. *J. Biomed. Res. Rev.* **2018**, *1*, 16–19.
45. AlOtaibi, M.; De Marco, M.; Venneri, A. Measuring Olfactory-related Brain Region Volume Loss in MCI and AD Using Structural MRI. *Alzheimer's Dement.* **2023**, *19*, e060723. [CrossRef]
46. Su, M.-W.; Ni, J.-N.; Cao, T.-Y.; Wang, S.-S.; Shi, J.; Tian, J.-Z. The Correlation between Olfactory Test and Hippocampal Volume in Alzheimer's Disease and Mild Cognitive Impairment Patients: A Meta-Analysis. Front. *Aging Neurosci.* **2021**, *13*, 755160. [CrossRef]
47. Parvand, M.; Rankin, C.H. Is There a Shared Etiology of Olfactory Impairments in Normal Aging and Neurodegenerative Disease? *J. Alzheimer's Dis.* **2020**, *73*, 1–21. [CrossRef]
48. Jobin, B.; Zahal, R.; Bussières, E.-L.; Frasnelli, J.; Boller, B. Olfactory Identification in Subjective Cognitive Decline: A Meta-Analysis. *J. Alzheimer's Dis.* **2021**, *79*, 1497–1507. [CrossRef]
49. Windon, M.J.; Kim, S.J.; Oh, E.S.; Lin, S.Y. Predictive Value of Olfactory Impairment for Cognitive Decline among Cognitively Normal Adults. *Laryngoscope* **2020**, *130*, 840–847. [CrossRef]

50. Reid, L.M.; Maclullich, A.M.J. Subjective Memory Complaints and Cognitive Impairment in Older People. *Dement. Geriatr. Cogn. Disord.* **2006**, *22*, 471–485. [CrossRef]
51. Albert, M.S.; DeKosky, S.T.; Dickson, D.; Dubois, B.; Feldman, H.H.; Fox, N.C.; Gamst, A.; Holtzman, D.M.; Jagust, W.J.; Petersen, R.C.; et al. The Diagnosis of Mild Cognitive Impairment Due to Alzheimer's Disease: Recommendations from the National Institute on Aging-Alzheimer's Association Workgroups on Diagnostic Guidelines for Alzheimer's Disease. *Focus* **2013**, *11*, 96–106. [CrossRef]
52. Pereiro, A.X.; Ramos-Lema, S.; Lojo-Seoane, C.; Guàrdia-Olmos, J.; Facal-Mayo, D.; Juncos-Rabadán, O. Normative data for the Montreal Cognitive Assessment (MOCA) in a Spanish sample of community-dweller adults. *Eur. Geriatr. Med.* **2017**, *8*, 240–244. [CrossRef]
53. Nasreddine, Z.S.; Phillips, N.A.; Bédirian, V.; Charbonneau, S.; Whitehead, V.; Collin, I.; Cummings, J.L.; Chertkow, H. The Montreal Cognitive Assessment, MoCA: A Brief Screening Tool for Mild Cognitive Impairment: Moca: A Brief Screening Tool for MCI. *J. Am. Geriatr. Soc.* **2005**, *53*, 695–699. [CrossRef] [PubMed]
54. Delgado-Losada, M.L.; Delgado-Lima, A.H.; Bouhaben, J. Spanish Validation for Olfactory Function Testing Using the Sniffin' Sticks Olfactory Test: Threshold, Discrimination, and Identification. *Brain Sci.* **2020**, *10*, 943. [CrossRef]
55. Delgado-Losada, M.L.; Bouhaben, J.; Delgado-Lima, A.H. Development of the Spanish Version of Sniffin's Sticks Olfactory Identification Test: Normative Data and Validity of Parallel Measures. *Brain Sci.* **2021**, *11*, 216. [CrossRef]
56. Delis, D.C.; Kramer, J.H.; Kaplan, E.; Ober, B.A. *California Verbal Learning Test*, 2nd ed.; Pearson Education: Upper Saddle River, NJ, USA, 2016.
57. Wechsler, D. *Wechler Adult Intelligence Scales-IV*; Pearson Education: Upper Saddle River, NJ, USA, 2008.
58. Huppert, F.A.; Gardener, E.; McWilliams, B. *Cognitive Function. En. Retirement, Health and Relationships of the Older Population in England: The 2004 English Longitudinal Study of Ageing (Wave 2)*; Banks, J., Breeze, E., Lessof, C., Nazroo, J., Eds.; Patersons: Tunbridge Wells, UK, 2006; pp. 217–242, ISBN 9781903274460.
59. Teófilo-Rodríguez, J.; González-Cabezas, A.N.; Díaz-Veiga, P.; Rodríguez-Rodríguez, V. *Estudio Longitudinal Envejecer en España: El proyecto ELES*; Instituto de Mayores y Servicios Sociales (España): Madrid, Spain, 2011.
60. Meyers, J.E.; Meyers, R.K. *RCFT. Test de la Figura Compleja de Rey y Prueba de Reconocimiento*; TEA Ediciones: Madrid, Spain, 2009.
61. Lezak, M.D. *Neuropsychological Assessment*, 3rd ed; Oxford University Press: Nueva York, NY, USA, 1995.
62. Reitan, R.M.; Wolfson, D. *The Halstead-Reitan Neuropsychological Test Battery. En The Neuropsychology Handbook: Behavioral and Clinical Perspectives*; Wedding, D., Horton, J., MacNeill, A., Webster, J., Eds.; Springer: Nueva York, NY, USA, 1986; pp. 134–160, ISBN 9780826146502.
63. R Core Team. *R: A Language and Environment for Statistical Computing*; R Foundation for Statistical Computing: Vienna, Austria, 2018; Available online: https://www.R-project.org/ (accessed on 31 October 2024).
64. Bouhaben, J.; Delgado-Lima, A.H.; Delgado-Losada, M.L. The Role of Olfactory Dysfunction in Mild Cognitive Impairment and Alzheimer's Disease: A Meta-Analysis. *Arch. Gerontol. Geriatr.* **2024**, *123*, 105425. [CrossRef]
65. Doty, R.L.; McKeown, D.A.; Lee, W.W.; Shaman, P. A Study of the Test-Retest Reliability of Ten Olfactory Tests. *Chem. Senses* **1995**, *20*, 645–656. [CrossRef]
66. Doty, R.L.; Kamath, V. The Influences of Age on Olfaction: A Review. *Front. Psychol.* **2014**, *5*, 20. [CrossRef]
67. Rahayel, S.; Frasnelli, J.; Joubert, S. The Effect of Alzheimer's Disease and Parkinson's Disease on Olfaction: A Meta-Analysis. *Behav. Brain Res.* **2012**, *231*, 60–74. [CrossRef]
68. Knight, J.E.; Yoneda, T.; Lewis, N.A.; Muniz-Terrera, G.; Bennett, D.A.; Piccinin, A.M. Transitions between Mild Cognitive Impairment, Dementia, and Mortality: The Importance of Olfaction. *J. Gerontol. A Biol. Sci. Med. Sci.* **2023**, *78*, 1284–1291. [CrossRef]
69. Li, J.; Jiang, Z.; Duan, S.; Zhu, X. Multiple Early Biomarkers to Predict Cognitive Decline in Dementia-Free Older Adults. *J. Geriatr. Psychiatry Neurol.* **2024**, *37*, 395–402. [CrossRef] [PubMed]
70. Papadatos, Z.; Phillips, N.A. Olfactory Function Reflects Episodic Memory Performance and Atrophy in the Medial Temporal Lobe in Individuals at Risk for Alzheimer's Disease. *Neurobiol. Aging* **2023**, *128*, 33–42. [CrossRef] [PubMed]
71. Park, S.-J.; Lee, J.-E.; Lee, K.-S.; Kim, J.-S. Comparison of Odor Identification among Amnestic and Non-Amnestic Mild Cognitive Impairment, Subjective Cognitive Decline, and Early Alzheimer's Dementia. *Neurol. Sci.* **2018**, *39*, 557–564. [CrossRef] [PubMed]
72. Tahmasebi, R.; Zehetmayer, S.; Pusswald, G.; Kovacs, G.; Stögmann, E.; Lehrner, J. Identification of Odors, Faces, Cities and Naming of Objects in Patients with Subjective Cognitive Decline, Mild Cognitive Impairment and Alzheimer´s Disease: A Longitudinal Study. *Int. Psychogeriatr.* **2019**, *31*, 537–549. [CrossRef] [PubMed]
73. Wheeler, P.L.; Murphy, C. Olfactory Measures as Predictors of Conversion to Mild Cognitive Impairment and Alzheimer's Disease. *Brain Sci.* **2021**, *11*, 1391. [CrossRef]
74. Sohrabi, H.R.; Bates, K.A.; Rodrigues, M.; Taddei, K.; Laws, S.M.; Lautenschlager, N.T.; Dhaliwal, S.S.; Johnston, A.N.B.; Mackay-Sim, A.; Gandy, S.; et al. Olfactory Dysfunction Is Associated with Subjective Memory Complaints in Community-Dwelling Elderly Individuals. *J. Alzheimer's Dis.* **2009**, *17*, 135–142. [CrossRef]
75. Olofsson, J.K.; Ekström, I.; Larsson, M.; Nordin, S. Olfaction and Aging: A Review of the Current State of Research and Future Directions. *Iperception* **2021**, *12*, 20416695211020331. [CrossRef]
76. Ribeiro, J.C.; Simões, J.; Silva, F.; Silva, E.D.; Hummel, C.; Hummel, T.; Paiva, A. Cultural Adaptation of the Portuguese Version of the «Sniffin' Sticks» Smell Test: Reliability, Validity, and Normative Data. *PLoS ONE* **2016**, *11*, e0148937. [CrossRef]

77. Dulay, M.F.; Murphy, C. Olfactory Acuity and Cognitive Function Converge in Older Adulthood: Support for the Common Cause Hypothesis. *Psychol. Aging* **2002**, *17*, 392–404. [CrossRef]
78. Conti, M.Z.; Vicini-Chilovi, B.; Riva, M.; Zanetti, M.; Liberini, P.; Padovani, A.; Rozzini, L. Odor Identification Deficit Predicts Clinical Conversion from Mild Cognitive Impairment to Dementia Due to Alzheimer's Disease. *Arch. Clin. Neuropsychol.* **2013**, *28*, 391–399. [CrossRef]
79. Devanand, D.P.; Liu, X.; Tabert, M.H.; Pradhaban, G.; Cuasay, K.; Bell, K.; de Leon, M.J.; Doty, R.L.; Stern, Y.; Pelton, G.H. Combining Early Markers Strongly Predicts Conversion from Mild Cognitive Impairment to Alzheimer's Disease. *Biol. Psychiatry* **2008**, *64*, 871–879. [CrossRef] [PubMed]
80. Dulay, M.F.; Gesteland, R.C.; Shear, P.K.; Ritchey, P.N.; Frank, R.A. Assessment of the Influence of Cognition and Cognitive Processing Speed on Three Tests of Olfaction. *J. Clin. Exp. Neuropsychol.* **2008**, *30*, 327–337. [CrossRef] [PubMed]
81. Seubert, J.; Laukka, E.J.; Rizzuto, D.; Hummel, T.; Fratiglioni, L.; Bäckman, L.; Larsson, M. Prevalence and Correlates of Olfactory Dysfunction in Old Age: A Population-Based Study. *J. Gerontol. A Biol. Sci. Med. Sci.* **2017**, *72*, 1072–1079. [CrossRef] [PubMed]
82. Deary, I.J.; Corley, J.; Gow, A.J.; Harris, S.E.; Houlihan, L.M.; Marioni, R.E.; Penke, L.; Rafnsson, S.B.; Starr, J.M. Age-Associated Cognitive Decline. *Br. Med. Bull.* **2009**, *92*, 135–152. [CrossRef] [PubMed]
83. Hedner, M.; Larsson, M.; Arnold, N.; Zucco, G.M.; Hummel, T. Cognitive Factors in Odor Detection, Odor Discrimination, and Odor Identification Tasks. *J. Clin. Exp. Neuropsychol.* **2010**, *32*, 1062–1067. [CrossRef]
84. Melero, H.; Borromeo, S.; Cristobal-Huerta, A.; Manzanedo, E.; Luna, G.; Toledano, A.; Hernández-Tamames, J.A. Sex Differences in the Olfactory System: A Functional MRI Study. *Chemosens. Percept.* **2019**, *12*, 50–58. [CrossRef]
85. Sorokowska, A.; Schriever, V.A.; Gudziol, V.; Hummel, C.; Hähner, A.; Iannilli, E.; Sinding, C.; Aziz, M.; Seo, H.S.; Negoias, S.; et al. Changes of Olfactory Abilities in Relation to Age: Odor Identification in More than 1400 People Aged 4 to 80 Years. *Eur. Arch. Otorhinolaryngol.* **2015**, *272*, 1937–1944. [CrossRef]
86. Chasles, M.-J.; Tremblay, A.; Escudier, F.; Lajeunesse, A.; Benoit, S.; Langlois, R.; Joubert, S.; Rouleau, I. An Examination of Semantic Impairment in Amnestic MCI and AD: What Can We Learn from Verbal Fluency? *Arch. Clin. Neuropsychol.* **2019**, *35*, 22–30. [CrossRef]
87. Delage, E.; Rouleau, I.; Akzam-Ouellette, M.-A.; Roy-Côté, F.; Joubert, S.; CIMA-Q. An Examination of Semantic Performance in Mild Cognitive Impairment Progressors and Nonprogressors. *Neuropsychology* **2024**, *38*, 309–321. [CrossRef]
88. Jobin, B.; Roy-Côté, F.; Frasnelli, J.; Boller, B. Olfaction and Declarative Memory in Aging: A Meta-Analysis. *Chem. Senses* **2023**, *48*, bjad045. [CrossRef]
89. Olofsson, J.K.; Josefsson, M.; Ekström, I.; Wilson, D.; Nyberg, L.; Nordin, S.; Nordin Adolfsson, A.; Adolfsson, R.; Nilsson, L.-G.; Larsson, M. Long-Term Episodic Memory Decline Is Associated with Olfactory Deficits Only in Carriers of ApoE-∈4. *Neuropsychologia* **2016**, *85*, 1–9. [CrossRef] [PubMed]
90. Swan, G.E.; Carmelli, D. Impaired Olfaction Predicts Cognitive Decline in Nondemented Older Adults. *Neuroepidemiology* **2002**, *21*, 58–67. [CrossRef] [PubMed]
91. Schipolowski, S.; Wilhelm, O.; Schroeders, U. On the nature of crystallized intelligence: The relationship between verbal ability and factual knowledge. *Intelligence* **2014**, *46*, 156–168. [CrossRef]
92. Han, P.; Croy, I.; Raue, C.; Bensafi, M.; Larsson, M.; Cavazzana, A.; Hummel, T. Neural Processing of Odor-Associated Words: An fMRI Study in Patients with Acquired Olfactory Loss. *Brain Imaging Behav.* **2020**, *14*, 1164–1174. [CrossRef]
93. Bahar-Fuchs, A.; Moss, S.; Rowe, C.; Savage, G. Can I Smell Gas (or Is It Lilac)? Olfactory Semantic Deficits in Mild Cognitive Impairment and Alzheimer's Disease. *Chemosens. Percept.* **2010**, *3*, 118–128. [CrossRef]
94. Dhilla Albers, A.; Asafu-Adjei, J.; Delaney, M.K.; Kelly, K.E.; Gomez-Isla, T.; Blacker, D.; Johnson, K.A.; Sperling, R.A.; Hyman, B.T.; Betensky, R.A.; et al. Episodic Memory of Odors Stratifies Alzheimer Biomarkers in Normal Elderly. *Ann. Neurol.* **2016**, *80*, 846–857. [CrossRef]
95. Frank, C.; Albertazzi, A.; Murphy, C. The Effect of the Apolipoprotein E E4 Allele and Olfactory Function on Odor Identification Networks. *Brain Behav.* **2024**, *14*, e3524. [CrossRef]
96. Ramirez-Gomez, L.; Albers, M.W.; Baena, A.; Vila-Castelar, C.; Fox-Fuller, J.T.; Sanchez, J.; Jain, F.; Albers, A.D.; Lopera, F.; Quiroz, Y.T. Olfactory Function and Markers of Brain Pathology in Non-Demented Individuals with Autosomal Dominant Alzheimer's Disease. *J. Alzheimer's Dis.* **2022**, *88*, 721–729. [CrossRef]
97. Tabert, M.H.; Liu, X.; Doty, R.L.; Serby, M.; Zamora, D.; Pelton, G.H.; Marder, K.; Albers, M.W.; Stern, Y.; Devanand, D.P. A 10-Item Smell Identification Scale Related to Risk for Alzheimer's Disease. *Ann. Neurol.* **2005**, *58*, 155–160. [CrossRef]
98. Kirova, A.-M.; Bays, R.B.; Lagalwar, S. Working Memory and Executive Function Decline across Normal Aging, Mild Cognitive Impairment, and Alzheimer's Disease. *Biomed. Res. Int.* **2015**, *2015*, 748212. [CrossRef]
99. Challakere, V.M.; Schofield, P.W. Olfaction and Executive Cognitive Performance: A Systematic Review. *Front. Psychol.* **2022**, *13*, 871391. [CrossRef] [PubMed]
100. Uchida, S.; Shimada, C.; Sakuma, N.; Kagitani, F.; Kan, A.; Awata, S. The Relationship between Olfaction and Cognitive Function in the Elderly. *J. Physiol. Sci.* **2020**, *70*, 48. [CrossRef] [PubMed]

101. Fornazieri, M.A.; Doty, R.L.; Bezerra, T.F.P.; de Rezende Pinna, F.; Costa, F.O.; Voegels, R.L.; Silveira-Moriyama, L. Relationship of Socioeconomic Status to Olfactory Function. *Physiol. Behav.* **2019**, *198*, 84–89. [CrossRef] [PubMed]
102. James, J.; Tsvik, A.M.; Chung, S.Y.; Usseglio, J.; Gudis, D.A.; Overdevest, J.B. Association between Social Determinants of Health and Olfactory Function: A Scoping Review. *Int. Forum Allergy Rhinol.* **2021**, *11*, 1472–1493. [CrossRef]

European Journal of
Investigation in Health, Psychology and Education

MDPI

Article

Sexual Well-Being and Aging Patterns: Findings of a Cluster Analysis among Older Adults in Portugal and Spain

Sofia von Humboldt [1,*], Emilia Cabras [2], Gail Low [3] and Isabel Leal [1]

1 William James Center for Research, ISPA–Instituto Universitário, Rua Jardim do Tabaco, 34, 1149-041 Lisbon, Portugal; ileal@ispa.pt
2 Department of Education, Universidad Alfonso X EI Sabio, 28691 Madrid, Spain; ecabras@hotmail.it
3 Faculty of Nursing, University of Alberta, Edmonton, AB T6G 1C9, Canada; gaill@ualberta.ca
* Correspondence: sofia.humboldt@gmail.com; Tel.: +351-218811700; Fax: +351-218860954

Abstract: Objectives: From a cross-cultural perspective, aging well may encompass pertinent challenges in terms of adjustment, sexual well-being, and satisfaction with life in the late years. Considering the paucity of empirical data concerning cultural diversity of experiencing aging, this study aims to help fill this gap by assessing the specific patterns of sexual satisfaction, adjustment to aging (AtA), and life satisfaction with life (SwL) of older adults in Portugal and Spain. Methods: This cross-national study included 326 older adults, age 65 and older, from Portugal and Spain. Five instruments were applied: (a) Adjustment to Aging Scale (ATAS); (b) Satisfaction with Life Scale (SwLS); (c) New Sexual Satisfaction Scale-Short (NSSS-S); (d) Mini-Mental State Exam; and (e) Sociodemographic, Health and Lifestyle questionnaire. K-means cluster analysis was employed to identify and characterize the clusters considering adjustments to aging, sexual satisfaction, and life satisfaction. One-way ANOVAs were conducted to analyze differences in sexual well-being among clusters. Results: Findings indicated three clusters, which explained 77.7% ($R\text{-}sq = 0.777$) of the total variance: Cluster 1: "Most skilled" ($n = 26$, 8.0%), Cluster 2: "Least adjusted" ($n = 115$, 35.3%), and Cluster 3: "Aging strivers" ($n = 185$, 56.7%). Participants in Cluster 1 were mostly Portuguese, with high levels of AtA, sexual satisfaction, and SWL. Conversely, Cluster 2 included mostly Portuguese participants with moderate sexual satisfaction and lower levels of AtA and SwL. Participants from Cluster 3 were mostly Spanish, with moderate levels of AtA and reduced sexual satisfaction and SwL. Conclusions: This study innovates by exploring the elaborate interplay among sexual satisfaction, AtA, and SwL in a cross-cultural perspective, with implications for tailoring interventions, service planning, development, and evaluation of culturally diverse older populations.

Keywords: adjustment to aging; cluster analysis; older adults; satisfaction with life; sexual satisfaction

1. Introduction

Countries worldwide are facing significant challenges in adapting their health and social systems to accommodate the aging of the population [1]. Portugal ranks as the third-oldest country among the 27 European Union (EU), while Spain holds the eighth position [2]. In 2021, Portugal (22.4%) and Spain (19.8%) stood out as countries with the highest proportions of people aged 65 or older in their populations [3].

The aging of the population has implied the need for a comprehensive understanding of aging, considering the complex interconnection of variables, such as adjustment to aging (AtA), sexual well-being, and overall satisfaction with life (SwL). Moreover, an inclusive approach underlines the importance of understanding the multifaceted dynamics of aging [4–7].

Old age is frequently associated with dependence, apathy, illness, and diminished sexual allure [8]. An increasing body of literature often promotes a youthful image, rather than one of aging, to emphasize sexual attractiveness. Additionally, the media frequently show ideals for beauty and sexual attractiveness by portraying young and wrinkle-free bodies [8,9]. A youthful appearance is closely tied to increased sexual desire interest and attractiveness, with diverse effects on sexual satisfaction [8,9]. Indeed, older adults frequently face ageist stereotyping of both their sexuality and their aging bodies [7,8]. Moreover, in some cultures, sexual activity is seen as energy-intensive and unnecessary for maintaining health and well-being. Indeed, some cultural standards tend to view older individuals as devoid of sexuality, emotions, and sensations [9]. Conversely, recent decades have witnessed shifting attitudes regarding sexual engagement in older life. The majority of older individuals remain sexually active, and sexual interactions and emotional intimacy significantly seem to contribute to their overall well-being [10].

Sexual well-being has been indicated as the emotional, physical, and cognitive assessment of an individual's sexual life, including relationship quality, sexual satisfaction, activity, attraction, pleasure, intimate relationships, self-esteem, and other psychosexual factors [10,11], and it is an important component of overall well-being [9,12]. The term *sexual satisfaction* refers to the appraisal of one's sexual life, both physically and non-physically [13].

A significant proportion of older individuals view sexual satisfaction as pivotal to a satisfying relationship and overall SwL [13]. Recent research has expanded the knowledge, revealing a connection between positive well-being and sexual satisfaction in older adulthood [14]. Moreover, literature has indicated associations between regular sexual activity and reduced relationship tension [15], as well as positive correlations between the frequency and significance of sexual experiences and sexual satisfaction for both partnered and single older adults [16,17]. Additionally, emotional intimacy, personal communication, and relationship happiness are all positively correlated with higher levels of sexual satisfaction [11].

Research about sexual satisfaction in the Spanish [18] and Portuguese [19] older populations is scarce. Almost 50% of the Spanish older adults reported being sexually activity, but sexual activity decreased with age [20]. This highlights that a significant portion of the older population still values and engages in sexual activity, emphasizing its importance despite age-related declines. Moreover, older Portuguese individuals display an interest in sexuality, and in one study, one-third of the participants expressed a need to express their sexuality [19]. Additionally, 16.6% of older participants believe they should engage in more sexual experiences, reflecting favorable attitudes toward sexuality in old age [19], indicating that many still see it as an important part of life.

In a different study, Portuguese older adults primarily associated their sexual well-being with self-reported good health and demonstrations of love. However, the unavailability of a partner emerged as the most prevalent theme (17.9%) contributing to their sexual dissatisfaction [21], suggesting that while health and emotional connection are crucial, social factors like partner availability significantly impact sexual well-being.

Among older Spanish adults, the primary reasons for low sexual well-being were the death of a spouse (31%), loss of sexual desire (29%), and health considerations (17%) [20]. For Spanish people, health status is essential apart from age, so older people who reported good health and vitality were more likely to be sexually active [20] and showed better sexual satisfaction [22]. This finding reinforces the idea that maintaining good health is vital for continued sexual activity and satisfaction in older age.

Despite recognizing the importance of sexual satisfaction and physical intimacy for older adults' well-being, the role of sexuality in aging well has been largely overlooked [23].

Moreover, cultural norms and gender expectations also shape the sexual experiences of older individuals. For example, in Nordic cultures, sexual interactions between men and women are negotiated with relatively more equality compared to Southern cultures. Despite this, women historically occupied subordinate roles to men in these societies. The contemporary emphasis on gender equality may have empowered women to feel more in control of their sexuality, potentially leading to a shift in traditional gender dynamics where men may feel disempowered and insecure about their roles [24]. The extent to which older individuals feel comfortable expressing their sexuality and advocating for resources promoting sexual health depends on the prevailing culture and its associated gender roles, health accessibility, and affordability [24].

As people get older, SwL becomes increasingly more important [25]. Satisfaction with life may be characterized as people's opinions about the worth or goodness of their lives, their overall level of happiness, or occasionally how satisfied they are with their lives in general. Other terms for this description include subjective well-being and happiness with life [26]. Literature also highlighted the link between sexual satisfaction and SwL in both older men and women. Across age groups, SwL is closely intertwined with contentment in one's sex life and forms an integral aspect of SwL for older adults. Additionally, enhancing sexual satisfaction might indeed have a positive influence on the process of aging well [27].

Aging is an enduring process that requires continuous adjustment [7]. von Humboldt et al. considered AtA to be a critical aspect of the well-being of older adults [28]. Furthermore, consistent evidence indicates that older adults develop active and purposeful strategies for AtA, by including psychological factors, interactions with significant others, sexual intimacy, and social comparisons [7,29–31]. AtA is a dynamic process that involves the alignment of personality, social environment, and well-being, with implications for aging well [28]. Moreover, AtA, well-being and health of older individuals are affected by love, intimacy, and sexual satisfaction [7,27,32]. Considering health as the pursuit of maximum individual functionality, AtA is relevant for a health-focused approach to aging well [30].

Aging is a multifaceted process influenced by cultural, ethnic, and gender differences. Variations in the perception of well-being, satisfaction, adjustment, and sexuality between different cultures and genders are substantial [33,34]. Modern societal views of old age now acknowledge the possibility of older individuals experiencing joy, satisfaction, adjustment, vitality, and health while engaging in sexual activity; however, age-related differences in love and sexuality may be influenced by culture [33]. Despite the connection between AtA, SwL, and sexual satisfaction, there is a noticeable lack of comprehensive cross-cultural studies about the intricate relationships among these constructs [34,35].

Additionally, while there have been studies on sexual activity, there has been a lack of cross-cultural comparisons of older individuals in different countries utilizing consistent measurements, sociodemographic variables, and data collection techniques.

This study aims to address these gaps by using a cluster analysis approach to examine specific patterns of sexual satisfaction, AtA, and SwL among older adults in Portugal and Spain.

2. Materials and Methods

2.1. Participants

Our sample included 326 older people ($M = 70.59$; $SD = 5.24$). Among them, 54.3% were Portuguese and 45.7% were Spanish. The age of participants varied between 65 and 92 years old; 51.5% were female. Our sample is well educated, with 50% having a bachelor's/master's/doctoral degree, 12.3% having completed secondary school, and 37.7% of the individuals having only completed elementary school. Furthermore, a substantial 78.8% of participants reported good health. Less than 10% of participants disclosed recent psychological concerns, with a predominant focus on issues related to anxiety and depression. Including these demographic characteristics is essential for identifying distinct clusters and patterns in sexual satisfaction, AtA, and SwL among older adults and for providing a comprehensive understanding of the factors influencing the aging process. Table 1 lists the sociodemographic details of the participants.

Participants were recruited from senior universities, message boards, emails, community center lists, and network contacts. Different recruitment sources contributed to the sample diversification, with senior universities targeting lifelong learners, message boards and emails reaching a broader audience, and network contacts accessing existing social networks, ensuring a varied pool of participants. The eligibility criteria encompassed the following requirements: (a) Participants were required to be a minimum of 65 years old, (b) possess a clear understanding of their voluntary participation in the study, and (c) have no prior history of cognitive impairments, psychiatric or neurological disorders, substance abuse, or similar conditions. Additionally, participants were expected to possess proficiency in utilizing contemporary technologies, such as smartphones, tablets, computers, and apps. For queries or assistance, participants were encouraged to seek support either through phone or online channels. Participants were screened to ensure their eligibility based on their capacity for decision-making and cognitive abilities.

Table 1. Sociodemographic and health characteristics of the participants.

Characteristics	Portuguese 177 (54.3%)	Spanish 149 (45.7%)	Total (%) 326 (100%)
Age, Average ± SD			M = 70.59 ± 5.24
Gender, *n* (%)			
Female	88 (49.7%)	80 (53.7%)	168 (51.5%)
Male	89 (50.3%)	69 (46.3%)	158 (48.5%)
Educational level, *n* (%)			
<Secondary	118 (66.7%)	5 (3.4%)	123 (37.7%)
Secondary	19 (10.7%)	21 (14.1%)	40 (12.3%)
>Secondary	40 (22.6%)	123 (82.5%)	163 (50.0%)
Marital status, *n* (%)			
Single	15 (8.5%)	8 (5.4%)	23 (7.1%)
Married/de facto union	95 (53.7%)	110 (73.8%)	205 (62.9%)
Divorced/separated	20 (11.3%)	16 (10.7%)	36 (11.0%)
Widow	47 (26.6%)	15 (10.1%)	62 (19.0%)
Household, *n* (%)			
Living with someone	125 (70.6%)	133 (89.3%)	258 (79.1%)
Living alone	52 (23.4%)	16 (10.7%)	68 (20.9%)
Family Annual Income, *n* (%)			
≤25,000 €	119 (67.2%)	41 (27.5%)	160 (49.1%)
>25,000 €	58 (32.8%)	108 (72.5%)	166 (50.9%)
Perceived health, *n* (%)			
Good	132 (74.6%)	133 (89.3%)	265 (81.3%)
Poor	45 (25.4%)	16 (10.7%)	61 (18.7%)

2.2. *Instruments*

2.2.1. Adjustment to Aging Scale (AtAS)

The Adjustment to Aging Scale (AtAS) comprised five different subscales, and the internal reliability of the scale and its five subscales proved to be strong: sense of purpose and ambitions (0.874); zest and spirituality (0.927); body and health (0.904); aging in place and stability (0.862); and social support (0.932). Cronbach's alpha coefficient indicated an internal consistency of 0.891 for the overall scale. Respondents used a 7-point Likert-type scale, ranging from 1, which indicates "Not at all important", to 7, which indicates "Very important". This measure proved good psychometric properties, and the low cross-national invariance of this measure highlights its cross-cultural character [28], further underscoring its suitability for cross-cultural assessments, aligning with our study's aim to explore AtA across different cultural contexts.

2.2.2. New Sexual Satisfaction Scale-Short (NSSS-S)

The 12-item New Sexual Satisfaction Scale-Short (NSSS-S) has a two-dimensional factor structure, assessing self-centrality and partner and sexual activity centrality. It may be utilized with individuals from both genders and has recently been verified in Spanish and Portuguese samples [36,37]. The NSSS-S is composed of five 5-point ordinal items, with higher scores on the scale indicating higher levels of sexual satisfaction. The NSSS-S shows strong psychometric qualities in terms of validity and reliability. Furthermore, internal consistency was evidenced by Cronbach's alpha of 0.94, which assured confidence in its ability to provide robust measurements of sexual satisfaction among older adults, enhancing the reliability of our study's findings.

2.2.3. Satisfaction with Life Scale (SwLS)

The Satisfaction with Life Scale (SwLS), developed by Larsen et al. [38], was designed as a quick assessment of a person's overall level of satisfaction with life. The SwLS has only five items but has been shown to be a useful instrument for assessing the mental population and to have high psychometric qualities [39]. The SwLS has been used in several cross-cultural studies investigating life satisfaction and SWB in general. In addition to its demonstrated validity and reliability of the life satisfaction component, the SwLS scale's strong internal consistency (r = 0.78) [39,40] further supports its suitability for assessing overall life satisfaction among older adults, reinforcing the robustness of our measurement approach.

2.2.4. Sociodemographic, Health and Lifestyle Questionnaire

Key sociodemographic, health, and lifestyle details of the participants were analyzed. It included information on age, gender, education level, income, employment, and marital status, among others. The health and lifestyle component of the questionnaire included the participant's current state of health, medication lifestyle decisions, and access to medical treatment.

2.3. *Procedure*

The objectives of the study were explained to the participants. Every participant was made aware that their participation was entirely free and that they might quit at any time. Confidentiality and anonymity of the data were guaranteed. Data collection took place from 1 October to 30 December 2022. No compensation was given to respondents for completing the questionnaires. The ISPA-Instituto Universitário and the Research Ethics Committee of the William James Center for Research gave their approval to all procedures. The ethical principles outlined in the Helsinki Declaration and the Code of Ethics of the Portuguese Psychologists were followed in this study. In addition, other precautions to handle sensitive issues included ensuring anonymity and confidentiality, providing informed consent, and offering support resources for participants who may experience discomfort or distress during the study. We also employed measures to ensure the participants' ease and privacy, such as offering the option to withdraw from the study at any time, without consequences, and providing clear communication about the nature and purpose of the research.

2.4. *Data Analysis*

The 326 respondents were divided into different groups using cluster analysis based on their scores in various measures, which included AtA (sense of purpose and ambitions, zest and spirituality, body and health, aging in place and stability, and social support), sexual satisfaction (ego-centered and partner/sexual activity centered), and SwL. The sample size was determined based on a power analysis to ensure sufficient statistical power to detect expected effect sizes in our analyses. With an error probability of 0.05, the power analysis indicated that a total sample size of 326 showed a power of 0.95, for an effect size of 0.50. The final sample size is lower than the initially proposed sample size of 400 participants, which corresponded to an approximately 20% expected attrition rate due to participants that did not match eligibility criteria or decided to withdraw from the study.

We aimed to identify distinct groups based on specific measures, and for this purpose, we used hierarchical cluster analysis with the Ward technique, which, in turn, used squared Euclidean distance as a measure of subject difference. This approach was favored over other possible methods due to its ability to handle large datasets and its capability to produce well-separated and interpretable clusters; hence, it is suitable for providing a comprehensive understanding of the underlying patterns within the data.

The R^2 evaluation, as indicated by Marôco [41], was utilized to establish the correct number of clusters. The analysis identified three homogenous clusters, accounting for around 77.7% of the total variance. The classification of each subject within these clusters was then further refined using the non-hierarchical *k-Means* approach.

Following the methodology outlined in Marôco [41], the significance of each variable in each of the three clusters was assessed using the *F* statistics of the clusters ANOVA. Chi-square analysis was used to investigate how people in each of the three clusters differed in terms of sociodemographic, health, and lifestyle variables.

Additionally, mean differences between cluster groups were evaluated using Analysis of Variance (ANOVA) and Tukey HSD tests, with sexual well-being indicators as the dependent variables. Statistical significance was determined to be $p < 0.05$ for all analyses. To describe the sample, descriptive statistics were utilized. All analyses were made with IBM SPSS Statistics for Windows, version 29.

3. Results

This study aimed to examine specific patterns of sexual satisfaction, AtA, and SwL among older adults in Portugal and Spain.

Using R^2 criterion, findings indicated the retention of three clusters, which together accounted for 77.7% (*R-sq* = 0.777) of the total variance. This R^2 criterion indicates that approximately 77.7% of the variance of the dependent variable is explained by the independent variables in the model; that is, this model provides a robust explanation for the patterns observed in the data. The dendrogram representing the hierarchical relationships shows the three clusters (see Figure 1).

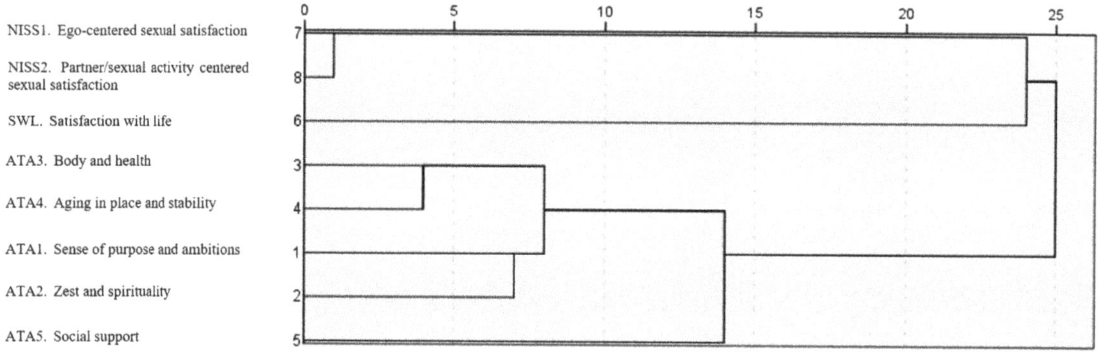

Figure 1. Dendrogram: Hierarchical clustering with single linkage.

The centers of the clusters and the *F* statistics for each variable are presented in Table 2. The *F*-statistic determines whether the model as a whole is statistically significant, indicating that the observed relationships are unlikely to be random. Among the dimensions analyzed, those that most differentiate the clusters are related to AtA. Specifically, "body and health" (*F* = 309.887) has the highest differentiating effect, followed by "aging in place and stability" (*F* = 262.061), "social support" (*F* = 196.478), "zest and spirituality" (*F* = 192.719) and "sense of purpose and ambitions" (*F* = 161.274). Both ego-centered sexual satisfaction (*F* = 149.102) and partner/sexual activity-centered sexual satisfaction (*F* = 148.255) also contribute to differentiating the clusters. On the other hand, satisfaction with life (*F* = 81.302) is the dimension that least differentiates the clusters.

This study aimed to identify clusters that were characterized by varying levels of AtA, sexual satisfaction, and SwL, which supported our hypothesis regarding the intricate relationships among these constructs in the context of aging.

Table 2. Clusters centers, frequencies, and F statistics for each variable.

	Cluster 1 (n = 26)	Cluster 2 (n = 115)	Cluster 3 (n = 185)	F
1. Sense of purpose and ambitions	2.058	0.300	0.475	161.274 ***
2. Zest and spirituality	2.269	0.213	0.451	192.719 ***
3. Body and health	2.642	0.067	0.413	309.887 ***
4. Aging in place and stability	2.585	0.031	0.383	262.061 ***
5. Social support	2.006	0.414	0.539	196.478 ***
6. Ego-centered sexual satisfaction	1.053	0.726	0.599	149.102 ***
7. Partner/sexual activity-centered sexual satisfaction	0.967	0.748	0.601	148.255 ***
8. Satisfaction with life	1.239	0.484	0.475	81.302 ***

*** $p < 0.001$.

The three distinct clusters were retained based on participants' scores in various dimensions. The first cluster (Cluster 1: "most skilled"; high AtA/high sexual satisfaction/high SwL) included 26 participants who exhibited relatively high levels of AtA, sexual satisfaction, and SwL. The second cluster (Cluster 2: "least adjusted"; low AtA/moderate sexual satisfaction/low SwL) comprised 115 participants with low levels of AtA and SwL and moderate sexual satisfaction. Finally, the third cluster (Cluster 3: "aging strivers"; moderate AtA/low sexual satisfaction/low SwL) included 185 participants with moderate levels of AtA and low levels of sexual satisfaction and SwL.

The results indicate that the three clusters showed specific sociodemographic features, which support our hypothesis regarding the variations in sociodemographic, health, and lifestyle factors among the participants in each of the three clusters.

In this context, chi-square tests (χ^2) were performed to examine the variations in sociodemographic, health, and lifestyle traits among the participants in each of the three clusters (see Table 3).

The results of the study revealed significant differences among the three clusters in terms of nationality [χ^2 (2) = 17.572, $p < 0.001$]. Cluster 1 ("most skilled") included mostly Portuguese participants, while Cluster 3 ("aging strivers") included mostly Spanish people. In terms of sex [χ^2 (2) = 3.273, $p = 0.195$], Cluster 1 exhibits a greater prevalence of women, whereas Cluster 3 shows a higher incidence of men.

Furthermore, there were significant differences in terms of education [χ^2 (12) = 45.111, $p < 0.001$]. Interestingly, participants with lower educational levels were mostly in Cluster 1 ("most skilled"). In contrast, participants with higher levels of education were mainly in Cluster 2 ("least adjusted") and Cluster 3 ("aging strivers"). This result may indicate that factors beyond education contribute significantly to the highest levels of AtA, SwL, and sexual satisfaction, prompting further investigation to understand the additional influences that may be affecting these aspects of well-being. Significant differences were also found in marital status [χ^2 (6) = 45.225, $p < 0.001$]. Cluster 1 ("most skilled") showed more married participants than the other clusters.

In addition, being a spiritual person [χ^2 (2) = 2.646, $p = 0.266$] appeared to be associated with a high level of AtA, sexual satisfaction, and satisfaction with life in Cluster 1 ("most skilled"). Participants in Cluster 2 ("least adjusted") were more likely to report perceived poor general health [χ^2 (2) = 29.556, $p < 0.001$].

Additionally, having a positive love experience in life [χ^2 (2) = 43.461, $p < 0.001$] and engaging in leisure activities [χ^2 (2) = 4.332, $p = 0.115$] were mostly shown by participants in Cluster 1 ("most skilled").

Last, results indicated that the three clusters showed specific sexual well-being features, which support our hypothesis regarding the variations in sexuality-related items among the participants in each of the three clusters.

Table 3. Three cluster solutions according to sociodemographic and lifestyle characteristics.

	N	*Cluster 1* *High AtA/High SS/High SwL* *n = 26 (%)*	*Cluster 2* *Low AtA/Moderate SS/Low SwL* *n = 115 (%)*	*Cluster 3* *Moderate AtA/Low SS/Low SwL* *n = 185 (%)*	χ^2	*df*	*sig.*
Nationality							
Portuguese	177	24 (92.3%)	63 (54.8%)	90 (48.6%)	17.572	2	<0.001
Spanish	149	2 (7.7%)	52 (45.2%)	95 (51.4%)			
Biological sex							
Female	168	13 (50.0%)	67 (58.3%)	88 (47.6%)	3.273	2	0.195
Male	158	13 (50.0%)	48 (41.7%)	97 (52.4%)			
Educational level							
<Secondary	123	23 (88.5%)	47 (40.9%)	53 (28.6%)	45.111	12	<0.001
Secondary	40	0 (0.0%)	13 (11.3%)	27 (14.6%)			
>Secondary	163	3 (11.5%)	55 (47.8%)	105 (56.8%)			
Marital status							
Single	23	4 (15.4%)	8 (7.0%)	11 (5.9%)	45.225	6	<0.001
Married/de facto union	205	17 (65.4%)	69 (60.0%)	119 (64.3%)			
Divorced/separated	36	2 (7.7%)	16 (13.9%)	18 (9.7%)			
Widow	62	3 (11.5%)	22 (19.1%)	37 (20.0%)			
Spiritual person							
Yes	212	19 (73.1%)	69 (60.0%)	124 (67.0%)	2.646	2	0.266
No	114	7 (26.9%)	46 (40.0%)	61 (33.0%)			
Perceived general health							
Good	265	20 (76.9%)	80 (69.6%)	164 (88.6%)	29.556	2	<0.001
Poor	61	6 (23.1%)	35 (30.4%)	21 (11.4%)			
Love experience in life							
Good	234	21 (80.8%)	64 (55.7%)	134 (72.4%)	43.461	2	<0.001
Bad	92	5 (19.2%)	51 (44.3%)	51 (27.5%)			
Leisure activity							
Yes	161	20 (76.9%)	51 (44.3%)	90 (48.6%)	4.332	2	0.115
No	165	6 (23.1%)	64 (55.7%)	95 (51.4%)			

The findings of group differences are summarized in Table 4. Cluster membership was associated with significant variations in participants' perceived overall sexual well-being [$F_{(2174)} = 16.987$, $p < 0.001$], sexual attractiveness [$F_{(2,322)} = 23.694$, $p < 0.001$], sexual openness and communication [$F_{(2,323)} = 93.160$, $p < 0.001$], and sexual satisfaction [$F_{(2,323)} = 93.233$, $p < 0.001$]. The distinct clusters identified in our study, distinguished by sociodemographic, health, and lifestyle traits and sexual well-being variables among participants, contribute to our research aims concerning the multifaceted influences on aging experiences.

Post hoc multiple comparisons using the Tukey HSD test were employed due to its ability to effectively control the family-wise error rate while facilitating comprehensive comparisons among group means. In relation to this, participants in Cluster 1 ("most skilled") showed the highest levels of the sexual items when compared to participants in the other clusters; that is, these participants indicated the highest scores regarding overall sexual well-being, sexual attractiveness, sexual openness and communication, and sexual satisfaction when compared to the other clusters. The observed clusters, differentiated by sexual well-being items, provide crucial insights into the nuanced dynamics of sexual experiences in aging individuals.

While the statistical analysis yielded robust findings, it is essential to acknowledge potential limitations associated with the assumptions underlying cluster analysis, including the assessment of the number of clusters.

Table 4. Three cluster groups according to sexual well-being items: Descriptives and univariate tests.

	Cluster	*M*	*DP*	*F*	*p*
How do you classify your sexual well-being?	1	4.40 a	1.90	16.987	<0.001
	2	2.94 b	1.69		
	3	2.50 c	1.96		
How do you classify your sexual attractiveness?	1	4.62 a	1.51	23.694	<0.001
	2	3.09 b	3.23		
	3	2.19 b	1.81		
How do you classify your sexual openness and communication?	1	5.15 a	1.54	93.160	<0.001
	2	2.84 b	1.68		
	3	2.19 b	1.83		
How do you classify your sexual satisfaction?	1	4.96 a	1.61	93.233	<0.001
	2	2.68 b	1.48		
	3	2.08 c	1.76		

Note: Measures marked with different letters differ statistically, at the level of $\alpha < 0.05$, according to the Tukey HSD test.

4. Discussion

This study aimed to identify clusters that were characterized by varying levels of AtA, sexual satisfaction, and SwL, which supported our hypothesis regarding the relationships between these constructs. The three distinct clusters showed specific characteristics: Cluster 1 ("most skilled") with high AtA, high sexual satisfaction, and high SwL; Cluster 2 ("least adjusted") with low levels of AtA and SwL, and moderate sexual satisfaction; and Cluster 3 ("aging strivers"), with moderate levels of AtA and low levels of sexual satisfaction and SwL. The three clusters also exhibit distinct sociodemographic, health, lifestyle characteristics, and variations in terms of sexual well-being items.

Furthermore, results indicated that the three clusters showed specific sociodemographic sexual well-being features, which support our hypothesis regarding the variations in sociodemographic, health, and lifestyle factors and sexuality-related items among the participants in each of the three clusters.

Cluster 1 ("most skilled") reflected a strong alignment of different variables, with high levels of AtA, sexual satisfaction, and SwL. These participants displayed a comprehensive sense of well-being, encompassing purpose, spirituality, health, stability, social support, fulfillment in both individual and partnered sexual experiences, and a high satisfaction with life. Literature indicated that older adults with higher SwL exhibited more positive health outcomes, such as physical health indicators, health behaviors, and psychosocial well-being in subsequent evaluations [42,43]. Moreover, a higher level of sexual well-being has been correlated with greater overall SwL [12,44]. Indeed, perspectives about the importance of maintaining a satisfying sex life in later years have been leading to relations with psychological variables that subsidize sexual satisfaction [45].

This cluster predominantly comprises older adults in a relationship, mostly from Portugal, and predominantly consisting of older women with varying levels of education. These participants self-perceive themselves as spiritual and consider their general health to be good. Moreover, these older adults show diverse experiences of love and engagement in leisure activities. Literature highlights the influence of education, leisure, and spirituality on older adults' sexual well-being since these factors play a crucial role in the cultural context of older individuals' sexual perspectives and their sexual satisfaction [46–49].

Cluster 1 is also distinguished by its higher scores on sexual well-being items. Within this cluster, individuals consistently express a profound sense of positive sexual experiences, marking a noteworthy level of satisfaction with their sexual lives. Their sense of sexual well-being encompasses positive sexual attractiveness, open communication about sex, and overall satisfaction. This cluster represents individuals who find contentment and fulfillment in their sexual experiences, and their positive self-perception contributes to their robust sexual well-being. The literature indicates that open communication about sexuality is strongly associated with higher levels of sexual satisfaction [50]. In a study conducted by Velten and Margraf [51], various factors contributing to sexual satisfaction in stable relationships included partner-related aspects, relationship dynamics, effective sexual communication, and the individual's SwL.

Participants in Cluster 1 may present higher levels of all variables due to their diverse experiences of love, engagement in leisure activities, and self-perceived spirituality, which contribute to their sense of fulfillment. Additionally, their positive sexual experiences and open communication about sex highlight the importance of interpersonal dynamics and cultural attitudes toward sexuality in shaping sexual satisfaction and overall well-being in older adulthood.

Participants in Cluster 2 ("least adjusted") demonstrated low AtA, moderate sexual satisfaction, and relatively low SwL. Despite facing challenges, these participants are motivated to find a balance between relatively positive sexual satisfaction and overall satisfaction and adjustment. Studies indicate that SwL played a significant role in predicting AtA [7]. Furthermore, sexual well-being and experiencing happiness and SwL were linked to aging well [44,52].

The second cluster includes both Portuguese and Spanish older adults, with a slightly higher proportion of women with varied educational levels. While this cluster predominantly consists of married participants, it also has a notable percentage of divorced individuals. A significant portion of participants in this cluster identify as spiritual; most report good health and showed varied experiences in love. Interestingly, older adults in this cluster tend not to engage in leisure activities despite the widely recognized benefits of such activities for older people, including the maintenance of cognitive function, physical and mental health, and overall successful aging [47].

Furthermore, older adults in Cluster 2 show a moderate classification of sexual well-being items. Indeed, individuals in this cluster maintain a balanced perspective of their sexual experiences, and their assessment of sexual attractiveness is moderate, reflecting their nuanced perception of their sexual appeal. Considering the average levels of sexual openness and communication, as well as moderate satisfaction with sexual experiences observed in this group, further exploration is needed to understand the underlying factors influencing these aspects of sexual well-being and how they relate to overall SwL. Studies show that successful aging is significantly influenced by sexual desire and being sexually satisfied [23,53,54], and sexual expression may be beneficial to physical and mental health [55]. Additionally, the multifaceted concept of positive attractiveness, which encompasses aspects such as body appreciation and acceptance, has been shown to have an impact on sexual well-being [56,57].

In Cluster 2, despite lower AtA and SwL, individuals maintain moderate levels of sexual satisfaction. Their balanced perspective on sexual experiences suggests a nuanced psychological resilience, emphasizing the importance of individual coping mechanisms in navigating aging-related challenges.

Older participants in Cluster 3 ("aging strivers") show moderate AtA, low sexual satisfaction, and relatively low SwL. These older adults show a balance between AtA and experiencing limited sexual satisfaction. Their overall SwL is comparatively lower, indicating room for improvement. Prior research revealed a strong connection between sexual satisfaction and contentment in various life domains, such as the ability to take care of oneself, partnership satisfaction, and family life satisfaction [52,58,59]. More recent studies have also demonstrated that sexual satisfaction has been linked to successful aging [44,58], as well as to overall SwL and well-being [60].

Cluster 3 contains a diverse group with an equal mix of Portuguese and Spanish individuals. The majority of participants in this cluster have higher educational attainment and are married, with a significant proportion of widowed individuals. Additionally, these older adults identify themselves as spiritual and report good health. Within this cluster, participants reported positive experiences in love and active engagement in leisure activities. Existing research has indicated a positive relationship between marital status, spirituality, education, and sexual well-being [27,52]. Given the existing evidence indicating a positive association between general well-being, sexual well-being, and SwL, further research on these constructs is warranted to explore how these positive constructs interact and influence each other, especially when considering sociocultural variations across diverse old populations.

Older adults in Cluster 3 exhibited a lower classification of sexual well-being items. Individuals within this cluster express a more restrained sense of satisfaction with their sexual lives. Their sexual attractiveness is relatively low, and their sexual openness and communication are limited, potentially affecting their overall sexual experiences. This cluster included mostly older men with challenges concerning their sexual well-being, likely stemming from issues related to self-perception and communication. In a previous study, among the motivations for a poor sex life among older adults were not having a partner (12.7%), not having desire (9.32%), and physical difficulties (7.62%) [18]. Enhancing sexual well-being may involve efforts to improve self-confidence and foster open conversations about their sexual experiences [27]. Research and clinical data have indicated that couples experiencing sexual difficulties often report poor sexual communication. Positive correlations have been observed between sexual communication, attractiveness, and various facets of sexual function, including desire, arousal, erection, lubrication, orgasm, and reduced pain [61].

In Cluster 3, older adults exhibit moderate AtA but experience low sexual satisfaction and relatively low satisfaction with life. Despite positive attributes such as higher education, marriage, and engagement in leisure activities, they report limited sexual well-being, potentially influenced by issues with self-perception and communication. Efforts to enhance sexual well-being in this group may involve improving self-confidence and fostering open conversations about sexual experiences. Despite similarities in educational attainment and marital status, cultural nuances may also influence perceptions of aging, sexual satisfaction, and overall well-being.

The three clusters were culturally diverse. Cluster 1 comprised mostly Portuguese older adults with high levels of AtA, sexual satisfaction, and SwL. Conversely, Cluster 2 integrated mostly Portuguese participants with moderate sexual satisfaction and lower levels of AtA and SwL. Cluster 3 encompassed mostly Spanish men with moderate levels of AtA and reduced sexual satisfaction and SwL. The significant differences in nationality among the clusters highlight the potential influence of cultural factors on the AtA, SwL, and sexual satisfaction in two different geographic areas in Europe [24,34]. These findings underscore the importance of considering the cultural context in understanding the variability in well-being outcomes among older adults in different geographical regions. The literature highlights the importance of cultural values, such as religious beliefs, in expressing sexuality, attractiveness, intimacy, gender roles, and sexual health [24,34].

Moreover, these results support the multidimensional AtA theoretical framework [32], in which AtA constitutes a multifactor adjustment process with dimensions involving sexuality and intimacy, with implications on well-being, satisfaction with life, and, ultimately, aging well [7,9,32].

This study contains several limitations. While our study comprehensively compiles responses highlighting cultural differences, the oldest-old adults, especially those in their late 80s and 90s were poorly represented. Moreover, there is a lack of diversity in terms of sexual orientation and gender identity within the sample. It is equally critical to distinguish between nationality and cultural identity, which can be nuanced and not necessarily related to a specific nationality. These qualities have specific displays and should be carefully considered, even though there may be situations in which they intersect [24,34]. Connections may also exist between academic education (e.g., risk factors, health promotion) and sexual education, for example, through the promotion of open discussions in the community or psychoeducational programs; however, these two areas cover different topics. Further investigation of these factors in larger-scale and qualitative research may provide insightful information to older populations and health professionals.

Another limitation concerns the reliance on self-reported measures. Older adults could present their perceptions positively, which could further have biased responses, as older individuals might have avoided sharing unfavorable sexual experiences. Because measures were mainly quantitative, these instruments might not fully encompass the intricate experiences of older individuals or possess the necessary precision to detect meaningful changes over time. The use of cross-sectional data limits the ability to establish causality, allowing for unmeasured factors and contextual elements to influence the observed correlations. Factors such as interpersonal relationships, religious beliefs, and access to healthcare could significantly shape perceptions of sexual well-being among older adults. Additionally, cluster analysis primarily serves an exploratory purpose, and different clustering strategies might yield distinct outcomes. It is also important to recognize that the assessment of clusters relies on predefined criteria, which may not fully capture the complexity of the data. Additionally, due to the limited existing research in this field, making potential comparisons based on demographics and outcomes became a challenging endeavor. These limitations underscore the need for cautious interpretation and suggest avenues for future research to address these methodological constraints. Future studies could consider incorporating qualitative data and longitudinal designs to provide deeper insights into the dynamics of aging, sexual satisfaction, and overall well-being among older adults.

Notwithstanding these limitations, our findings have significant implications for both policy development and practical applications in the field of public health. Public health practitioners can prioritize interventions aimed at promoting sexual well-being and overall satisfaction with life among older adults, addressing barriers to sexual communication and openness. In relation to this, psychoeducational interventions may strongly contribute to sharing difficulties and building important resources for older adults and public health practitioners dealing with these. Moreover, policymakers could integrate sexual health education into existing aging programs, while community leaders can facilitate open discussions in the community and promote clear information that endorses healthy attitudes toward sexuality, risk prevention, and, ultimately, aging well. Indeed, prior research has already highlighted that a substantial number of older adults, regardless of gender, often refrain from seeking help for their sexual issues [12]. This study emphasizes the relevance of knowing more about older adults' sexual well-being and how it relates to SwL and AtA from a cultural perspective. There is a pressing need for healthcare providers to take a proactive role in assisting older adults in achieving positive sexual experiences [24]. These findings not only contribute to academic understanding but also have practical implications. Up to now, interventions rarely focus on sexual well-being and even less on the relation between sexual well-being and aging well [58]. In this context, these results can be an important means for guiding healthcare providers and policymakers in developing tailored interventions to promote a comprehensive approach to well-being among older adults, which includes targeted support programs and community interventions focused on the interaction between sexual satisfaction, adjustment to aging, and overall satisfaction with life.

This study sheds light on the intricate relationship between sexual satisfaction, AtA, and SwL. Our findings indicate that older adults approach these constructs differently. Hence, future interventions with older adults from different cultural contexts should be tailored to their specific needs. Promoting sexual well-being and providing resources to support sexual functioning hold the potential to enhance overall SwL and AtA among older adults. Similarly, initiatives focused on nurturing positive perceptions of AtA and fortifying resilience against age-related changes could facilitate sexual well-being, ultimately contributing to aging well.

In addition to declining health, multiple factors influence sexual activity and satisfaction in later life, as indicated by prior research [24]. Effectively addressing sexual concerns in older adults requires a comprehensive approach that considers not only their needs concerning sexual activity but also various aspects of their lifestyle and the challenges of living well.

This study underscores the critical importance of challenging age-related biases regarding sexuality in older adults. Literature reiterates the importance of sexual well-being for aging well; however, negative stereotypes can hinder the so-needed support available for sexual health concerns and contribute to feelings of isolation and despair. Building knowledge in the sphere of sexual well-being, particularly from a cross-cultural perspective, plays a pivotal role in combating detrimental social stereotypes. These findings shed light on recognizing the strong connection between sexual satisfaction and AtA and SwL has the potential to reshape attitudes, fostering inclusivity that transcends age boundaries. Moreover, this study highlighted the importance of acknowledging the culturally diverse experiences and needs of older adults.

Older adults perceive and prioritize sexual satisfaction, AtA, and SwL differently. Indeed, older populations are demographic heterogeneous, encompassing individuals from different cultural backgrounds, varying socioeconomic statuses, and distinct health conditions. Acknowledging and appreciating this diversity are fundamental steps toward formulating interventions and policies that effectively cater to the unique needs of the various subgroups within the older adult population.

It is imperative to elucidate the intricate relationships among the variables of sexuality, aging, and satisfaction while concurrently investigating intercultural variations [62,63]. The significance of conducting comprehensive cross-cultural studies that scrutinize these dynamics across diverse cultural contexts cannot be overstated [6,7,31,58]. Cultural nuances significantly shape individuals' perceptions and experiences of aging and sexuality, influencing the generalizability of our findings. By undertaking a study with two different older samples, we aimed to explore cultural differences and to understand how the assessment of these cultural influences is crucial for interpreting and applying our research findings appropriately within their contexts. Considering the cross-cultural nature of our study, it would be advantageous for future research to explore larger older cohorts to identify patterns and assess their stability or evolution over time. Furthermore, considering the anticipated generational differences due to evolving lifestyles, it is important to account for potential shifts in the perceptions of sexual well-being along the life cycle [34,63].

Future approaches to older adults from various cultures benefit from a tailored comprehension of sexual well-being, AtA, and SwL [63]. Different cultures ascribe unique meanings to these concepts and, thus, a nuanced understanding is crucial [33,63].

5. Conclusions

In sum, there is a significant shortage of cross-cultural research on these topics, particularly utilizing cluster analysis. This study intended to fill this gap by exploring in detail three patterns of the intricate relation between sexual well-being, AtA, and SwL among older adults. Cluster 1 ("most skilled") embodied participants with a positive alignment, with high levels of AtA, sexual satisfaction, and SwL. Cluster 2 ("least adjusted") showed participants with low AtA, moderate sexual satisfaction, and relatively low SwL. Finally, participants from Cluster 3 ("aging strivers") placed a central focus on AtA, while presenting low sexual satisfaction and SwL. These participants showed significant challenges to their sexual well-being. These findings contributed to scientific knowledge in an insufficient research area, with inconsistencies within the existing literature. Future interventions and policy programs with different cultures and older populations benefit from including sexual well-being, in all its complexity, as an integral and inseparable dimension of the lives of older individuals. By doing so, older adults may be truly empowered to embrace their sexual well-being as an enduring and meaningful part of their aging well. In conclusion, our study adds to the literature by exploring the importance of addressing the multifaceted interaction of sexual satisfaction, adjustment to aging, and overall well-being among older adults, advocating for tailored interventions and further research in multi-cultural contexts, which actively include sexual variables and its relation to satisfaction with life and AtA, among older populations.

Author Contributions: Contributions: S.v.H.: study concept and design, analysis and interpretation of data, recruitment of subjects, preparation of manuscript; E.C.: analysis and interpretation of data, recruitment of subjects, preparation of manuscript; G.L.: study concept and design, interpretation of data; I.L.: study concept and design, interpretation of data. All authors have read and agreed to the published version of the manuscript.

Funding: This research was funded by the Fundação para a Ciência e Tecnologia, I.P., under Grant [number SFRH/BPD/116114/2016]. This work is funded with national funds from FCT—Fundação para a Ciência e Tecnologia, I.P., in the context of the project UID/04810/2020, https://doi.org/10.54499/UIDB/04810/2020 (accessed on 14 January 2024).

Institutional Review Board Statement: The study was conducted according to the guidelines of the Declaration of Helsinki, and approved by the Ethics Committee of ISPA–Instituto Universitário (Protocol code: SFRH/BPD/116114/2016; Date of approval: 11 July 2016).

Informed Consent Statement: Informed consent was obtained from all subjects involved in the study.

Data Availability Statement: The data presented in this study are available on request from the corresponding author. The data are not publicly available due to privacy and ethical restrictions.

Conflicts of Interest: The authors declare no conflict of interest. The authors alone are responsible for the content and writing of the paper.

References

1. Ageing and Health. Available online: https://www.who.int/news-room/fact-sheets/detail/ageing-and-health (accessed on 14 January 2024).
2. Aging Europe: Looking at the Lives of Older People in the EU. Available online: https://ec.europa.eu/eurostat/documents/3217494/11478057/KS-02-20-655-EN-N.pdf (accessed on 15 January 2024).
3. Population Structure and Ageing. Available online: https://ec.europa.eu/eurostat/statistics-explained/index.php?title=Population_structure_and_ageing#The_share_of_elderly_people_continues_to_increase (accessed on 15 January 2024).
4. Marzo, R.R.; Khanal, P.; Shrestha, S.; Mohan, D.; Myint, P.K.; Su, T.T. Determinants of active aging and quality of life among older adults: Systematic review. *Front. Public Health* **2023**, *11*, 1193789. [CrossRef]
5. Asejeje, F.O.; Ogunro, O.B. Deciphering the mechanisms, biochemistry, physiology, and social habits in the process of aging. *Arch. Gerontol. Geriatr. Plus* **2024**, *1*, 100003. [CrossRef]
6. von Humboldt, S.; Leal, I. The Orientation to Life Questionnaire: Validation of a Measure to Assess Older Adults' Sense of Coherence. *Educ. Gerontol.* **2015**, *41*, 451–465. [CrossRef]
7. von Humboldt, S.; Leal, I. Correlates of adjustment to aging among the young-old and the oldest-old: A comparative analysis. *Educ. Gerontol.* **2017**, *43*, 175–185. [CrossRef]
8. Schaller, S.L.; Kvalem, I.L.; Træen, B. Constructions of Sexual Identities in the Ageing Body: A Qualitative Exploration of Older Norwegian Adults' Negotiation of Body Image and Sexual Satisfaction. *Sex. Cult.* **2023**, *27*, 1369–1402. [CrossRef]
9. Flynn, T.J.; Gow, A.J. Examining associations between sexual behaviours and quality of life in older adults. *Age Ageing* **2015**, *44*, 823–828. [CrossRef]
10. Štulhofer, A.; Jurin, T.; Graham, C.; Janssen, E.; Træen, B. Correction to: Emotional intimacy and sexual well-being in aging European couples: A cross-cultural mediation analysis. *Eur. J. Ageing* **2020**, *17*, 139–150. [CrossRef] [PubMed]
11. Ménard, A.D.; Kleinplatz, P.J.; Rosen, L.; Lawless, S.; Paradis, N.; Campbell, M.; Huber, J.D. Individual and relational contributors to optimal sexual experiences in older men and women. *Sex. Relatsh. Ther.* **2015**, *30*, 78–93. [CrossRef]
12. DeLamater, J. Sexual Expression in Later Life: A Review and Synthesis. *J. Sex Res.* **2012**, *49*, 125–141. [CrossRef]
13. Træen, B.; Carvalheira, A.; Kvalem, I.L.; Štulhofer, A.; Janssen, E.; Graham, C.A.; Hald, G.M.; Enzlin, P. Sexuality in Older Adults (65+)—An Overview of The Recent Literature, Part 2: Body Image and Sexual Satisfaction. *Int. J. Sex. Health* **2017**, *29*, 11–21. [CrossRef]
14. Orr, J.; Layte, R.; O'Leary, N. Sexual activity and relationship quality in middle and older age: Findings from the Irish Longitudinal Study on Ageing (TILDA). *J. Gerontol. B Psychol. Sci. Soc. Sci.* **2019**, *74*, 287–297. [CrossRef] [PubMed]
15. Gillespie, B.J. Correlates of sex frequency and sexual satisfaction among partnered older adults. *J. Sex Marital Ther.* **2017**, *43*, 403–423. [CrossRef]
16. Soysal, P.; Smith, L. Sexual activity and successful aging. *Eur. Geriatr. Med.* **2022**, *13*, 1235–1238. [CrossRef] [PubMed]
17. Carrasco, M.H.; de la Fuente Ballesteros, S.L.; Granja, N.G.; Benito, A.H.; Álvarez, I.G.; Pazos, M.C. Characteristics of the sexual sphere in elderly patients. *Semergen* **2019**, *45*, 37–43. [CrossRef]
18. Monteiro, A.; von Humboldt, S.; Leal, I. How do formal caregivers experience the sexuality of older adults? Beliefs and attitudes towards older adults' sexuality. *Psychol. Community Health* **2017**, *6*, 77–92. [CrossRef]

19. Palacios-Ceña, D.; Carrasco-Garrido, P.; Hernández-Barrera, V.; Alonso-Blanco, C.; Jiménez-García, R.; Fernández-de-las-Peñas, C. Sexual behaviors among older adults in Spain: Results from a population-based national sexual health survey. *J. Sex. Med.* **2012**, *9*, 121–129. [CrossRef] [PubMed]
20. von Humboldt, S.; Leal, I.; Pimenta, F.; Maroco, J. Assessing Adjustment to Aging: A Validation Study for the Adjustment to Aging Scale (AtAS). *Soc. Indic. Res.* **2014**, *119*, 455–472. [CrossRef]
21. Sánchez-Fuentes, M.M.; Sierra, J.C. Sexual satisfaction in a heterosexual and homosexual Spanish sample: The role of socio-demographic characteristics, health indicators, and relational factors. *Sex. Relat. Ther.* **2015**, *30*, 226–242. [CrossRef]
22. Štulhofer, A.; Hinchliff, S.; Jurin, T.; Carvalheira, A.; Træen, B. Successful aging, change in sexual interest and sexual satisfaction in couples from four European Countries. *Eur. J. Ageing* **2019**, *16*, 155–165. [CrossRef]
23. Træen, B.; Štulhofer, A.; Janssen, E.; Carvalheira, A.A.; Hald, G.M.; Lange, T.; Graham, C. Sexual Activity and Sexual Satisfaction Among Older Adults in Four European Countries. *Arch. Sex. Behav.* **2019**, *48*, 815–829. [CrossRef]
24. Blanchflower, D.G. Is happiness U-shaped everywhere? Age and subjective well-being in 145 countries. *J. Popul. Econ.* **2021**, *34*, 575–624. [CrossRef] [PubMed]
25. Tavares, A.I. Health and life satisfaction factors of Portuguese older adults. *Arch. Gerontol. Geriatr.* **2022**, *99*, 104600. [CrossRef] [PubMed]
26. Buczak-Stec, E.; König, H.-H.; Hajek, A. The link between sexual satisfaction and subjective well-being: A longitudinal perspective based on the German Ageing Survey. *Qual. Life Res.* **2019**, *28*, 3025–3035. [CrossRef] [PubMed]
27. Zhang, K.; Kan, C.; Luo, Y.; Song, H.; Tian, Z.; Ding, W.; Xu, L.; Han, F.; Hou, N. The promotion of active aging through older adult education in the context of population aging. *Front. Public Health* **2022**, *10*, 998710. [CrossRef]
28. von Humboldt, S.; Leal, I.; Pimenta, F. Analyzing Adjustment to Aging and Subjective Age from Angolan and Portuguese Community-dwelling Older Adults' Perspectives. *Int. J. Gerontol.* **2013**, *7*, 209–215. [CrossRef]
29. von Humboldt, S.; Leal, I. Adjustment to Aging in Late Adulthood: A Systematic Review. *Int. J. Gerontol.* **2014**, *8*, 108–113. [CrossRef]
30. von Humboldt, S.; Monteiro, A.; Leal, I. How do older adults experience intergenerational relationships? Different cultures, ambivalent feelings. *Educ. Gerontol.* **2018**, *44*, 501–513. [CrossRef]
31. Ornat, L.; Martínez-Dearth, R.; Muñoz, A.; Franco, P.; Alonso, B.; Tajada, M.; Pérez-López, F.R. Sexual function, satisfaction with life and menopausal symptoms in middle-aged women. *Maturitas* **2013**, *75*, 261–269. [CrossRef]
32. Santos Pechorro, P.; Almeida, A.I.; Soares Figueiredo, C.; Monteiro Pascoal, P.; Xavier Vieira, R.; Neves Jesus, S. Validação portuguesa da Nova Escala de Satisfação Sexual. *Rev. Int. Androl.* **2015**, *13*, 47–53. [CrossRef]
33. Strizzi, J.; Fernández-Agis, I.; Alarcón-Rodríguez, R.; Parrón-Carreño, T. Adaptation of the New Sexual Satisfaction Scale-Short Form Into Spanish. *J. Sex Marital Ther.* **2016**, *42*, 579–588. [CrossRef]
34. Larsen, R.J.; Diener, E.; Emmons, R.A. An evaluation of subjective well-being measures. *Soc. Indic. Res.* **1985**, *17*, 1–17. [CrossRef]
35. Pavot, W.; Diener, E. The Satisfaction With Life Scale and the emerging construct of life satisfaction. *J. Posit. Psychol.* **2008**, *3*, 137–152. [CrossRef]
36. Vázquez, C.; Duque, A.; Hervás, G. Satisfaction with life scale in a representative sample of Spanish adults: Validation and normative data. *Span. J. Psychol.* **2013**, *16*, E82. [CrossRef] [PubMed]
37. Marôco, J. *Análise de Equações Estruturais: Fundamentos Teóricos, Software e Aplicações [Structural Equation Analysis: Theoretical Fundamentals, Software and Applications]*, 3rd ed.; Pero Pinheiro: Lisbon, Portugal, 2021.
38. Kim, E.; Delaney, S.; Tay, L.; Chen, Y.; Diener, E.; VanderWeele, T. Life Satisfaction and Subsequent Physical, Behavioral, and Psychosocial Health in Older Adults. *Milbank Q.* **2021**, *99*, 209–239. [CrossRef] [PubMed]
39. Hopper, S.; Hammond, N.G.; Stinchcombe, A. Satisfaction with life in mid-age and older Canadians in the CLSA: Examining personality and minority stress. *Appl. Res. Qual. Life* **2022**, *17*, 3455–3473. [CrossRef]
40. Erens, B.; Mitchell, K.R.; Gibson, L.; Datta, J.; Lewis, R.; Field, N.; Wellings, K. Health status, sexual activity and satisfaction among older people in Britain: A mixed methods study. *PLoS ONE* **2019**, *14*, e0213835. [CrossRef] [PubMed]
41. Srinivasan, S.; Glover, J.; Tampi, R.R.; Tampi, D.J.; Sewell, D.D. Sexuality and the Older Adult. *Curr. Psychiatry Rep.* **2019**, *21*, 97. [CrossRef] [PubMed]
42. Ricoy-Cano, A.J.; Obrero-Gaitán, E.; Caravaca-Sánchez, F.; De La Fuente-Robles, Y.M. Factors Conditioning Sexual Behavior in Older Adults: A Systematic Review of Qualitative Studies. *J. Clin. Med.* **2020**, *9*, 1716. [CrossRef] [PubMed]
43. Sala, G.; Jopp, D.; Gobet, F.; Ogawa, M.; Ishioka, Y.; Masui, Y.; Inagaki, H.; Nakagawa, T.; Yasumoto, S.; Ishizaki, T.; et al. The impact of leisure activities on older adults' cognitive function, physical function, and mental health. *PLoS ONE* **2019**, *14*, e0225006. [CrossRef]
44. Vasconcelos, P.; Paúl, C.; Serruya, S.; Ponce de León, R.G.; Nobre, P. A systematic review of sexual health and subjective well-being in older age groups. *Rev. Panam. Salud. Publica* **2022**, *46*, e179. [CrossRef]
45. Faílde Garrido, J.M.; Dapía Conde, M.D.; Vázquez Vázquez, M.Á.; Vázquez Rodríguez, L. Are Older Adults' Leisure Patterns Consistent with the Active Ageing Model? The Influence of the Ageist Stereotypes. *Soc. Policy Soc.* **2022**, *21*, 575–596. [CrossRef]
46. Øverup, C.S.; Hald, G.M.; Pavan, S. Sociodemographic predictors of sexual communication and sexual communication as a predictor of sexual, relationship, and life satisfaction in Denmark, Finland, France, Norway, Sweden, and the UK. *Sex. Cult.* **2024**, 1–30. [CrossRef]

47. Velten, J.; Margraf, J. Satisfaction guaranteed? How individual, partner, and relationship factors impact sexual satisfaction within partnerships. *PLoS ONE* **2017**, *12*, e0172855. [CrossRef] [PubMed]
48. Teater, B.; Chonody, J.M. How Do Older Adults Define Successful Aging? A Scoping Review. *Int. J. Aging Hum. Dev.* **2020**, *91*, 599–625. [CrossRef]
49. Štulhofer, A.H.; Hinchliff, S.; Jurin, T.; Hald, G.M.; Træen, B. Successful aging and changes in sexual interest and enjoyment among older European men and women. *J. Sex Med.* **2018**, *15*, 1393–1402. [CrossRef] [PubMed]
50. Bauer, M.H.; Haesler, E.; Fetherstonhaugh, D. Let's talk about sex: Older people's views on the recognition of sexuality and sexual health in the health-care setting. *Health Expect.* **2016**, *19*, 1237–1250. [CrossRef] [PubMed]
51. Fisher, L.; Anderson, G.O.; Chapagain, M.; Montenegro, X.; Smoot, J.; Takalkar, A. *Sex, Romance, and Relationships: AARP Survey of Midlife and Older Adults*; AARP: Washington, DC, USA, 2010.
52. Ramseyer Winter, V.; O'Neill, E.A.; Cook, M.; Rose, K.L.; Hood, A. Sexual function in hook-up culture: The role of body image. *Body Image* **2020**, *34*, 135–144. [CrossRef] [PubMed]
53. Rao, T.S.S.; Tripathi, A.; Manohar, S.; Tandon, A. Promoting sexual well-being. *Indian J. Psychiatry* **2024**, *66*, S262–S271. [CrossRef]
54. Lee, D.M.; Nazroo, J.; O'Connor, D.B.; Blake, M.; Pendleton, N. Sexual health and well-being among older men and women in England: Findings from the English Longitudinal Study of Ageing. *Arch. Sex. Behav.* **2016**, *45*, 133–144. [CrossRef]
55. Doerwald, F.; Albrecht, B.M.; Stalling, I.; Bammann, K. Domain-specific life satisfaction among older adults with and without children: The role of intergenerational contact. *PLoS ONE* **2021**, *16*, e0257048. [CrossRef]
56. Træen, B.; Villar, F. Sexual well-being is part of aging well. *Eur. J. Ageing* **2020**, *17*, 135–138. [CrossRef] [PubMed]
57. Mallory, A.B.; Stanton, A.M.; Handy, A.B. Couples' sexual communication and dimensions of sexual function: A meta-analysis. *J. Sex Res.* **2019**, *56*, 882. [CrossRef] [PubMed]
58. DeLamater, J.; Koepsel, E. Relationships and sexual expression in later life: A biopsychosocial perspective. *Sex Relat. Ther.* **2015**, *30*, 37–59. [CrossRef]
59. Gore-Gorszewska, G.; Ševčíková, A.; Gottfried, J. Predicting changes to sexual activity in later life: A longitudinal study. *Sex Res. Soc. Policy* 2023. [CrossRef]
60. Syme, M.L.; Cohn, T.J.; Stoffregen, S.; Kaempfe, H.; Schippers, D. "At my age…": Defining sexual wellness in mid-and later life. *J. Sex Res.* **2019**, *56*, 832–842. [CrossRef]
61. Ji, L.J.; Imtiaz, F.; Su, Y.; Zhang, Z.; Bowie, A.C.; Chang, B. Culture, aging, self-continuity, and life satisfaction. *J. Happiness Stud.* **2022**, *23*, 3843–3864. [CrossRef] [PubMed]
62. Kolodziejczak, K.; Drewelies, J.; Deeg, D.J.H.; Huisman, M.; Gerstorf, D. Perceived Importance and Enjoyment of Sexuality in Late Midlife: Cohort Differences in the Longitudinal Aging Study Amsterdam (LASA). *Sex Res. Soc. Policy* **2021**, *18*, 621–635. [CrossRef]
63. Towler, L.B.; Graham, C.A.; Bishop, F.L.; Hinchliff, S. Sex and Relationships in Later Life: Older Adults' Experiences and Perceptions of Sexual Changes. *J. Sex Res.* **2022**, *60*, 1318–1331. [CrossRef]

European Journal of
Investigation in Health, Psychology and Education

MDPI

Article

Technological Perception with Rural and Urban Differentiation and Its Influence on the Quality of Life of Older People with Age-Related Macular Degeneration

Angel Parra-Sanchez [1], Vanessa Zorrilla-Muñoz [2,3,*], Gema Martinez-Navarrete [1,*] and Eduardo Fernandez [1,4]

1 Neuroprosthesis and Visual Rehabilitation Laboratory, Bioengineering Institute, University Miguel Hernández of Elche, 03202 Elche, Spain; a.parra@umh.es (A.P.-S.); e.fernandez@umh.es (E.F.)
2 Bioengineering Institute, University Miguel Hernández of Elche, 03202 Elche, Spain
3 Institute on Gender Studies, University Carlos III of Madrid, Getafe, 28903 Madrid, Spain
4 Biomedical Research Network Center (CIBER-BBN), 28029 Madrid, Spain
* Correspondence: vzorrilla@umh.es (V.Z.-M.); gema.martinezn@umh.es (G.M.-N.); Tel.: +34-685727950 (V.Z.-M.); +34-657137673 (G.M.-N.)

Abstract: The past decade has seen a global increase in population age, especially in developed countries, where aging involves visual diseases such as age-related macular degeneration (AMD), which severely affect quality of life (QoL) and mental health, as well as increase isolation and care costs. This study investigated how persons with AMD perceive the impact of technology use on their QoL, focusing on potential disparities between urban and rural contexts in Spain. Using a cross-sectional observational design, data from the 2020 National Statistics Institute's Disability, Personal Autonomy, and Dependency Situations Survey were analyzed, focusing on QoL aspects based on the WHO items of the WHOQOL-100 scale. The results revealed a generally positive perception of technology among participants, with urban residents perceiving technology's positive impact more favorably. Sex discrepancies in technology perception were also observed, as women exhibited a more positive outlook on technology's influence on QoL. The analysis of QoL aspects, such as 'Visibility', 'Learning', 'Mobility', and 'Domestic life', highlighted distinct challenges faced by rural and urban populations, underscoring the importance of context-specific approaches in technology interventions. However, these perceptions were intertwined with comorbidities, which can exacerbate AMD-related issues. Furthermore, this study explored the role of technology in enhancing QoL among older adults with AMD, examining how it influences daily activities and independence, particularly in the context of AMD management. This study concluded that developing more-inclusive policies tailored to the specific needs of persons with AMD, with special attention to environmental and sex differences, is imperative to enhance the positive impact of technology on their QoL.

Keywords: AMD; rural; sex; older people; self-perceived health; new technologies; quality of life

1. Introduction

In the last decade, there has been an increase in the global population's age, especially in developed countries, such as the European community, where more than 17% of the total population is over 65 years old [1]. This increase in age has led to the emergence of diseases related to visual impartments and blindness (Figure 1). Visual impairment and blindness in older adults significantly impact quality of life (QoL) and mental health and may lead to anxiety and depression [2–5]. Moreover, persons with visual disabilities and/or blindness may experience isolation, stigma and self-stigma, discrimination, and other social conditions affecting well-being [6–8]. For older adults, visual impairment can reduce physical activity [9], increase the risk of hip fracture [10], and contribute to social isolation [11]. Additionally, older people with low vision are more likely to be admitted to nursing homes, increasing the cost of care [10,12] and the burden related to informal support/care by relatives [13]. This represents a significant global burden, with an estimated annual loss of worldwide productivity amounting to approximately USD 411.3 million. This figure far exceeds the estimated cost for addressing the needs of visual impairment [14,15].

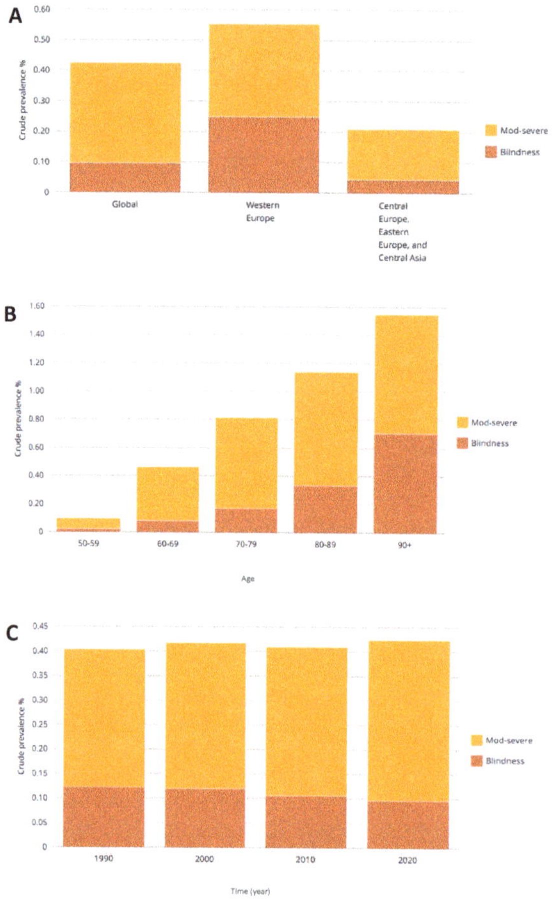

Figure 1. Crude prevalence of vision loss due to age-related macular degeneration by location (**A**), age (**B**), and time period (**C**). Adults $\geq$ 50 years old, men and women. Source: Data from VLEG/GBD 2020 model, accessed via the IAPB Vision Atlas (https://www.iapb.org/learn/vision-atlas/magnitude-and-projections/gbd-super-regions/, accessed on 2 February 2024).

Visual impairment and blindness in aging is associated with main diseases such as glaucoma, diabetic retinopathy, and age-related macular degeneration (AMD). AMD is the most common cause of blindness in developed countries, accounting for 8.7% of all blindness worldwide [16–19], reaching around 196 million cases in 2020, a figure expected to increase to 288 million by 2040 [20]. AMD is a chronic and progressive degenerative disorder that primarily affects the central part of the retina known as the macula. It is characterized by the loss of central vision due to abnormalities in the photoreceptor/retinal pigment epithelium/Bruch's membrane/choroid complex, often leading to geographic atrophy and/or neovascularization. AMD can be classified into dry and wet forms, with the latter being responsible for the majority of the severe vision loss [21]. The prevalence of AMD-related vision loss is higher in western Europe than in other regions and countries worldwide, with a greater prevalence among older people. Over the past decade, the prevalence of AMD has slightly increased. In Spain, data from the National Institute of Statistics (INE) disabilities database [22] indicate that AMD disproportionately affects women as they age, with a prevalence of 6.09 per 1000 inhabitants among those aged 65 to 69 years and 27.22 per 1000 inhabitants aged 80 and older. In comparison, the prevalence among men in the corresponding age group is 3.09 per 1000 and 17.35 per 1000 inhabitants, respectively. Therefore, AMD is a disease that is more closely associated with women, placing them at a higher risk, thus suggesting the need for a sex-based analysis. According to sex in AMD, some authors such as Lin et al. suggested sex disparities and inequality burdens associated with such diseases [23].

The risk factors for AMD can be broadly classified into two main groups: (1) environmental factors and (2) personal factors. Environmental factors include (a) smoking, (b) exposure to sunlight, and (c) nutritional factors such as a lack of micronutrients, fish-poor diets, and alcohol consumption. Environmental factors encompass not only external physical elements, such as pollution and climate, but also aspects of the social and cultural environment that significantly affect individual decisions and behaviors. For example, the practice of smoking is influenced by the social and cultural environment, such as advertising and social norms. Additionally, smoking introduces toxins that are known risks to ocular health [24]. On the other hand, personal factors can be further subdivided into (a) sociodemographic factors (age, sex, race/ethnicity, heredity, and socioeconomic level), (b) ocular factors (mainly iris color, optical density of the macular pigment, cataracts and their surgery, refractive error, and cup/disc ratio), and (c) systemic factors (suffering cardiovascular disease, reproductive system disorders, hormonal problem, elastotic degeneration of the skin, and antioxidant enzyme scarcity) [21]. Focusing on the risk factors evaluated in this study, Święch et al. found that the place of residence (urban or rural) and sex can influence the perception of the exudative form of AMD [25]. This perception can impact the QoL and well-being of older people, especially those over the age of 50 years. Additionally, AMD has been found to be associated with rural regions [26,27], especially when comparing urban and rural populations for an intervention. These personal factors include demographics, health literacy, cultural beliefs and attitudes, psychological factors, lifestyle and behavior, economic stability and technological proficiency. Overall, while sex-related factors may contribute to AMD risk, the interplay between genetic, lifestyle, and environmental factors likely plays a more significant role in determining individual risk profiles [28].

AMD, an irreversible condition, is currently addressed with innovative technologies with therapies like ultra-wide-field fundus ophthalmoscopy-assisted deep learning [29] and microarray technology [30], alongside established treatments such as photodynamic and anti-VEGF therapies [31], which aim to mitigate vision loss. Despite these advancements, not all forms of vision loss are preventable, and disparities in access to treatments like anti-VEGF injections persist [32,33]. Consequently, there is an increasing focus on the socio-health impacts of technology [34] and the need for research into the usability and acceptability of these technologies, particularly in patients with AMD [35,36], to enhance QoL and safety. Given these factors, it is likely that disruptive technologies and new therapies and drugs will be developed in the future for the treatment of AMD with the potential to improve QoL. In this context, authors from the last century, such as Williams (1998), found that persons affected by AMD experience emotional distress and a reduced QoL in their daily activities. Moreover, these persons usually report lower self-rated general health due to their low visual acuity [37]. Mitchell and Bradley (2006) highlighted the significant decrease in QoL experienced by persons with AMD when there is a delay in diagnosis and a lack of ongoing medical support. They concluded that investing in rehabilitation, low-vision aids, training, and ongoing support could have a significant impact on QoL [38]. More recently, COVID-19 has served as an example of the lack of support and delays in medical treatments for conditions like AMD. Sanabria et al. (2023) demonstrated a worsening perception of QoL in those with AMD [39]. According to Van Hu et al. (2023), comorbidities are factors influencing QoL, with the presence of $\geq$3 chronic diseases in addition to AMD being associated with lower evaluations of the mental health component. This can lead to depressive symptoms and a deterioration in basic activities of daily living [40]. A series of studies have explored the impact of AMD on QoL using different methodologies, consistently revealing significant declines in QoL among affected patients. A study employing the National Eye Institute Visual Function Questionnaire-25 (NEI-VFQ-25) found that patients with AMD reported lower scores across all domains of the questionnaire, highlighting a substantial negative impact on their QoL [41]. Similarly, research utilizing the International Index of Quality of Life (IQoL) observed that patients with AMD scored lower in both the physical and emotional domains, further emphasizing the profound effects on the overall quality of life [42]. Additionally, an analysis focusing on the correlation between visual acuity and QoL in Patients with AMD revealed that those with lower visual acuity experienced significantly reduced QoL, underscoring the direct relationship between the severity of vision loss and QoL degradation in these individuals [43].

In summary, previous studies have examined the concept of QoL from multiple and interdisciplinary perspectives, considering various factors that impact the daily activities and independence of patients with AMD. However, it remains unclear whether persons affected by AMD perceive the positive impact on their QoL when using technology as a means of support and assistance. Therefore, it is essential to gain a comprehensive understanding of the overall perception of these people in order to develop technologies that can facilitate the management and support of their condition, ultimately improving their QoL.

Taking this perspective into account, the assessment of QoL among older people affected by AMD becomes significant in relation to the role of technology and sociodemographic variables. Based on these previous considerations, the objective of this study was to determine the perspective and influence of technology on QoL determinants among adults and older persons ($\geq$50 years old) with AMD, residing in both rural and urban areas of Spain, using data obtained from the Survey of Disability, Personal Autonomy and Dependency Situations, collected by the National Statistics Institute (INE).

2. Materials and Methods

This research was based on examining technological perception and its influence on the quality of life among people 50 years and older affected by AMD.

2.1. Data Collection

This study was based on data from the "Survey of Disability, Personal Autonomy and Dependency Situations" (AGE) [22] developed by the National Institute of Statistics (INE). All ethical considerations and data protection measures were handled and documented by the INE. Also, this study received approval from the Ethics Committee of the Miguel Hernández University of Elche (code UT.IB.GCMN.240202). AGE encompasses a comprehensive macro-survey that specifically targets persons residing in private households within Spain. The questionnaire was administered during the year 2020 and has already undergone rigorous validation processes conducted by the INE. The data collected included as criteria for disability or limitation needed to be current and have a duration at least one year. The sample size consisted of 68,000 Spanish households. Furthermore, in order to achieve the survey's objectives and ensure reliable estimations at the national and regional levels, the INE determined an initial sample size of 110,130 households distributed across 3671 census sections. This decision to consider a sample of 110,130 households was based on the sample obtained from a previous disability survey conducted in 2008. Each section had thirty households selected as titular units [22]. Data collection involved a two-stage stratified approach, employing a multidata collection method that included computer-assisted web interviewing (CAWI) and computer-assisted personal interviewing (CATI) collection, and a paper questionnaire sent by regular mail. When persons with disabilities were identified, their information was collected through a CAPI interview using an individual questionnaire, which means that each respondent answered questions in a personalized interview. However, due to the outbreak of the COVID-19 pandemic during the field work, the data had to collected through CAPI and CATI in a second phase, resulting in a reduction in the initial sample (from 110,130 to 68,000 Spanish households). The survey aimed to capture the experiences of approximately 4.38 million people (equivalent to 94.9 per 1000 inhabitants) who had reported having some form of disability. The figure of 4.38 million individuals reporting some form of disability is an estimate applied to the sample data, adjusted for the probability of selection, nonresponse, and poststratification factors to ensure that the estimates were representative of the national population. This was calculated with a precision of 4.3 decimals, as indicated by the INE in its methodology (https://www.ine.es/metodologia/t15/meto_edad_2020.pdf, accessed on 2 February 2024, https://www.ine.es/daco/daco42/discapa/faltar_2020.pdf, accessed on 2 February 2024) to ensure the accuracy of these adjustments. The detailed level of precision helped to accurately scale the sample data to reflect the entire population, taking into account the complex survey design.

2.2. Sampling

The total sample size corresponded to 2405 individuals (see Table 1). The sample size was justified as follows: the prevalence of AMD in the Spanish population was 3.4% in 2022 [44], while data collected by the INE in 2020 included a total of 21,021,128 individuals aged 50 years or older [22]. Considering 21,021,128 individuals with a prevalence rate of 3.4%, there were 714,718 individuals affected by AMD and 20,306,410 individuals at risk of developing AMD in 2020. Based on this, the sample of 367 individuals with AMD was obtained with a confidence level (1–α) of 95% (with noncritical consideration), a precision (d) of 3%, a probability (p) of 0.3, and an expected loss proportion (R) of 12% for 714,718 persons with AMD. The calculated sample size for 20,306,410 persons without AMD was 2038 individuals for 1-α = 95%, d = 3%, p = 0.5, and R = 47.64%.

For the AMD sampling, we assumed 367 persons with a standard deviation of 10. First, we calculated the power obtained for sample size increases by 20, 40, 60, and 80 points when population increases 100, 200, 300, 400, and 500. The power range obtained was 0.92–1 (Figure 2A). Second, the power calculation was performed to detect the increased population with a standard deviation of 10 at power levels of 0.8 and 0.9 (Figure 2B).

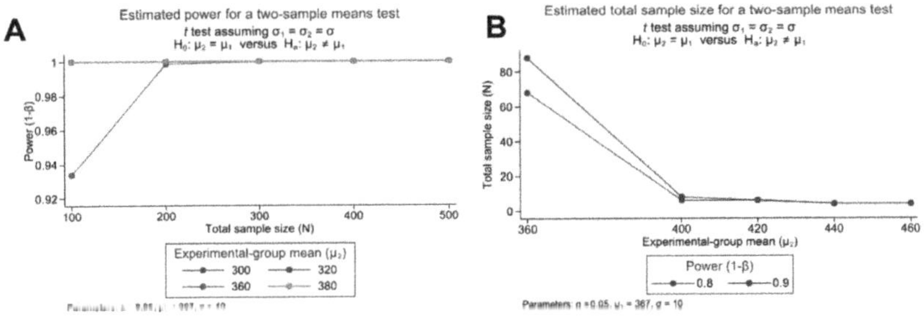

Figure 2. Power range (**A**) and total sample size representation (**B**) for the AMD sampling.

Data were extracted regarding persons aged 50 years or more and persons aged more than 50 years at risk of developing AMD. For this reason, the sample included diagnosed and undiagnosed persons 50 years and older living in rural and urban areas, diagnosed with AMD by a health professional, with their relationship to other visual pathologies and other diagnoses related or unrelated to vision pathologies in rural and urban areas (see Table 2). The total sample included 2405 persons, where a total of 53.13% of persons with AMD had been diagnosed with cataracts. Moreover, there were more comorbidities for persons with AMD, such as osteoarthritis (60.22% of persons diagnosed with AMD) and arthritis (33.79%). Regarding rural persons affected by AMD, cataracts cover a total of 51.38%, osteoarthritis 55.96%, and arthritis the 33.11%. In comparison, the percentage of these diseases was slightly higher for persons who were living with AMD in urban areas: cataracts in 55.88%, osteoarthritis percentage in 62.02%, and arthritis in 34.50% (Table 2).

Table 1. Sociodemographic variables in older people with or without AMD distributed in rural and urban areas.

Sociodemographics Variables		**Totals (n = 2405)**			**Rural Areas (n = 855) < 20,000 Habitants**		**Urban Areas (n = 1550) ≥ 20,000 Habitants**	
		Totals (n = 2405)	**AMD (n = 367)**	**Non-AMD (n = 2038)**	**AMD Persons (n = 109)**	**Non-AMD Persons (n = 746)**	**AMD Persons (n = 258)**	**Non-AMD Persons (n = 1292)**
		[Mean ± SD]	**[Mean ± SD]**	**[Mean ± SD]**	**[Mean ± SD]**	**[Mean ± SD]**	**[Mean ± SD]**	**[Mean ± SD]**
		[N(%)]	**[N(%)]**	**[N(%)]**	**[N(%)]**	**[N(%)]**	**[N(%)]**	**[N(%)]**
AMD diagnosis	**Persons with AMD diagnosis**	367 (15.26)	367 (100)	--	109 (100)		258 (100)	--
	Persons with non-AMD diagnosis	2038 (84.74)	--	2038 (100)	--	746 (100)	--	1292 (100)
Sex	**Men**	870 (36.55)	110 (29.97)	760 (37.29)	33 (30.28)	292 (39.14)	77 (29.84)	468 (36.22)
	Women	1535 (63.83)	257 (70.03)	1278 (62.71)	76 (69.72)	454 (60.86)	181 (70.16)	824 (63.78)
Age (≥50 years)	**Total (n = 2405)**	79.20 ± 0.27	79.29 ± 0.63	73.27 ± 0.29	77.38 ± 1.18	74.77 ± 0.47	80.24 ± 0.74	72.40 ± 0.36
	Women (n = 1535)	72.81 ± 0.43	77.94 ± 1.14	72.08 ± 0.46	79.22 ± 1.33	75.32 ± 0.61	80.34 ± 0.92	73.23 ± 0.45
	Men (n = 870)	74.99 ± 0.34	80.01 ± 0.76	73.97 ± 0.37	73.12 ± 2.27	73.91 ± 0.73	80.01 ± 1.25	70.93 ± 0.59

AMD: age-related macular degeneration. --: Not applicable.

Table 2. Diagnoses related or unrelated to vision pathologies in rural and urban areas.

		Total (n = 2405)						**Rural Areas (n = 855)**				**Urban Areas (n = 1550)**			
		Total (n = 2405)		**AMD (n = 367)**		**Non-AMD (n = 2038)**		**AMD Persons (n = 109)**		**Non-AMD Persons (n = 746)**		**AMD Persons (n = 258)**		**Non-AMD Persons (n = 1292)**	
		N	% total	N	% AMD	N	% Non-AMD	N	% AMD	N	% Non-AMD	N	% AMD	N	% Non-AMD
Diagnosis related to vision	*Retinitis pigmentosa*	74	3.08	15	4.09	59	2.89	6	5.50	25	3.35	9	3.49	34	2.63
	Magma myopia	257	10.69	56	15.26	201	9.86	17	15.60	74	9.92	39	15.12	127	9.83
	Diabetic retinopathy	150	6.24	21	5.72	129	6.33	5	4.59	45	6.03	16	6.20	84	6.50
	Glaucoma	345	14.35	73	19.89	272	13.35	26	23.85	94	12.60	47	18.22	178	13.78
	Cataract	1207	50.19	195	53.13	1012	49.66	56	51.38	381	51.07	139	53.88	631	48.84

Table 2. *Cont.*

		Total (n = 2405)						Rural Areas (n = 855)				Urban Areas (n = 1550)			
		Total (n = 2405)		AMD (n = 367)		Non-AMD (n = 2038)		AMD Persons (n = 109)		Non-AMD Persons (n = 746)		AMD Persons (n = 258)		Non-AMD Persons (n = 1292)	
		N	% total	N	% AMD	N	% Non-AMD	N	% AMD	N	% Non-AMD	N	% AMD	N	% Non-AMD
Diagnosis non-related to vision	*Cancer/malignant tumor*	268	11.14	50	13.62	218	10.70	16	14.68	76	10.19	34	13.18	142	10.99
	Diabetes	678	28.19	83	22.62	595	29.20	31	28.44	221	29.62	42	16.28	374	28.95
	Chronic depression	464	19.29	72	19.62	392	19.23	25	22.94	118	15.82	47	18.22	274	21.21
	Chronic anxiety	423	17.59	53	14.44	370	18.16	21	19.27	110	14.75	32	12.40	260	20.12
	Parkinson	80	3.33	13	3.54	67	3.29	5	4.59	16	2.14	8	3.10	51	3.95
	Alzheimer	260	10.81	27	7.36	233	11.43	10	9.17	46	6.17	17	6.59	87	6.73
	Muscular dystrophy	149	6.20	25	6.81	124	6.08	10	9.17	37	4.96	15	5.81	87	6.73
	Stroke	250	10.40	36	9.81	214	10.50	13	11.93	86	11.53	23	8.91	128	9.91
	Myocardial infarction	222	9.23	38	10.35	184	9.03	12	11.01	72	9.65	26	10.08	112	8.67
	Arthritis	720	29.94	124	33.79	596	29.24	35	32.11	228	30.56	89	34.50	368	28.48
	Osteoarthritis	1242	51.64	221	60.22	1021	50.10	61	55.96	382	51.21	160	62.02	369	28.56

AMD: Age-related macular degeneration.

2.3. Method Description

The methodology employed for the questionnaire encompassed various aspects related to QoL based on the WHO items of the WHOQOL-100 scale (https://www.who.int/tools/whoqol/whoqol-100, accessed on 5 February 2024). This questionnaire primarily aims to elucidate an individual's physical health, physiological state, independence level, and social relationships and their environment (https://www.ine.es/metodologia/t15/meto_edad_2020.pdf, accessed on 2 February 2024). Specifically, this questionnaire examines the domains of the level of independence, which consists of mobility, self-care, and domestic life, as well as social relationships, which encompass interpersonal relationships related to communication and learning.

The questionnaire variables were measured using a Likert scale, with varying levels as follows: The dependent variable on the perception of technology and its relationship with the improvement in the QoL was formulated in this way: 'Do you think that the use of new technologies has improved aspects of your daily life?' This question could be answered 1 to 4 points, with 1 indicating 'Yes, it has improved a lot', 2 indicating "Yes, it has improved something my daily life", 3 indicating "Technology has not gotten better or worse my daily life", and 4 indicating 'No, daily life has worsened'.

Moreover, the questionnaire also incorporates independents variables: 'Do you find difficulties for/to...' for activities related to the items 'Visibility', 'Communication', 'Learning', 'Mobility', 'Self-care', 'Domestic Life', and 'Interpersonal Relationships (see Table S1). A Likert scale, ranging from 1 to 3 points, was employed to measure responses, where 1 indicated a significant improvement, while a response of 3 suggested a maximum difficulty value.

2.4. Statistical Analysis

First, internal consistency was measured by Cronbach's alpha coefficient, which was measured as 0.79. Second, nonparametric and parametric test was used: The Spearman correlation was used prior to applying parametric tests in order to verify the relationship between two variables when it could not be assumed that they followed a normal distribution. This evaluates the monotonic relationship between variables, meaning it does not assume a linear relationship and is less sensitive to outliers and deviations from normality in the data. The results allow confirming that the variables are monotonically correlated, establishing a stronger basis for applying parametric tests and making assumptions about the distribution of the data. This helps ensure the validity of results obtained through subsequent parametric tests. Spearman correlation nonparametric test showed that population data were normally distributed. That confirmed the validity of the use of parametric tests. Third, the Pearson correlation matrix and one-way analysis of variance (ANOVA) were analyzed for each independent variable and the dependent variable related to the specified items: 'Visibility', 'Communication', 'Learning', 'Mobility', 'Self-care', 'Domestic Life', and 'Interpersonal Relationships'. All independent variables without significant Pearson and ANOVA values were excluded from the next analysis. Fourth, the significant variables ($p < 0.05$) in the Pearson and ANOVA tests were distributed across item variables. Fifth, Pearson correlation and ANOVA were applied between the dependent variable and each independent item formed. Significance levels of $p < 0.01$ and $p < 0.05$ are marked in the results. Sixth, the average covariance between items was measured with an average interitem covariance between 0.15 and 0.5. Seventh, the scale reliability coefficient was considered acceptable with a value of between 0.6 and 0.7 and greater than 0.8; Cronbach's alpha coefficient, which assesses the internal consistency of the scale, was calculated based on these interitem covariances. This coefficient quantifies the extent to which all items of the scale measure the same underlying construct, with values falling within the specified ranges indicating acceptable to excellent reliability. Finally, missing data were not imputed in the model but were excluded from the analysis. This decision was made to avoid potential biases that could arise from imputing values that may not accurately represent the true responses of the participants.

All the independents variables were tested with the dependent variable 'Do you think new technology use has improved aspects of your daily life?' with 6 possibilities: Persons with AMD (n = 367), non-AMD persons (n = 2038), persons with AMD in rural areas (n = 109), non-AMD persons in rural areas (n = 746), persons with AMD in urban areas (n = 258,) and non-AMD persons in urban areas (n = 1292). The statistical analysis was conducted, employing STATA software (version MP 17.0, developed by Statacorp).

3. Results

The analysis of the data from 2405 participants demonstrated significant patterns in the perception of technology and its influence on the quality of life for people over 50 years old, with special attention to those affected by AMD. The participants were classified based on whether they lived in rural or urban areas and whether they had AMD or not.

Among the respondents, 14.51% (349 persons) of the total sample firmly believed that technology had greatly improved their daily life. This positive perception was more prevalent in the non-AMD group, where 14.82% (302 persons) expressed this view, compared to 12.81% (47 persons) of those with AMD (Figure 3A,B). The differences between rural and urban areas were also notable. In rural areas, only 10.09% (11 persons) of respondents with AMD considered that technology had significantly improved their daily life, in contrast to 13.95% (36 persons) in urban areas. Among non-AMD participants, this perception increased to 17.18% (222 persons) in urban areas, compared to 10.72% (80 persons) in rural areas (Figure 3C,D).

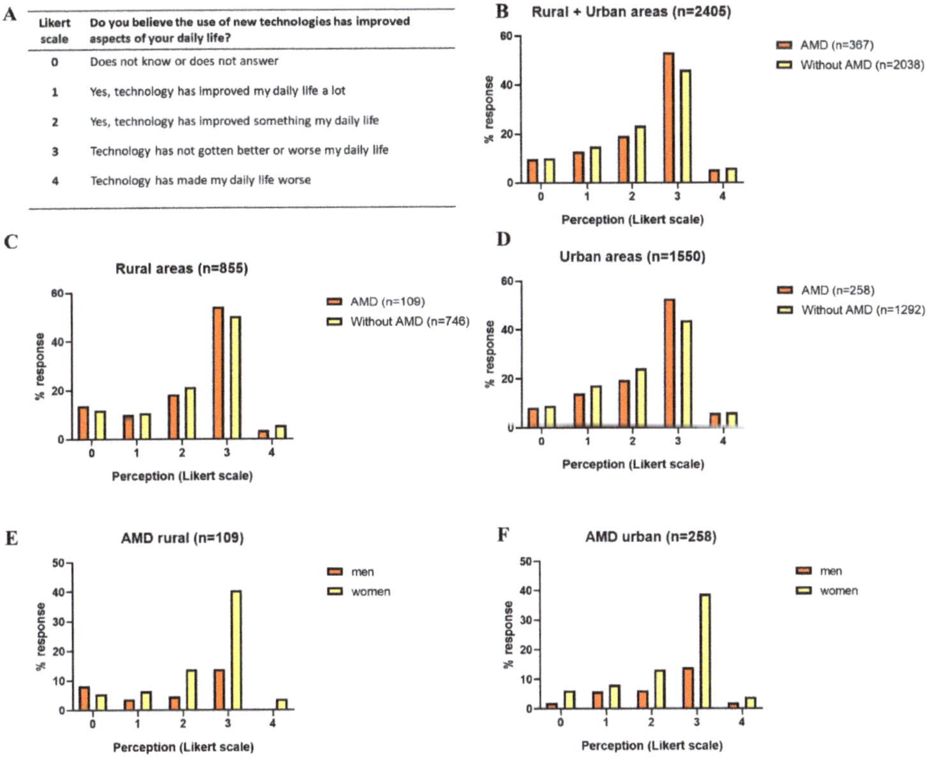

Figure 3. Perception of quality of life with the use of technologies in people with or without AMD in rural and urban areas in Spain. (**A**) Likert scale, (**B**) response rate in rural + urban areas, (**C**) response rate in rural areas, (**D**) response rate in urban areas, (**E**) response rate by sex in rural areas (n = 109), (**F**) response rate by sex in urban areas (n = 258).

Moreover, 22.54% (542 persons) of the 2405 participants indicated technology had somewhat improved their daily life. This trend remained consistent among groups with and without AMD, as well as between rural and urban areas, suggesting a generally positive perception of technology. Across all scenarios, it is noteworthy that the impact of new technologies had a more pronounced positive or negative influence in urban areas than in rural ones, with a significant portion of the AMD population in urban settings reporting such effects. These results underscored the importance of technology in improving the quality of life of older adults, with a more positive perception in urban areas and among those without AMD. However, they also highlighted the necessity of addressing disparities in perception and access to technology among these groups, particularly for the purpose of improving the lives of older adults with AMD in rural areas.

Figure 3E,F illustrate the differences in technological perception between women and men, both in persons with AMD and in those without this condition. In general, women usually reported a more positive perception of the influence of technology on their quality of life compared to men. For instance, in the group of persons with AMD, there was higher percentage of women who expressed that technology had significantly improved their daily life compared to men. This trend remained constant in both urban and rural environments.

Table 3 provides data on the average interitem covariance, number of items, and scale reliability coefficients for items related to QoL, such as 'Visibility', 'Communication', 'Learning', 'Mobility', 'Selfcare', 'Domestic life', and 'Interpersonal relationships'. The average interitem covariance for AMD items (n = 367) achieved acceptable levels, with the 'Domestic life' item exhibiting a coefficient of 0.3815. However, the items 'Communication', 'Selfcare', and 'Interpersonal relationships' were excluded from the analysis due to having only one variable remaining for the AMD group. Moreover, the scale reliability coefficients obtained were as follows: (1) For the item 'Visibility', the reliability coefficient was 0.6314. This value falls within the range considered acceptable for the internal consistency of the scale (0.6–0.7), suggesting that items related to visibility were moderately related and measured the same construct coherently. (2) For the item 'Learning', the reliability coefficient was 0.8642. This value is greater than 0.8, indicating high internal consistency among the items related to learning. This suggests that these items were highly related and measured the same construct consistently and reliably. (3) For the item 'Mobility', the reliability coefficient was 0.8511. Similar to the 'Learning' item, this value also exceeds 0.8, indicating high internal consistency among the items related to mobility. (4) For the item 'Domestic Life', the reliability coefficient was 0.7744. Although this value is above 0.7, it does not reach the threshold of 0.8 to be considered excellent. However, it remains acceptable and suggests moderate internal consistency among items related to domestic life. (5) Interestingly, the rural population (n = 109) considered the 'Domestic Life' item with two variables, resulting in an average interitem covariance of 0.2966 and a scale reliability coefficient of 0.7428. These values suggest moderate internal consistency, which is relatively acceptable.

For AMD people living in urban areas (n = 258), only the 'Mobility' item was considered, with an accepted average interitem covariance of 0.2753 and a scale reliability coefficient of 0.7243. Table 3 also indicates differences between older participants with AMD and older people not affected by AMD. For example, the analysis for persons without AMD in rural areas (n = 746) excluded the 'Learning' item. In contrast, urban areas excluded the items 'Communication' and 'Learning'. However, 'Communication' was included in the rural and urban analyses.

Table 3. Average interitem covariance, number of items, and scale reliability coefficients.

ITEM	Total (n = 2405)						Rural Areas (n = 855) < 20,000 Habitants						Urban Areas (n = 1550) $\geq$ 20,000 Habitants					
	AMD (n = 367)			Non-AMD (n = 2038)			AMD Persons (n = 109)			Non-AMD Persons (n = 746)			AMD Persons (n = 258)			Non-AMD Persons (n = 1292)		
	Average Interitem Covariance	Number of Items in the Scale	Scale Reliability Coefficient	Average Interitem Covariance	Number of Items in the Scale	Scale Reliability Coefficient	Average Interitem Covariance	Number of Items in the Scale	Scale Reliability Coefficient	Average Interitem Covariance	Number of Items in the Scale	Scale Reliability Coefficient	Average Interitem Covariance	Number of Items in the Scale	Scale Reliability Coefficient	Average Interitem Covariance	Number of Items in the Scale	Scale Reliability Coefficient
Visibility	0.1938 [1]	3	0.6314 [2]	0.2628 [1]	3	0.7353 [2]	---	1	---	0.0742	6	0.2628	---	1	---	0.2560 [1]	3	0.7181 [2]
Communication	---	1	---	0.3244 [1]	6	0.8741 [3]	---	0	---	0.3816 [1]	5	0.8886 [3]	---	0	---	---	0	---
Learning	0.3410 [1]	7	0.8642 [3]	0.2225 [1]	4	0.7573 [2]	---	0	---	---	1	---	---	0	---	---	0	---
Mobility	0.2799 [1]	8	0.8511 [3]	0.2781 [1]	14	0.9119 [3]	---	1	---	0.2494 [1]	10	0.8812 [3]	0.2753 [1]	4	0.7243 [2]	0.2881 [1]	9	0.8772 [3]
Selfcare	---	1	---	0.3573 [1]	9	0.8806 [3]	---	0	---	0.5014	6	0.8535 [3]	---	1	---	0.2651 [1]	3	0.7213 [2]
Domestic life	0.3815 [1]	3	0.7744 [2]	0.3983 [1]	6	0.8474 [3]	0.2966 [1]	2	0.7428 [2]	0.3848 [1]	5	0.8314 [3]	---	1	---	0.4026 [1]	6	0.8490 [3]
Interpersonal relationships	---	0	---	0.2399 [1]	4	0.7646 [2]	---	0	---	0.3043 [1]	3	0.7937 [2]	---	0	---	0.2882 [1]	2	0.8094 [3]

Note: [1] Average interitem covariance: 0.15 to 0.5; scale reliability coefficient: [2] acceptable = 0.6–0.8. [3] Value > 0.8. AMD: Age-related macular degeneration. ---: excluded from the analysis.

4. Discussion

This study aimed to investigate how adults aged 50 and above—diagnosed with AMD and residing in rural and urban areas of Spain—perceived the impact of new technologies on the QoL items. The main findings focused on the response to the statement 'Do you believe the use of new technologies has improved aspects of your daily life?'

Firstly, it has been well documented that aging is associated with an increase in diseases or issues related to mobility [45–47]. Our findings revealed a higher prevalence of AMD among women than men. While the distribution of ocular conditions such as glaucoma, cataracts, or diabetic retinopathy varies by sex, women with visual impairments constituted the majority. Approximately two out of every three persons in these categories were women with visual impairments [48]. This sex difference may be partly attributed to women's longer life expectancy, which averages five years more than that of men [49]. Other factors, including disparities in the significance of optimal vision in daily activities, variations in the inclination to seek medical attention, and sex and/or gender disparities in access to healthcare services, could have also contributed to this disparity. Furthermore, lifestyle-related factors such as smoking habits and sun exposure may differ by sex, influencing the risk and distribution of ocular diseases among men and women. Moreover, sex-linked biological differences can influence the underlying pathogenic mechanisms of diseases [50]. Lastly, a technological divide was observed among older persons, and there were sex inequalities influenced by differences in biases. This disparity is particularly evident in women with disabilities. This study's results revealed that how women perceive technologies has the potential to enhance their QoL and overall well-being, specifically in relation to AMD. Women see technological advancements as mitigating the impacts on autonomy and independence and improving their ability to manage their health. Additionally, women often engage in more caregiving activities, which can be physically and emotionally demanding. Technologies assisting in these areas provide significant relief and support [36]. For example, technologies such as Instead Technologies for Helping People (see EGARA handle) or rehabilitation neurorobotics for people that experienced stroke (see iDRhA) are specialized by grouping by sex [51].

Despite this positive outlook, prevailing social stereotypes and images present a conflicting narrative. These societal views often depict women, especially older women, as less capable of using or benefiting from new technologies [36]. This contradiction highlights the gap between women's actual perceptions and experiences and the cultural, educational, and societal expectations. This also indicates the importance of rethinking about how new generations and intergenerational programs interact with older women, their demands, and the necessity for various technologies. This discrepancy influences how technologies are developed and scaled, potentially ignoring the real needs and insights offered by women about their health management and caregiving roles [52,53] in patients with AMD and family caregivers. For instance, social images and representations of older women tend to be characterized by stereotypes and discriminatory idealizations in relation to the understanding and use of technologies. As a result, older women are often rendered invisible in society and from its own images [52–54].

Another factor to take into consideration is the age-related sociocultural discrimination and antifeminist bias that women face in caregiving roles. Women continue to bear the greatest burden of care, with very few men participating in caregiving activities. These burden extent thought a woman's life, including during old age and disability. Consequently, older women have a tendency to minimize the impact of their health and inequalities they face in comparison to older men. This phenomenon is evident in the responses provided on the Likert scale, where older women expressed that technology had no significant impact on either improving or worsening their daily lives. This limitation is also reflected in the current study, given that the number of male participants was smaller than that of women, potentially influencing the outcomes of the independent variables concerning sex differences. A second phase of this questionnaire that includes sex differences based on stratifying the analysis by age group would be helpful. This segmentation process can yield a more profound comprehension of how age impacts the associations between variables and uncover age-specific trends or patterns within the dataset. Moreover, expanding the male sample size will ensure a more equitable sex distribution, thereby proving advantageous. This would help mitigate the potential biases arising from the unequal representation of the sexes in the sample and enhance the generalizability of the findings. Furthermore, it is important to highlight that this research specifically concentrated on physiological sex distinctions and did not encompass a wider exploration of gender-related issues, encompassing social, cultural, and identity aspects.

On the other hand, our findings indicate that the majority of respondents, both in rural and urban areas, believed that new technologies' use had not significantly altered their daily lives. However, a larger proportion of persons residing in urban areas claimed technology had improved certain aspects of their daily life compared to those in rural areas, which aligns with our expectations. AMD significantly impacts multiple aspects of daily functioning and the ability to live independently, encompassing essential activities such as reading, shopping, driving, and self-sufficient cooking [55]. The differences found between rural and urban areas were consistent with the results of a study conducted by Święch et al. 2021, which identified variations among subpopulations of patients with AMD residing in rural and urban environments [25]: persons with disabilities in rural areas frequently reported difficulties in reading. This suggests that the prescription of low-vision devices might be less frequent in rural areas, possibly due to a lack of detailed information provided to patients in these areas. Additionally, rural patients perceived that their vision loss significantly impacted their QoL more than persons living in urban areas. This difference may be attributed to urban areas being better adapted to persons with low vision, likely due to the widespread use of new technologies [25,56]. Rural areas present a multitude of additional challenges. Hence, our results indicate that in rural zones, a lower percentage of persons responded affirmatively to the question 'Yes, technology has improved my daily life a lot' and a higher percentage of persons who asserted that 'Technology has not significantly changed my daily life'. This contrast is explained by the unequal access to advanced health services, which are more accessible in urban areas and may include telehealth and remote monitoring technologies, essential elements for the effective management of AMD. Additionally, internet connectivity, which facilitates access to information and online health services, tends to be more robust and reliable in urban areas. The complexity of rural challenges in medical aid are increased by insufficient internet connectivity and the persistent digital divide, which impact older people residing outside urban regions. These medical aids include mobility issue opportunities and risks. These risks encompass not only healthcare disparities for older people [57] but also the profound impacts of issues such as loneliness, isolation, and the various social challenges arising from the broader context of social distancing [58]. The sociocultural environment also influences the acceptance and adoption of new technologies and varies considerably between these areas, with those in rural areas often showing greater reluctance to adopt technological innovations due to cultural norms and resistance to change [57]. These multifaceted problems underscore the complex landscape faced by persons in rural settings, where a combination of factors, including limited healthcare access, technological disparities, and the broader sociocultural environment, collectively contribute to a distinct set of challenges that significantly influence the well-being of the population. Nevertheless, persons with low vision may experience increased insecurity in urban areas due to the increased mobility in urban settings.

More women expressed that new technologies improved their QoL than men. However, more women also believed that their daily life activities had neither improved nor worsened. This may also have been due to a limitation of this study, as there were more women than men included in the survey. For that reason, sex differences and a gendered approach may play a crucial role in how technology is perceived and used among older adults, underscoring the importance of considering gender differences in future research and in the development of technological interventions.

On the other hand, the findings of this study highlight significant differences in the perception of new technologies intended to enhance the daily QoL among older persons affected by AMD in urban and rural settings. Specifically, there was a notable positive impact observed in QoL aspects such as 'Domestic life', 'Learning', and 'Mobility', though with a less pronounced impact on the 'Visibility' item. In rural areas, a particularly positive perception was emphasized for 'Domestic life', reflecting the importance and demand for this item in such environments. Moreover, technology plays a crucial role in transforming domestic life. Although technological advancement has improved the living conditions for people in rural areas, there is still a significant gap in technology access and adoption, especially among older populations. This paper demonstrates that in rural older people affected by AMD, technology was positively impacting their learning abilities. This suggests that the digital divide may be narrowing in this population. On the other hand, according to the results obtained, there was no evidence that other factors such as mobility or communication impacted the QoL of people with AMD, consequently reducing the digital divide experienced by these persons.

Conversely, in urban areas, 'Mobility' emerged as the sole item considered in the analysis, underscoring the differences in the needs and priorities of persons according to their geographical context. In urban areas where there is the constant movement of people, mobility was a key factor intertwined with technology, which positively affected the QoL of older individuals with AMD. However, a different kind of divide was found, one centered around communication and learning, as observed in the results of this study.

For individuals aged 50 years and over in both rural and urban environments, the results showed that technological inclusion may have been favorably impacting learning and mobility, bridging the digital divide among older people with this condition. Addressing this challenge will require efforts by policymakers, public institutions, educators, and technology providers to emphasize solutions based on specific educational initiatives, accessible technology training programs [59,60], and inclusive design principles, aimed at empowering older people with technology. This suggests that future research on technology use and its impact on QoL in terms of mobility items should be related to the type of technological aid/device, which could be beneficial in uncovering the differences between areas and from a gender perspective.

Moreover, the data revealed that while older persons with AMD valued items related to 'Learning', those without this condition did not perceive a significant impact in this area. This finding suggests that AMD might specifically influence the perception and value placed on learning ability in adults and older adults, emphasizing the need for personalized and individually adapted strategies and training tailored to improve intrinsic capacity in promoting healthy aging. The necessity for personalized approaches becomes evident when considering these differences, both in the comparison between urban and rural settings and among persons with and without AMD. Therefore, previous studies analyzed technological opportunities for blind and visually impaired people [61]. This highlighted the specific impact of AMD on QoL and the importance of considering the individual and intrinsic capacity context when designing and implementing support technologies and programs, as stated by LaMonica et al., 2021 [62]. There are several strategies that can enhance the acceptance and effectiveness of technologies by the older adult community, including the use of codesign methodologies to ensure technology usability, acceptability, and efficiency. Telemedicine (e.g., virtual consultations, virtual rehabilitation programmes, remote diagnosis and patient monitoring and, emergency assistance) has emerged as an effective alternative for managing AMD, leveraging telecommunication technologies for remote treatment and patient assessment. This method includes synchronous and asynchronous care, communication between doctors and patients, and remote monitoring, allowing physicians to make accurate diagnoses and manage treatment from a distance [63] Additionally, the integration of mobile applications for visual self-monitoring and artificial intelligence for early detection has strengthened this strategy, enhancing diagnostic efficiency and access to medical care, reducing costs, and optimizing clinical time for cases requiring more intensive direct intervention [64].

During the COVID-19 pandemic, the emerging need to utilize technological services for socio-healthcare services, such as telemedicine, which has played a significant role, was clearly demonstrated, impacting patients with AMD. However, the current challenge extends beyond the immediate health crisis and calls for a holistic approach that exploits technology's capabilities to enhance medical care and the QoL for patients, particularly those with chronic conditions like AMD. In this context, it is important to highlight that COVID-19 has underscored the significance in ensuring uninterrupted and safe medical care, reducing virus exposure, and improving healthcare accessibility [34].

The pandemic has indeed heightened concerns regarding the emergence of comorbidities. For individuals already afflicted with chronic ailments like AMD, the repercussions can be more severe as they encounter a heightened risk of complications and a potential decline in QoL [65–67].

The current challenge extends further, and it is necessary to continue promoting new technological advancements in healthcare, beyond telemedicine. This could encompass the development and implementation of artificial intelligence algorithms [51] based on machine learning and deep learning, aiding in the early detection, precise diagnosis, and personalized treatment of diseases like AMD. Moreover, disruptive technologies such as quantum computing open new possibilities for research and the development of more effective treatments.

Our study's reliance on self-reported data potentially introduced biases, as participants may have inaccurately represented their technology usage and perceptions. The cross-sectional design additionally restricted our ability to establish causality between technology use and QoL improvements in older patients with AMD. Additionally, the representativeness of our sample may have affected the generalizability of our findings due to potential demographic and regional disparities. To address these issues, future research should include longitudinal studies to evaluate the long-term effects of technology interventions on QoL among older adults with AMD. Moreover, qualitative research is needed to uncover the reasons behind the sex differences in technology perception and usage, which will help tailor more effective interventions for this population in the clinic context. These interventions could include tailored technological solutions that are sensitive to the unique needs of this population, potentially influencing policy and practice in healthcare settings focused on aging populations [61,62]. To improve technology access in rural areas, strategies could include enhancing broadband infrastructure, providing incentives for technology companies, and increasing digital literacy through targeted education programs. Additionally, fostering partnerships between technology firms and healthcare providers and advocating for policies that promote technological equity are essential. These measures aim to bridge the gap in technology utilization, ensuring better health outcomes and QoL for rural communities.

Finally, our results underscore the importance of public policies and intervention strategies tailored to sex differences and geographic dispersion. Designing accessible technological solutions is crucial for promoting autonomy and enhancing the QoL among older adults, irrespective of their location. Moreover, gaining a comprehensive understanding of their perception is essential for developing supportive technologies that improve QoL. By considering these factors, technologies to facilitate interventions should be designed to be more aligned with the needs of older adults, promoting the management of their conditions and ultimately enhancing their overall well-being. In the future, addressing these gaps and harnessing technology's capabilities will require coordinated efforts from policymakers, healthcare providers, educators, and technology developers. This collaboration should aim to ensure equal access to technology and personalized interventions for older adults with AMD. By prioritizing inclusivity and innovation, we can effectively use technology to improve the overall well-being and independence of older populations, promoting healthy aging for all.

5. Conclusions

This research demonstrated a correlation between technology perception and the improvement in the QoL of adults and older people. The distinction between urban and rural settings suggests substantial discrepancies in accessibility and technological impact. The greater appreciation for technology in persons affected by AMD and urban residents highlights the need for inclusive policies to enhance access to and utility of technologies in rural areas and for people with AMD. Although there was generally a positive perception of technology, the variations based on the presence of AMD and geographical location emphasize the importance of considering these differences in the development of technological interventions. Significant sex differences in technology perception were observed, with women reporting a more positive impact. This suggests that interventions should be sex-sensitive to maximize effectiveness.

This study revealed that those with AMD perceived technology as improving their condition, which was associated with various aspects of QoL, particularly affecting 'Visibility', 'Learning', 'Mobility', and 'Domestic life'. Notably, rural populations assessed 'Domestic life' with two variables, while urban areas focused primarily on 'Mobility'. These findings underscore the need for context-specific evaluations in QoL assessments, taking into account geographic location and AMD status. However, these perceptions are also influenced by the presence of comorbidities, which can exacerbate the problems associated with AMD.

Finally, this research provides a basis for future studies to explore the barriers and facilitators of technological adoption among older adults with AMD, with a particular focus on the intersection of sex, technology, and rural residence. Implementing these findings into practical applications and policy development would greatly aid in the inclusion of this demographic group into digital and social spheres, aligning with the Sustainable Development Goals focused on ensuring a dignified and high-quality life for all older people.

Supplementary Materials: The following supporting information can be downloaded at: https://www.mdpi.com/article/10.3390/ejihpe14050097/s1, Table S1: Items: 'Difficulty level, difficulty level for/to'.

Author Contributions: Conceptualization, A.P.-S., V.Z.-M., G.M.-N. and E.F.; methodology, V.Z.-M.; software, V.Z.-M.; validation, V.Z.-M., formal analysis, A.P.-S., V.Z.-M. and G.M.-N.; investigation A.P.-S., V.Z.-M. and G.M.-N.; resources, V.Z.-M., G.M.-N. and E.F.; data curation, V.Z.-M.; writing—original draft preparation, A.P.-S., V.Z.-M. and G.M.-N.; writing—review and editing, A.P.-S., V.Z.-M., G.M.-N. and E.F.; visualization, A.P.-S., V.Z.-M., G.M.-N. and E.F; supervision, V.Z.-M., G.M.-N. and E.F.; project administration, V.Z.-M., G.M.-N. and E.F.; funding acquisition, A.P.-S., V.Z.-M., G.M.-N. and E.F.; All authors have read and agreed to the published version of the manuscript.

Funding: This research was funded in part by the International Center for Aging Research Foundation (ICAR) 2023, cofinanced by ICAR Foundation and, INNTA1/2022/23 Project 'Innovation Agent for the Bioengineering Institute, Miguel Hernandez University' (2022–2024), co-financed by Valencian Community EU-FEDER Program, 2021–2027. It was also supported by a FPU grant from the Spanish 'Ministerio de Ciencia, Innovación y Universidades' published by the Order of 12 November 2021 (FPU21/04360).

Institutional Review Board Statement: This study was conducted in accordance with the ethical guidelines of the Miguel Hernandez University of Elche (protocol code 240202121250, approved on 2 March 2024). Institutional Review Board (IRB). Based on the nature of the research, IRB review and approval were not required as per institutional policies. All procedures adhered to the ethical standards of the 1964 Helsinki declaration and its later amendments or comparable ethical standards. Informed consent was obtained from all subjects involved in the study.

Data Availability Statement: The data from the "Survey of Disability, Personal Autonomy and Dependency Situations (2020)", developed by the National Institute of Statistics (INE), are available at https://www.ine.es/dyngs/INEbase/en/operacion.htm?c=Estadistica_C&cid=1254736176782&idp=1254735573175, accessed on 2 February 2024. The methodology employed for the questionnaire encompassed various aspects related to QoL based on the WHO dimensions of the WHOQOL-100 scale, available at https://www.who.int/tools/whoqol/whoqol-100, accessed on 5 February 2024.

Conflicts of Interest: The authors declare no conflicts of interest.

References

1. The World Bank Data. Population Ages 65 and Above (% of Total Population). Available online: https://data.worldbank.org/indicator/SP.POP.65UP.TO.ZS (accessed on 23 November 2023).
2. Varadaraj, V.; Ehrlich, J.R.; Swenor, B.K. Vision Impairment Has Implications for Aging and Health Outcomes, Beyond Ophthalmology. *JAMA Netw. Open* **2022**, *5*, e2214610. [CrossRef] [PubMed]
3. Brunes, A.; Heir, T. Visual impairment and depression: Age-specific prevalence, associations with vision loss, and relation to life satisfaction. *World J. Psychiatry* **2020**, *10*, 139–149. [CrossRef] [PubMed]
4. Parravano, M.; Petri, D.; Maurutto, E.; Lucenteforte, E.; Menchini, F.; Lanzetta, P.; Varano, M.; van Nispen, R.M.A.; Virgili, G. Association Between Visual Impairment and Depression in Patients Attending Eye Clinics. *JAMA Ophthalmol.* **2021**, *139*, 753. [CrossRef] [PubMed]
5. Demmin, D.L.; Silverstein, S.M. Visual Impairment and Mental Health: Unmet Needs and Treatment Options. *Clin. Ophthalmol.* **2020**, *14*, 4229–4251. [CrossRef] [PubMed]
6. Heinze, N.; Davies, F.; Jones, L.; Castle, C.L.; Gomes, R.S.M. Conceptualizations of well-being in adults with visual impairment: A scoping review. *Front. Psychol.* **2022**, *13*, 964537. [CrossRef] [PubMed]
7. Partow, S.; Cook, R.; McDonald, R. Coping with stigmatization and discrimination related to blindness and low vision. *Rehabil. Psychol.* **2021**, *66*, 576–588. [CrossRef] [PubMed]
8. Kong, L.; Gao, Z.; Xu, N.; Shao, S.; Ma, H.; He, Q.; Zhang, D.; Xu, H.; Qu, H. The relation between self-stigma and loneliness in visually impaired college students: Self-acceptance as mediator. *Disabil. Health J.* **2021**, *14*, 101054. [CrossRef]
9. Ong, S.R.; Crowston, J.G.; Loprinzi, P.D.; Ramulu, P.Y. Physical activity, visual impairment, and eye disease. *Eye* **2018**, *32*, 1296–1303. [CrossRef]
10. Hamedani, A.G.; VanderBeek, B.L.; Willis, A.W. Blindness and Visual Impairment in the Medicare Population: Disparities and Association with Hip Fracture and Neuropsychiatric Outcomes. *Ophthalmic. Epidemiol.* **2019**, *26*, 279–285. [CrossRef]
11. Kotwal, A.A.; Holt-Lunstad, J.; Newmark, R.L.; Cenzer, I.; Smith, A.K.; Covinsky, K.E.; Escueta, D.P.; Lee, J.M.; Perissinotto, C.M. Social Isolation and Loneliness among San Francisco Bay Area Older Adults during the COVID-19 Shelter-in-Place Orders. *J. Am. Geriatr. Soc.* **2021**, *69*, 20–29. [CrossRef]
12. Zhou, J.; Chang, H.; Leng, M.; Wang, Z. Intrinsic Capacity to Predict Future Adverse Health Outcomes in Older Adults: A Scoping Review. *Healthcare* **2023**, *11*, 450. [CrossRef] [PubMed]
13. Chuvarayan, Y.; Finger, R.P.; Köberlein-Neu, J. Economic burden of blindness and visual impairment in Germany from a societal perspective: A cost-of-illness study. *Eur. J. Health Econ.* **2020**, *21*, 115–127. [CrossRef] [PubMed]
14. GBD 2019 Blindness; Vision Impairment Collaborators; the Vision Loss Expert Group of the Global Burden of Disease Study. Causes of blindness and vision impairment in 2020 and trends over 30 years, and prevalence of avoidable blindness in relation to VISION 2020: The Right to Sight: An analysis for the Global Burden of Disease Study. *Lancet Glob. Health* **2021**, *9*, e144–e160. [CrossRef] [PubMed]
15. Burton, M.J.; Ramke, J.; Marques, A.P.; Bourne, R.R.A.; Congdon, N.; Jones, I.; Tong, B.A.M.A.; Arunga, S.; Bachani, D.; Bascaran, C.; et al. The Lancet Global Health Commission on Global Eye Health: Vision beyond 2020. *Lancet Glob. Health* **2021**, *9*, e489–e551. [CrossRef] [PubMed]
16. Klein, R.; Klein, B.E.K.; Cruickshanks, K.J. The prevalence of age-related maculopathy by geographic region and ethnicity1This paper has been edited by Neville N. Osborne, PhD, DSc, Nuffield Laboratory of Ophthalmology, University of Oxford, Walton Street, Oxford, UK; and Gerald J. Chader, The Foundation Fighting Blindness, Hunt Valley, MS.1. *Prog. Retin. Eye Res.* **1999**, *18*, 371–389. [CrossRef] [PubMed]
17. Mitchell, P.; Smith, W.; Attebo, K.; Wang, J.J. Prevalence of Age-related Maculopathy in Australia. *Ophthalmology* **1995**, *102*, 1450–1460. [CrossRef] [PubMed]
18. Kawasaki, R.; Yasuda, M.; Song, S.J.; Chen, S.-J.; Jonas, J.B.; Wang, J.J.; Mitchell, P.; Wong, T.Y. The Prevalence of Age-Related Macular Degeneration in Asians. *Ophthalmology* **2010**, *117*, 921–927. [CrossRef] [PubMed]
19. Wong, T.; Chakravarthy, U.; Klein, R.; Mitchell, P.; Zlateva, G.; Buggage, R.; Fahrbach, K.; Probst, C.; Sledge, I. The Natural History and Prognosis of Neovascular Age-Related Macular Degeneration. *Ophthalmology* **2008**, *115*, 116–126.e1. [CrossRef] [PubMed]
20. Wong, W.L.; Su, X.; Li, X.; Cheung, C.M.G.; Klein, R.; Cheng, C.Y.; Wong, T.Y. Global prevalence of age-related macular degeneration and disease burden projection for 2020 and 2040: A systematic review and meta-analysis. *Lancet Glob. Health* **2014**, *2*, e106–e116. [CrossRef]
21. Gheorghe, A.; Mahdi, L.; Musat, O. Age-Related Macular Degeneration. *Rom. J. Ophthalmol.* **2015**, *59*, 74–77.
22. Instituto Nacional de Estadística 2021; Encuesta de Discapacidad, Autonomía Personal y Situaciones de Dependencia 2020. Available online: https://www.ine.es/dyngs/INEbase/es/operacion.htm?c=Estadistica_C&cid=1254736176782&menu=resultados&idp=1254735573175#_tabs-1254736195764 (accessed on 2 February 2023).

23. Lin, X.; Lou, L.; Miao, Q.; Wang, Y.; Jin, K.; Shan, P.; Xu, Y. The pattern and gender disparity in global burden of age-related macular degeneration. *Eur. J. Ophthalmol.* **2021**, *31*, 1161–1170. [CrossRef] [PubMed]
24. Kansal, K.; Khan, H. Environmental factors and eye health: Protecting your vision in a changing world. *Int. J. Ophthalmol. Optometry* **2023**, *5*, 33–35. [CrossRef]
25. Swięch, A.; Dolar-Szczasny, J.; Wrobel-Dudzinska, D.; Kosior-Jarecka, E.; Mackiewicz, J. Quality of life among patients from urban and rural areas with advanced age-related macular degeneration assessed using the NEI-VFQ-25. *Ann. Agric. Environ. Med.* **2021**, *28*, 243–249. [CrossRef] [PubMed]
26. Bikbov, M.M.; Zainullin, R.M.; Gilmanshin, T.R.; Kazakbaeva, G.M.; Rakhimova, E.M.; Rusakova, I.A.; Bolshakova, N.I.; Safiullina, K.R.; Yakupova, D.F.; Uzianbaeva, Y.V.; et al. Prevalence and Associated Factors of Age-Related Macular Degeneration in a Russian Population: The Ural Eye and Medical Study. *Am. J. Ophthalmol.* **2020**, *210*, 146–157. [CrossRef] [PubMed]
27. Abdiyeva, Y.J. Prevalence of age-related macular degeneration of retina among rural and urban population of the western region of Azerbaijan. *Vestn. Oftalmol.* **2021**, *137*, 160. [CrossRef] [PubMed]
28. Ding, X.; Patel, M.; Chan, C.C. Molecular pathology of age-related macular degeneration. *Prog. Retin. Eye Res.* **2009**, *28*, 1–18. [CrossRef] [PubMed]
29. Matsuba, S.; Tabuchi, H.; Ohsugi, H.; Enno, H.; Ishitobi, N.; Masumoto, H.; Kiuchi, Y. Accuracy of ultra-wide-field fundus ophthalmoscopy-assisted deep learning, a machine-learning technology, for detecting age-related macular degeneration. *Int. Ophthalmol.* **2019**, *39*, 1269–1275. [CrossRef] [PubMed]
30. Schlecht, A.; Boneva, S.; Gruber, M.; Zhang, P.; Horres, R.; Bucher, F.; Auw-Haedrich, C.; Hansen, L.; Stahl, A.; Hilgendorf, I.; et al. Transcriptomic Characterization of Human Choroidal Neovascular Membranes Identifies Calprotectin as a Novel Biomarker for Patients with Age-Related Macular Degeneration. *Am. J. Pathol.* **2020**, *190*, 1632–1642. [CrossRef] [PubMed]
31. Sloan, F.A.; Hanrahan, B.W. The Effects of Technological Advances on Outcomes for Elderly Persons With Exudative Age-related Macular Degeneration. *JAMA Ophthalmol.* **2014**, *132*, 456. [CrossRef]
32. Wykoff, C.C.; Clark, W.L.; Nielsen, J.S.; Brill, J.V.; Greene, L.S.; Heggen, C.L. Optimizing Anti-VEGF Treatment Outcomes for Patients with Neovascular Age-Related Macular Degeneration. *J. Manag. Care Spec. Pharm.* **2018**, *24*, S3–S15. [CrossRef]
33. Prenner, J.L.; Halperin, L.S.; Rycroft, C.; Hogue, S.; Liu, Z.W.; Seibert, R. Disease Burden in the Treatment of Age-Related Macular Degeneration: Findings From a Time-and-Motion Study. *Am. J. Ophthalmol.* **2015**, *160*, 725–731.e1. [CrossRef] [PubMed]
34. Zorrilla-Muñoz, V.; Agulló-Tomás, M.S.; Forjaz, M.J.; Fernandez, E.; Rodriguez-Blazquez, C.; Ayala, A.; Fernandez-Mayoralas, G. Technology, Gender and COVID-19. Analysis of Perceived Health in Adults and Older People. In *Human Aspects of IT for the Aged Population. Supporting Everyday Life Activities*; Springer: Cham, Switzerland, 2021; pp. 363–379. [CrossRef]
35. O'connor, S.R.; Treanor, C.; Ward, E.; Wickens, R.A.; O'connell, A.; Culliford, L.A.; Rogers, C.A.; Gidman, E.A.; Peto, T.; Knox, P.C.; et al. Patient Acceptability of Home Monitoring for Neovascular Age-Related Macular Degeneration Reactivation: A Qualitative Study. *Int. J. Environ. Res. Public Health* **2022**, *19*, 13714. [CrossRef] [PubMed]
36. Deffler, R.A.; Xu, J.; Bittner, A.K.; Bowers, A.R.; Hassan, S.E.; Ross, N.; Cooley, S.-S.L.; Doubt, A.; Davidorf, F.H.; Dougherty, B.E. Use and Perceptions of Advanced Driver Assistance Systems by Older Drivers with and without Age-Related Macular Degeneration. *Transl. Vis. Sci. Technol.* **2022**, *11*, 22. [CrossRef] [PubMed]
37. Williams, R.A. The Psychosocial Impact of Macular Degeneration. *Arch. Ophthalmol.* **1998**, *116*, 514. [CrossRef] [PubMed]
38. Mitchell, J.; Bradley, C. Quality of life in age-related macular degeneration: A review of the literature. *Health Qual. Life Outcomes* **2006**, *4*, 97. [CrossRef] [PubMed]
39. Sanabria, M.R.; Calles-Monar, P.S.; Alonso-Tarancón, A.M.; Coco-Martín, R.M.; Mayo-Iscar, A. Impact of COVID-19 Confinement on Quality of Life of Patients with Age-Related Macular Degeneration: A Two-Wave Panel Study. *J. Clin. Med.* **2023**, *12*, 2394. [CrossRef] [PubMed]
40. Van Vu, K.; Mitchell, P.; Detaram, H.D.; Burlutsky, G.; Liew, G.; Gopinath, B. Risk factors for poorer quality of life in patients with neovascular age-related macular degeneration: A longitudinal clinic-based study. *Eye* **2023**, *37*, 2736–2743. [CrossRef] [PubMed]
41. Roque, A.B.; da Silva Borges, G.F.; Abe, R.Y.; de Souza, O.F.; Machado, M.C.; Ferreira, T.; José, N.K.; de Vasconcellos, J.P.C. The effects of age-related macular degeneration on quality of life in a Brazilian population. *Int. J. Retina Vitreous* **2021**, *7*, 20. [CrossRef] [PubMed]
42. Man, R.E.K.; Gan, A.T.L.; Fenwick, E.K.; Teo, K.Y.C.; Tan, A.C.; Cheung, G.C.M.; Teo, Z.L.; Kumari, N.; Wong, T.Y.; Lamoureux, E.L.; et al. Impact of incident age-related macular degeneration and associated vision loss on vision-related quality of life. *Br. J. Ophthalmol.* **2022**, *106*, 1063–1068. [CrossRef]
43. Van Nispen, R.M.; de Boer, M.R.; Hoeijmakers, J.G.; Ringens, P.J.; van Rens, G.H. Co-morbidity and visual acuity are risk factors for health-related quality of life decline: Five-month follow-up EQ-5D data of visually impaired older patients. *Health Qual. Life Outcomes* **2009**, *7*, 18. [CrossRef]
44. Marín, B.P.; Paniagua, N.M.G.; Gómez-Baldó, L.; Gallego-Pinazo, R. Burden of disease assessment in patients with neovascular age-related macular degeneration in Spain: Results of the AMD-MANAGE study. *Eur. J. Ophthalmol.* **2022**, *32*, 385–394. [CrossRef] [PubMed]
45. Cimas, M.; Ayala, A.; Sanz, B.; Agulló-Tomás, M.S.; Escobar, A.; Forjaz, M.J. Chronic musculoskeletal pain in European older adults: Cross-national and gender differences. *Eur. J. Pain* **2018**, *22*, 333–345. [CrossRef] [PubMed]
46. Metz, D.H. Mobility of older people and their quality of life. *Transp. Policy (Oxf.)* **2000**, *7*, 149–152. [CrossRef]

47. Zorrilla-Muñoz, V.; García-Sedano, T.; Agulló-Tomás, M.S. Análisis socio-ergonómico en la agricultura. Evaluación del sector oleico desde una perspectiva de género y envejecimiento. *Inf. Tec. Econ. Agrar.* **2019**, *115*, 83–104. [CrossRef]
48. Stevens, G.A.; White, R.A.; Flaxman, S.R.; Price, H.; Jonas, J.B.; Keeffe, J.; Leasher, J.; Naidoo, K.; Pesudovs, K.; Resnikoff, S.; et al. Global Prevalence of Vision Impairment and Blindness. *Ophthalmology* **2013**, *120*, 2377–2384. [CrossRef] [PubMed]
49. Møller, A.P.; Fincher, C.L.; Thornhill, R. Why men have shorter lives than women: Effects of resource availability, infectious disease, and senescence. *Am. J. Hum. Biol.* **2009**, *21*, 357–364. [CrossRef] [PubMed]
50. Zetterberg, M. Age-related eye disease and gender. *Maturitas* **2016**, *83*, 19–26. [CrossRef]
51. Zorrilla-Muñoz, V.; Veira-Ramos, A.; Agulló-Tomás, M.S.; Garcia-Aracil, N.; Fernandez, E. Effectiveness of Support Programmes for (in)Formal Caregivers of Older Dependent People to Design Technologies. In *Human Aspects of IT for the Aged Population*; Gao, Q., Zhou, J., Eds.; HCII 2023; Lecture Notes in Computer Science; Springer: Cham, Switzerland, 2023; Volume 14043. [CrossRef]
52. Cruceanu, G.L.; Clemente-Belmonte, S.; Herrero-Sanz, R.; Ayala, A.; Zorrilla-Muñoz, V.; Agulló-Tomás, M.S.; Martínez-Miguelez, C.; Fernández-Mayoralas, G. Evaluation of Older People Digital Images: Representations from a Land, Gender and Anti-ageist Perspective. *Land* **2022**, *12*, 18. [CrossRef]
53. Quesada, B.C.; Muñoz, V.Z.; Tomás, M.S.A. El uso de tecnologías de asistencia sanitaria digital por parte de la población mayor desde una perspectiva de género e intrageneracional. *Teknokultura. Rev. Cult. Digit. Mov. Soc.* **2021**, *18*, 103–113. [CrossRef]
54. Mikołajczyk, B. Universal human rights instruments and digital literacy of older persons. *Int. J. Hum. Rights* **2023**, *27*, 403–424. [CrossRef]
55. Orr, P.; Rentz, A.M.; Margolis, M.K.; Revicki, D.A.; Dolan, C.M.; Colman, S.; Fine, J.T.; Bressler, N.M. Validation of the National Eye Institute Visual Function Questionnaire-25 (NEI VFQ-25) in Age-Related Macular Degeneration. *Investig. Opthalmol. Vis. Sci.* **2011**, *52*, 3354. [CrossRef] [PubMed]
56. Mathew, R.S.; Delbaere, K.; Lord, S.R.; Beaumont, P.; Vaegan; Madigan, M.C. Depressive symptoms and quality of life in people with age-related macular degeneration. *Ophthalmic Physiol. Opt.* **2011**, *31*, 375–380. [CrossRef] [PubMed]
57. Henning-Smith, C. The Unique Impact of COVID-19 on Older Adults in Rural Areas. *J. Aging Soc. Policy* **2020**, *32*, 396–402. [CrossRef] [PubMed]
58. Fuller, H.R.; Huseth-Zosel, A. Older Adults' Loneliness in Early COVID-19 Social Distancing: Implications of Rurality. *J. Gerontol. Ser. B* **2022**, *77*, e100–e105. [CrossRef] [PubMed]
59. Zhao, Y.; Zhang, T.; Dasgupta, R.K.; Xia, R. Narrowing the age-based digital divide: Developing digital capability through social activities. *Inf. Syst. J.* **2023**, *33*, 268–298. [CrossRef]
60. Tirado-Morueta, R.; Rodríguez-Martín, A.; Álvarez-Arregui, E.; Ortíz-Sobrino, M.Á.; Aguaded-Gómez, J.I. The digital inclusion of older people in Spain: Technological support services for seniors as predictor. *Ageing Soc.* **2023**, *43*, 1409–1435. [CrossRef]
61. Hwang, J.; Kim, K.H.; Hwang, J.G.; Jun, S.; Yu, J.; Lee, C. Technological Opportunity Analysis: Assistive Technology for Blind and Visually Impaired People. *Sustainability* **2020**, *12*, 8689. [CrossRef]
62. LaMonica, H.M.; Davenport, T.A.; Roberts, A.E.; Hickie, I.B. Understanding Technology Preferences and Requirements for Health Information Technologies Designed to Improve and Maintain the Mental Health and Well-Being of Older Adults: Participatory Design Study. *JMIR Aging* **2021**, *4*, e21461. [CrossRef]
63. Armstrong, G.W.; Miller, J.B. Telemedicine for the Diagnosis and Management of Age-Related Macular Degeneration: A Review. *J. Clin. Med.* **2022**, *11*, 835. [CrossRef]
64. Perepelkina, T.; Fulton, A.B. Aplicaciones de inteligencia artificial (IA) para la degeneración macular relacionada con la edad (DMAE) y otras distrofias de retina. *Semin. Ophthalmol.* **2021**, *36*, 304–309. [CrossRef]
65. Russell, C.D.; Lone, N.I.; Baillie, J.K. Comorbidities, multimorbidity and COVID-19. *Nat. Med.* **2023**, *29*, 334–343. [CrossRef] [PubMed]
66. Chatterjee, S.; Nalla, L.V.; Sharma, M.; Sharma, N.; Singh, A.A.; Malim, F.M.; Ghatage, M.; Mukarram, M.; Pawar, A.; Parihar, N.; et al. Association of COVID-19 with Comorbidities: An Update. *ACS Pharmacol. Transl. Sci.* **2023**, *6*, 334–354. [CrossRef] [PubMed]
67. Florea, A.; Wu, J.; Qian, L.; Lewin, B.; Sy, L.S.; Lin, I.-C.; Ku, J.H.; Tseng, H.F. Risk of herpes zoster following mRNA COVID-19 vaccine administration. *Expert Rev. Vaccines* **2023**, *22*, 643–649. [CrossRef]

European Journal of
Investigation in Health, Psychology and Education

MDPI

Article

Associations of eHealth Literacy with Social Activity among Community-Dwelling Older Adults: A Cross-Sectional Study

Mamiko Eto [1] and Koji Yamatsu [1,2,3,*]

1 Graduate School of Medical Science, Saga University, Saga 849-8502, Japan; mamiko.eto@mark-lab.net
2 Graduate School of Advanced Health Sciences, Saga University, Saga 849-8502, Japan
3 Faculty of Education, Saga University, Saga 840-8502, Japan
* Correspondence: kyamatsu@cc.saga-u.ac.jp; Tel.: +81-952-28-8302

Abstract: Older adults who use digital technology are desired to adapt to digitalization and literacy. One required aspect is eHealth literacy, measured with the eHealth Literacy Scale (eHEALS). Many studies on eHealth literacy have used the eHEALS to examine the health behaviors of college students, relatively younger adults, and Internet users. However, the relevance of eHealth literacy to social activity has not yet been studied in older adults. The purposes of this study were to examine the relationship between eHealth literacy and health behaviors and social activities (community, cultural, and sports activities) and to investigate the factors associated with eHEALS scores among community-dwelling older adults. The mean eHEALS score was 12.4 points (SD 8.2), with the majority (73.3%) having the lowest score (the lowest score is 8 points). Males (17.6, SD 10.5) scored significantly higher than females (11.8, SD 7.7). The eHEALS score had a significant relationship with both cultural and community activity. Five factors significantly associated with having the lowest eHEALS score were cultural activity at least once a week, no cultural activity, no community activity, total IADL score, and intellectual activity. These results suggest that eHealth literacy is associated with community activity and cultural activity among older adults.

Keywords: digital health literacy; eHealth Literacy Scale; sports activity; cultural activity; community activity; health behavior; frailty; elderly

1. Introduction

The percentage of the global population aged 65 years and older is expected to increase from 10% in 2022 to 16% in 2050 [1]. The population of Japan was already 29% as of 2021 [2]. Advances in public health and medicine have helped many people to live longer and healthier lives [3]. However, not all older adults are healthy. In an aging society, healthy life expectancy is desired to extend while curbing rising healthcare expenditures without reducing the quality of healthcare services [4]. The increasing older adult population means that more people need healthcare simultaneously; this needs to be addressed using the benefits of digital technology [5]. Digital technology has great potential for addressing healthcare needs and transforming many aspects of geriatric care [6]. Older adults benefit from digital technology, including increased communication, increased activity, and improved health [7]. The COVID-19 pandemic has been a major turning point in the benefits of the use of digital technology by older adults, and the digitalization of everyday life has been accelerated. Since there is a possibility that a pandemic caused by such an infectious disease will occur in the future, it is necessary to urgently promote the acquisition and penetration of digital technology among older adults in order to be prepared. For community-dwelling older adults, digitization benefits healthcare, enhances daily life convenience, and helps to gather information during disasters [8]. Older adults need the skills and knowledge to use digital technologies [9].

Older adults are not proficient in using digital technology. According to a survey conducted by the Japan Ministry of Internal Affairs and Communications in 2020, the usage rate among older adults was low, at 86.8% for those aged 60–69, 65.5% for those aged 70–79, and 33.2% for those aged 80 and older, with over 80% of those aged 60–69 feeling uneasy about using the Internet [10]. Approximately 34% of older Internet users said they were not confident in their ability to use digital devices, and 48% said they needed someone to set up or teach them how to use them [11]. Despite the reported benefits of Internet use among older adults in improving cognitive function, social well-being [12], and loneliness [13], older adults have few opportunities to benefit from online digital technologies related to health maintenance. The disparity among older adults regarding access to and adaptation to digital technologies is known as the gray digital divide [14]. This gray digital divide constitutes a major concern shared by United Nations Economic Commission for Europe (UNECE) countries, affecting aging populations at both the individual and societal levels [15].

Older adults need eHealth literacy and digital abilities and skills to eliminate the digital divide in health. Acquiring eHealth literacy has an impact on individuals' treatment decision-making style [16]. As eHealth literacy improves, the ability to use online health resources improves [17]. eHealth literacy is a foundational competency in using digital technologies. In increasingly digitalized healthcare, individuals must manage and utilize electronic health records and welfare service information at the individual level, allowing them to take the initiative in making choices and managing their health [4]. Therefore, minimal eHealth literacy is necessary.

eHealth literacy refers to the ability to use digital health and electronic information. This is referred to as digital health literacy. Norman and Skinner defined "the concept of eHealth literacy as the ability to seek, find, understand, and appraise health information from electronic sources and apply the knowledge gained to address or solve health problems. eHealth literacy combines facets of different literacy skills and applies them to eHealth promotion and care. At its heart are six core skills (or literacies): traditional literacy, health literacy, information literacy, scientific literacy, media literacy, and computer literacy (the Lily Model) [18]". The eHealth Literacy Scale (eHEALS) is defined as a set of skills needed to use information technology for health effectively [19]. The eHEALS is often used as a measure of eHealth literacy [20]. The Japanese version of the eHEALS has also been developed and validated for reliability and validity [21].

Most studies on eHealth literacy have reported on health behaviors [20,22–27]. Many studies have found that eHealth literacy is associated with health behaviors, but many have focused on youth [22–25]. Despite the claimed need for digital health technologies, few studies on eHealth literacy exist for older adults. eHealth literacy is important for addressing health issues and supporting longevity through digital technologies. Therefore, this study investigated whether eHealth literacy among older adults is associated with health behaviors. Besides general health behaviors, the "Dietary Variety Score (DVS)" was added in this study. The DVS has been widely used to assess the eating behaviors of Japanese older adults [28]. The combination of food diversity, physical activity, and social interactions was highly effective in preventing disabilities in older adults [29], and ingesting various foods prevented a decrease in the independence of higher life functions of older adults living in the community [28].

eHealth literacy has also been associated with improved health status [30,31]. As decreased independence was associated with life expectancy [32], the 13 items of the Instrumental Activities of Daily Living (IADL) [33] developed by Koyano based on the Lawton assessment method [34] were employed in this study. Furthermore, we also investigated the association with frailty [35], a condition of increased vulnerability to health problems due to various age-related functional changes, and loss of reserve capacity using the revised Japanese version of the Cardiovascular Health Study (J-CHS) criteria [36]. In previous studies, the health status of older adults has mostly been determined by self-report [30,31,37]. Therefore, we adopted objective frailty assessments with confirmed validity and reliability to examine the relationship with eHealth literacy. This is a new finding, as no study has investigated an association between eHealth literacy and frailty.

In older adults, social activity effectively maintains health and improves health behaviors and statuses. Social activity prevented functional disability [38–42], cognitive decline [43,44], and mortality [42,45]. Although social activity has contributed to health outcomes in older adults, to our knowledge, no study has examined the association between eHealth literacy and social activities. Kanamori et al. classified social activities into eight types: neighborhood associations/senior citizen clubs/firefighting teams (local community), hobby groups (hobbies), sports groups or clubs (sports), political organizations or groups (politics), industrial or trade associations (industry), religious organizations or groups (religion), volunteer groups (volunteer), and citizen or consumer groups (citizen) [46]. Participation in local communities, hobbies, sports, or organizations may be especially effective in decreasing the risk of disability [46]. According to the Cabinet Office of Japan, social activities in older adults aged 65 and over include sports activities such as gymnastics and gateball, hobbies including haiku and shigin, and community activities including festivals [2]. These activities allow older adults to communicate with others and feel connected to society. Therefore, this study focused on three types of activities: sports, cultural activities including hobbies, and community activities. Findings from this study can provide basic information about future eHealth literacy among older adults. Moreover, the results of this study can provide basic information about eHealth literacy in the design of future health care, public policy, and programs for older adults, and can guide ways to improve eHealth literacy among older adults.

The purposes of this study were to investigate the relationship between eHealth literacy and health behaviors and social activities (community, cultural, and sports activities) among community-dwelling older adults in Japan and to identify factors associated with eHEALS scores among older adults. In particular, we hypothesized that eHealth literacy would be associated with all three types of social activities in community-dwelling older adults. Furthermore, we attempted to exploratorily examine predictors of eHealth literacy among many variables.

2. Research Methods

2.1. Study Design and Sampling

This cross-sectional study was conducted in Miyaki town, Saga Prefecture, Japan, a rural municipality with approximately 25,000 people. The participants in this study were 630 residents of Miyaki town aged 41–99 years. The recruitment method for this study was to provide information in the town newspaper, to participants in public health classes for older adults held in the town, and to general residents. eHealth literacy has never been explained or discussed in public health classes. Therefore, the target of this study was not a representative population of Miyaki town. All subjects received an explanation of the study and signed written consent. Of 630 residents, 561 aged 65 years or older were included in the analysis. Exclusion criteria were lack of consent, age 64 years or younger, missing eHEALS response items, missing social activity, health behavior, and health status items, and missing other variables. After excluding 69 participants with incomplete responses, data from 561 older adults were used for the analysis.

2.2. The Measurement Procedure

The measurement was conducted from October to December 2021 in 56 districts with small groups of 5 to 15 participants. The reason why the number of people to be measured was set at 5 people at a minimum and 15 people at a maximum was because the measurement location was sometimes a small community center, and consideration was given to the safety of the measurement and the waiting time of the subjects. All participants were asked to complete a questionnaire. Physical fitness and body composition were measured by trained research staff. At the end of the measurement, participants received a 10 min explanation so that they understood their own physical fitness and health status. Owing to the worldwide spread of COVID-19 in 2021, the measurement was conducted with thorough infection prevention measures in place.

2.3. Measurements

2.3.1. eHealth Literacy Level (eHEALS)

The Japanese version of the eHEALS [21] was used. The eHEALS was developed to measure consumers' combined knowledge, comfort, and perceived skills in finding, evaluating, and applying electronic health information to health problems [19]. The eHEALS consists of eight questions answered on a 5-point Likert scale ranging from "strongly disagree (1)" to "strongly agree (5)" for each question item. The total score of the eight items ranges from 8 [minimum] to 40 [maximum] points [21].

2.3.2. Social Activity

Social activity was divided into three categories based on the study by Kanamori et al. [46]. In this study, sports activity included ground golf, gateball, walking, and community-sponsored exercise classes for health, which were mainly physical activities. Cultural activity included karaoke, dance, computer classes, Go, calligraphy, cooking classes, and senior citizen colleges. Community activity, such as neighborhood and senior citizen associations, were defined as activities that occurred in the town. Social activity was converted into dummy variables and used in the analysis. Respondents were asked to select one of the following five options for frequency of participation: "almost every day", "a few times a week", "once a week", "once or twice a month", or "non". The responses obtained were divided into three categories: "at least once a week", "once or twice a month", or "non". In cultural activity example, cultural activity can be divided into two different variables (Figure 1). The first was to calculate the odds ratio using the variable "Cultural activity at least once a week" as an event and the variable "Cultural activity less than once a week" as a reference. Second, the variable "No cultural activity" was used as an event, and "almost every day", "at least once a week", "once or twice a month", and "non" are grouped together as a reference (Figure 1).

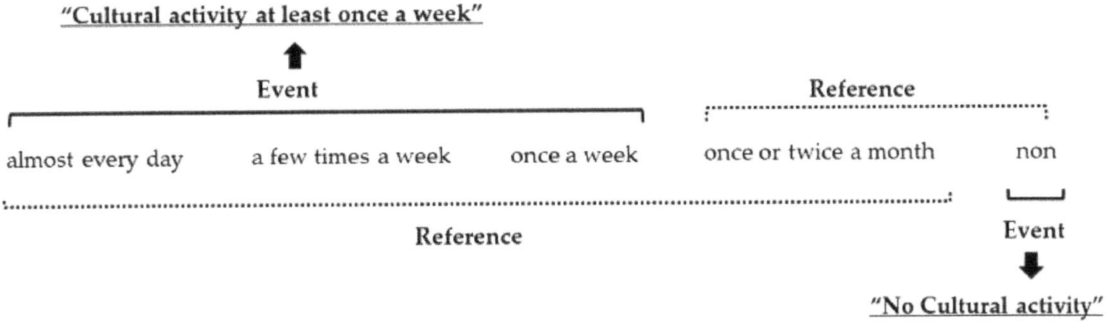

Figure 1. Definition when converting social activity into dummy variables.

2.3.3. Health Behavior

Health behaviors were assessed using questions on balanced food intake and smoking regarding previous studies that reported associations with eHealth literacy [22–25]. In addition, going out at least once a week (yes or no) and a sitting time of at least 8 h a weekday (yes or no) were added. The Japanese government advocates nutrition, food, physical activity, and smoking as important health behaviors for improving lifestyle and reducing risk factors in the policies of the Second National Health Promotion Campaign (Healthy Japan 21) [47]. Responses were dichotomized into yes or no for smoking, physical activity, going out once a week, and sitting time of at least 8 h a weekday according to the advice most commonly offered in Japanese public health settings [48]. Physical activity adopted sports activity in social activity.

The DVS was used to assess balanced foods. The DVS was assessed by the frequency of daily food intake of 10 selected food groups: meat, seafood, eggs, milk, soy products, green and yellow vegetables, seaweed, fruits, potatoes, and fats and oils [28]. The scores range from 0 to 10, with higher scores indicating greater dietary diversity [28].

Sitting time was asked: "How much time do you usually spend at rest without physical activity, sitting or lying down every day, in total per day?" Responses were answered yes or no to "Sitting time at least 8 hours a weekday".

2.3.4. Health Status

The IADL, body mass index (BMI), and frailty were assessed. Data on self-reported disease, single fall, and multiple falls were also included in the analysis.

The IADL is a 13-item index developed by Koyano [33] based on Lawton's evaluation method [34]. The IADL comprised five items for "Instrumental self-maintenance", four items for "Intellectual activity", and four items for "Social role". The 13 questions were self-administered and required a "yes (1 point)" or "no (0 point)" response; the higher the score, the more independent the IADL. The IADL refers to complex activities in daily life, such as shopping, coordination, laundry, telephone, medication management, property management, use of public transportation, etc. [47].

BMI was calculated as the weight divided by the height squared (kg/m^2) from actual height and weight measurements. BMI was used as a proxy for long-term health behavior. We categorized participants as "obesity ($\geq$25 kg/m^2)" or "non-obesity" based on BMI. We also used separate classifications of "thin (<18.5 kg/m^2)" or "non-thin" [49].

The J-CHS criteria were used as the diagnostic criteria for frailty. The J-CHS is based on the Fried phenotype model [50], modified for older Japanese individuals. The J-CHS includes five elements: (1) unintentional weight loss, (2) weakness (grip strength), (3) exhaustion, (4) slowness (normal gait speed), and (5) low physical activity [36]. (1) Unintentional weight loss was defined as a "yes" response to the question "Did you unintentionally lose 2 to 3 kg or more in 6 months?". (2) Weakness was assessed using grip strength. Grip strength was measured by having one person grip the measuring device twice on each side with maximum effort. A maximum of four grip strength values was used for the analysis. The cutoff values were 28 kg for males and 18 kg or less for females. (3) Exhaustion was defined as a "yes" response to the question "I feel tired for no reason for the past two weeks?". (4) Slowness was assessed using gait speed. The participants were asked to walk a distance of 11 m once at their usual walking speed. The measuring staff used a stopwatch to measure the time required to move 5 m on the way from the 3 m to the 8 m point. Normal gait speed was calculated as "5 m divided by the number of seconds required to move". (5) Low physical activity was defined as "Do you do light exercise or physical training?" and "Do you engage in regular exercise/sports?", and the two questions were asked. Both questions were applied to those who answered "no". In the J-CHS criteria, we categorized cases that apply answered "no" to all five items as "robust", cases that apply to one or two items as "pre-frailty", and cases that apply to three or more items as "frailty" [36].

Regarding pre-existing medical conditions, we asked if there were any diseases being treated and the types of diseases. When asked if they had fallen within the past year, those who answered no were treated as "no", those who had fallen once were treated as "single fall", and those who had fallen more than once were treated as "multiple falls".

3. Statistical Analysis

Comparisons of gender differences in participant characteristics were analyzed using Student's *t*-test or the chi-square test.

The association between the eHEALS and social activities was verified using logistic regression analysis. The independent variable was the eHEALS, which was used here as a continuous variable. The dependent variable was social activity, which is defined as a dummy variable. The associations between the eHEALS and health behaviors (dummy variable) or health status (dummy variable) were analyzed in the same way. Odds ratio (OR) and 95% confidence interval (95%CI) were calculated with logistic regression analysis.

In verifying the predictors of the eHEALS, 73.3% of all subjects had the lowest eHEALS score of 8 points, so a logistic regression analysis was performed using the lowest eHEALS score (dummy variable) as the dependent variable. At that time, those who did not have the lowest eHEALS score were used as reference. Because this analysis was an exploratory study, we examined a number of factors that could predict who would score the lowest on the eHEALS.

Logistic regression analysis first examined the association between the eHEALS and other factors (such as social activity) but ultimately statistically adjusted for age and gender (with males as the reference).

The significance level was set at less than 5%.

4. Results

4.1. Baseline Characteristics

The overall mean age was 76.9 years (SD 5.9), with males having a mean age of 75.3 years (SD 6.2) and females having a mean age of 77.1 years (SD 5.8), and females had a significantly higher mean age ($p < 0.05$) (Table 1). Participants were 561 older adults: 60 (10.7%) males and 501 (89.3%) females. The age distribution of the participants was 13 in the 65–69 age group, 335 in the 70–79 age group, 198 in the 80–89 age group, and 15 aged 90 or above.

In social activity, males were more likely than females to be involved in community activity at least once a week. There were no gender differences in sports activity and cultural activity. Sports activity was performed at least once a week by 356 respondents (63.5%). Cultural activity was answered "non" by 408 (72.7%) respondents.

The DVS had a mean score of 6.2 (SD 2.4). The DVS was 4.9 (SD 2.5) among males and 6.3 (SD 2.3) among females. Females' DVS was significantly higher than males ($p < 0.001$).

Regarding smoking habits, 548 participants (97.7%) were nonsmokers. Regarding the presence of diseases, 493 participants (87.9%) reported having chronic conditions. The types of diseases included 16 cases of cancer, 58 cases of heart disease, 5 cases of stroke, 238 cases of hypertension, 62 cases of diabetes, 22 cases of obesity, 169 cases of hyperlipidemia, 154 cases of osteoporosis, 73 cases of joint pain or neuropathy, 16 cases of injury or fracture, 40 cases of respiratory disease, 14 cases of gastrointestinal disease, and 4 cases of liver disease. However, no significant correlation was observed between the number of diseases and the eHEALS score.

Other characteristics of the subjects are also shown in the table (Table 1).

Table 1. Participant characteristics.

Characteristic	Total (n = 561)		Male (n = 60)		Female (n = 501)		
	Mean	(SD)	Mean	(SD)	Mean	(SD)	p
Age (years)	76.9	(5.9)	75.3	(6.2)	77.1	(5.8)	0.024
Dietary Variety Score (points)	6.2	(2.4)	4.9	(2.5)	6.3	(2.3)	<0.001
IADL Total score (points)	12.2	(1.5)	12.2	(1.4)	12.2	(1.5)	0.876
Instrumental Self-maintenance (points)	4.9	(0.6)	4.9	(0.6)	4.9	(0.6)	0.870
Intellectual Activity (points)	3.7	(0.7)	3.7	(0.7)	3.7	(0.7)	0.607
Social Role (points)	3.6	(0.8)	3.6	(0.7)	3.6	(0.8)	0.790
Body Mass Index (kg/m^2)	23.2	(3.3)	24.3	(2.9)	23.1	(3.3)	0.010
Grip strength (kg)	26.3	(6.7)	39.6	(6.9)	24.8	(4.7)	<0.001
Gait Speed (m/s)	1.30	(0.27)	1.34	(0.29)	1.29	(0.27)	0.251

Table 1. *Cont.*

	Characteristic	n	(%)	n	(%)	n	(%)	*p*
Gender	Male	60	(10.7)					
	Female	501	(89.3)					
Social Activity								
Cultural Activity	at least once a week	73	(13.0)	7	(11.7)	66	(13.2)	0.327
	once or twice a month	80	(14.3)	5	(8.3)	75	(15.0)	
	non (no activity)	408	(72.7)	48	(80.0)	360	(71.9)	
Community Activity	at least once a week	91	(16.2)	22	(36.7)	69	(13.8)	<0.001
	once or twice a month	206	(36.7)	27	(45.0)	179	(35.7)	
	non (no activity)	264	(47.1)	11	(18.3)	253	(50.5)	
Sports Activity	at least once a week	356	(63.5)	39	(65.0)	317	(63.3)	0.320
	once or twice a month	185	(33.0)	17	(28.3)	168	(33.5)	
	non (no activity)	20	(3.6)	4	(6.7)	16	(3.2)	
Health Behavior								
Going out at least once a week	Yes	553	(98.6)	60	(100.0)	493	(98.4)	0.324
	No	8	(1.4)	0	(0.0)	8	(1.6)	
Sitting time at least 8 hours a weekday	Yes	20	(3.6)	2	(3.3)	18	(3.6)	0.918
	No	541	(96.4)	58	(96.7)	483	(96.4)	
Smoking	Yes	13	(2.3)	3	(5.0)	10	(2.0)	0.144
	No	548	(97.7)	57	(95.0)	491	(98.0)	
Health Status								
Obesity	Yes	155	(27.6)	23	(38.3)	132	(26.3)	0.050
	No	406	(72.4)	37	(61.7)	367	(73.3)	
Thin	Yes	40	(7.1)	2	(3.3)	38	(7.6)	0.227
	No	521	(92.9)	58	(96.7)	463	(92.4)	
Robust	Yes	364	(64.9)	39	(65.0)	325	(64.9)	0.984
	No	197	(35.1)	21	(35.0)	176	(35.1)	
Pre-frailty	Yes	185	(33.0)	21	(35.0)	164	(32.7)	0.724
	No	376	(67.0)	39	(65.0)	337	(67.3)	
Pre-frailty or Frailty	Yes	197	(35.1)	21	(35.0)	176	(35.1)	0.984
	No	364	(64.9)	39	(65.0)	325	(64.9)	
Weakness	Yes	32	(5.7)	1	(13.3)	31	(11.4)	0.154
	No	529	(94.3)	59	(86.7)	470	(88.6)	
Slowness	Yes	67	(11.9)	6	(10.0)	61	(12.2)	0.623
	No	494	(88.1)	54	(90.0)	440	(87.8)	
Unintentional Weight loss	Yes	65	(11.6)	8	(13.3)	57	(11.4)	0.655
	No	496	(88.4)	52	(86.7)	444	(88.6)	
Exhaustion	Yes	82	(14.6)	8	(13.3)	74	(14.8)	0.766
	No	479	(85.4)	52	(86.7)	427	(85.2)	
Low physical activity	Yes	37	(6.6)	5	(8.3)	32	(6.4)	0.566
	No	524	(93.4)	55	(91.7)	469	(93.6)	
Desease	Yes	493	(87.9)	51	(85.0)	442	(88.2)	0.470
	No	68	(12.1)	9	(15.0)	59	(11.8)	
Single fall	Yes	146	(26.0)	11	(18.3)	135	(26.9)	0.151
	No	415	(74.0)	49	(81.7)	369	(73.7)	
Multiple falls	Yes	34	(6.1)	2	(3.3)	32	(6.4)	0.349
	No	527	(93.9)	58	(96.7)	469	(93.6)	

4.2. eHealth Literacy Level

The mean eHEALS score was 12.4 points (SD, 8.2) (Table 2). Males, at 17.6 points (SD 10.5), scored higher than females, at 11.8 points (SD 7.7) ($p < 0.001$). The mean scores for each eHEALS item ranged from 1.5 (0.9) to 1.6 points (1.2) (males: 2.1–2.3, females: 1.4–1.5). There were no differences in most questionnaire items. The eHEALS scores were significantly higher for males across all eight items ($p < 0.001$). From the reliability statistics, Cronbach's alpha for eight items in the eHEALS was 0.985.

Table 2. The eHEALS scores in this study.

Characteristic	Total (n = 561)		Male (n = 60)		Female (n = 501)		
	Mean	(SD)	Mean	(SD)	Mean	(SD)	*p*
eHEALS (points)	12.4	(8.2)	17.6	(10.5)	11.8	(7.7)	<0.001
Q1. I know what health resources are available on the internet.	1.6	(1.2)	2.3	(1.4)	1.5	(1.1)	<0.001
Q2. I know where to find helpful health resources on the internet.	1.6	(1.1)	2.3	(1.4)	1.5	(1.1)	<0.001
Q3. I know how to find helpful health resources on the internet.	1.6	(1.1)	2.2	(1.5)	1.5	(1.1)	<0.001
Q4. I know how to use the internet to answer my questions about health.	1.6	(1.1)	2.3	(1.4)	1.5	(1.1)	<0.001
Q5. I know how to use the health information I find on the internet to help me.	1.6	(1.1)	2.2	(1.4)	1.5	(1.0)	<0.001
Q6. I have the skills I need to evaluate the health resources I find on the internet.	1.5	(1.0)	2.2	(1.4)	1.4	(0.9)	<0.001
Q7. I can tell high-quality health resources from low-quality health resources on the internet.	1.5	(0.9)	2.1	(1.3)	1.4	(0.9)	<0.001
Q8. I feel confident in using information from the Internet to make health decisions.	1.5	(1.0)	2.1	(1.3)	1.4	(0.9)	<0.001
Characteristic	**n**	**(%)**	**n**	**(%)**	**n**	**(%)**	***p***
eHEALS Score 8 (Lowest point)	411	(73.3)	28	(46.7)	383	(76.4)	<0.001
9–40 (point)	150	(26.7)	32	(53.3)	118	(23.6)	

Overall, the number of participants with the lowest eHEALS score (8 points) was the majority (73.3%). Females (76.4%) were significantly more likely to have a lower eHEALS score than males (46.7%, $p < 0.001$). The highest eHEALS score (40 points) was obtained in four female participants.

4.3. Association of eHEALS Score with Social Activity

As a result of logistic regression analysis, significant associations were found between eHEALS score and two types of social activities (Table 3). The eHEALS score was positively associated with cultural activity at least once a week (OR: 1.037, 95%CI: 1.007–1.068) and negatively associated with no cultural activity (OR: 0.955, 95%CI: 0.933–0.977). Also, the eHEALS score was positively associated with community activity at least once a week (OR: 1.031, 95%CI: 1.003–1.059) and negatively associated with no community activity (OR: 0.971, 95%CI: 0.949–0.994). Regarding sports activity, no association with eHEALS score was observed.

Table 3. Relationship between eHEALS (continuous variable) and Social Activity.

Social Activity	Unadjusted OR (95%CI)	Adjusted $ OR (95%CI)
Cultural Activityat least once a week (No)	1.029 (1.002–1.057) *	1.037 (1.007–1.068) *
No Cultural Activity (At lesat once or twice a month)	0.962 (0.942–0.983) *	0.955 (0.933–0.977) *
Community Activity at least once a week (No)	1.040 (1.015–1.065) *	1.031 (1.003–1.059) *
No Community Activity (At lesat once or twice a month)	0.959 (0.938–0.980) *	0.971 (0.949–0.994) *
Sports Activity at least once a week (No)	1.020 (0.998–1.042)	1.019 (0.995–1.043)
No Sports Activity (At lesat once or twice a month)	1.010 (0.960–1.063)	1.009 (0.954–1.068)

OR, odds ratio; CI, confidence interval; * $p < 0.05$; $ Adjusted for age and gender; The notation in parentheses indicates a reference.

4.4. Association of eHEALS Score with Health Behavior

eHEALS score was not associated with the DVS (Table 4). There were no associations between eHealth literacy and health behaviors.

Table 4. Relationships between eHEALS (continuous variable) and Health Behavior or status.

	Unadjusted OR (95%CI)	Adjusted $ OR (95%CI)
Health Behavior		
Dietary Variety Score #	0.993 (0.973–1.014)	1.005 (0.983–1.028)
Going out at least once a week (No)	1.101 (0.919–1.318)	1.032 (0.862–1.235)
Sitting time at least 8 h a weekday (No)	0.970 (0.908–1.037)	0.960 (0.894–1.031)
Smoking (Yes)	1.016 (0.956–1.080)	1.004 (0.939–1.075)
Health Status		
IADL Total score #	1.045 (1.020–1.069) *	1.032 (1.006–1.058) *
Instrumental Self-maintenance #	1.072 (1.013–1.134) *	1.044 (0.984–1.107)
Intellectual Activity #	1.049 (1.017–1.083) *	1.040 (1.006–1.074) *
Social Role #	1.031 (1.004–1.059) *	1.021 (0.992–1.051)
Body Mass Index #	0.999 (0.979–1.019)	0.988 (0.966–1.010)
Obesity (No)	1.007 (0.985–1.029)	0.998 (0.974–1.022)
Thin (No)	0.995 (0.956–1.036)	1.008 (0.966–1.052)
Robust (No)	1.032 (1.009–1.057) *	1.016 (0.991–1.042)
Pre-frailty (No)	0.973 (0.951–0.996) *	0.985 (0.960–1.010)
Pre-frailty or Frailty (No)	0.969 (0.946–0.991) *	0.984 (0.960–1.009)
Weakness (No)	0.924 (0.856–0.998) *	0.967 (0.894–1.046)
Slowness (No)	0.944 (0.903–0.988) *	0.985 (0.939–1.033)
Unintentional Weight loss (No)	0.977 (0.943–1.013)	0.983 (0.946–1.022)
Exhaustion (No)	0.962 (0.928–0.997) *	0.975 (0.939–1.012)
Low physical activity (No)	1.016 (0.979–1.054)	1.012 (0.972–1.054)
Desease (No)	0.998 (0.968–1.029)	0.998 (0.965–1.031)
Single fall (No)	0.978 (0.954–1.003)	0.985 (0.960–1.012)
Multiple falls (No)	0.984 (0.940–1.031)	0.999 (0.951–1.050)

OR, odds ratio; CI, confidence interval; * $p < 0.05$; $ Adjusted for age and gender; # Used below average value as reference. The notation in parentheses indicates a reference.

4.5. eHEALS Score and Health Status

The eHEALS score had significant relationships between the IADL total score and intellectual activity in IADL (Table 4). The eHEALS score was positively related to the IADL total score (OR: 1.032, 95%CI: 1.006–1.058) and intellectual activity (OR: 1.040, 95%CI: 1.006–1.074). The eHEALS score was not significantly related to other health status variables.

4.6. Associated Factors with the Lowest eHEALS Score

The factors associated with having the lowest eHEALS score are shown (Table 5). Five items were found to have a significant relationship with the lowest eHEALS score: cultural activity at least once a week, no cultural activity, no community activity, the IADL total score, and intellectual activity.

Engaging in cultural activity once a week had a favorable influence on having the lowest eHEALS score, which was reduced by almost half (OR: 0.540, 95%CI: 0.307–0.948). "No cultural activity" had a negative influence, and was approximately 1.8 times higher than the lowest eHEALS score (OR, 1.845; 95%CI: 1.192–2.856). "No community activity" had a negative association, and had approximately a twofold increase in the lowest eHEALS score (OR: 1.946, 95%CI: 1.276–2.967). After statistically adjusting for age and gender, "no community activity" was still significant and community activity more than once a week was, oppositely, not significant.

Older adults with higher IADL total scores were less likely to have the lowest eHEALS score (OR, 0.819; 95%CI: 0.679–0.989). Intellectual activity also had a favorable influence on having the lowest eHEALS score (OR, 0.568; 95%CI: 0.377–0.855). Significant associations were found for some health statuses (ex, social role and robust), but all variables were no longer significant after adjusting for age and gender.

Table 5. Predictors of Being Lowest eHEALS Score.

	Unadjusted OR (95%CI)	Adjusted $ OR (95%CI)
Age #	1.142 (1.099–1.186) *	
Gender (Male)	3.709 (2.145–6.414) *	
Social Activity		
Cultural Activity at least once a week (No)	0.616 (0.366–1.036) *	0.540 (0.307–0.948) *
No Cultural Activity (At lesat once or twice a month)	1.699 (1.135–2.544) *	1.845 (1.192–2.856) *
Community Activity at least once a week (No)	0.549 (0.342–0.882) *	0.650 (0.386–1.095)
No Community Activity (At lesat once or twice a month)	2.354 (1.587–3.490) *	1.946 (1.276–2.967) *
Sports Activity at least once a week (No)	0.761 (0.512–1.132)	0.763 (0.499–1.166)
No Sports Activity (At lesat once or twice a month)	0.846 (0.319–2.244)	0.849 (0.293–2.462)
Health Behavior		
Dietary Variety Score #	1.018 (0.942–1.100)	0.957 (0.877–1.044)
Going out at least once a week (No)	0.912 (0.182–4.569)	2.812 (0.527–15.00)
Sitting time at least 8 h a weekday (No)	1.478 (0.486–4.495)	1.848 (0.535–6.380)
Smoking (No)	0.817(0.248–2.694)	1.015(0.276–3.725)
Health Status		
IADL Total Score #	0.750 (0.626–0.899) *	0.819 (0.679–0.989) *
Instrumental Self-maintenance #	0.447 (0.227–0.880) *	0.585 (0.303–1.129)
Intellectual Activity #	0.518 (0.347–0.772) *	0.568 (0.377–0.855) *
Social Role #	0.836 (0.644–1.086)	0.953 (0.714–1.273)
Body Mass Index #	0.987 (0.933–1.045)	1.032 (0.970–1.097)
Obesity (No)	0.975 (0.643–1.480)	1.193 (0.757–1.879)
Thin (No)	1.102 (0.525–2.314)	0.842 (0.388–1.829)
Robust (No)	0.588 (0.389–0.889) *	0.740 (0.473–1.156)
Pre-frailty (No)	1.568 (1.033–2.379) *	1.327 (0.846–2.083)
Frailty or Pre-frailty (No)	1.700 (1.125–2.569) *	1.352 (0.865–2.113)
Weakness (No)	3.720 (1.116–12.40) *	1.918 (0.549–6.701)
Slowness (No)	2.574 (1.242–5.335) *	1.322 (0.603–2.895)
Unintentional Weight loss (No)	1.703 (0.883–3.283)	1.758 (0.842–3.671)
Exhaustion (No)	1.602 (0.896–2.866)	1.233 (0.665–2.288)
Low physical activity (No)	0.654 (0.324–1.319)	0.713 (0.330–1.544)
Disease (No)	1.163 (0.665–2.034)	1.160 (0.634–2.123)
Single fall (No)	1.573 (0.999–2.477) *	1.397 (0.863–2.262)
Multiple falls (No)	1.755 (0.712–4.325)	1.514 (0.572–4.008)

OR, odds ratio; CI, confidence interval; * $p < 0.05$; $ Adjusted for age and gender; # Used as a continuous variable. The notation in parentheses indicates a reference.

Finally, in order to clarity which was the most powerful predictor, we performed multivariate logistic regression analysis using the variables in Table 5 that were significant even after adjusting for gender and age. "Cultural activity at least once a week" and "No cultural activity" were entered separately. As a result of inserting "cultural activity at least once a week", "no community activity", and "IADL total score" as independent variables (gender and age were also included as adjustment factors), only "no cultural activity" was significant. The OR for "no community activity" was 1.838 (95%CI: 1.201–2.814). Next, we entered "no cultural activity", "no community activity", and "IADL total score" as independent variables (gender and age were also included as adjustment factors). As a result, "no community activity" and "no cultural activity" were significant. The OR for "no community activities" was 1.780 (95%CI: 1.159–2.734) and the OR for "no cultural activities" was 1.595 (95%CI: 1.020–2.495).

5. Discussion

5.1. eHealth Literacy Level

The mean eHEALS score in this study was low at 12.4 points (SD 8.2). This score was relatively lower than 21.0 points for older adults (mean age 73.6) living in Shizuoka, Japan [51]. Another previous study reported the eHEALS scores of older adults overseas as follows: the US older adults mean of 24.5 points [52], Sweden's older adults mean of 27.5 points [37], and the Chinese older adults mean of 17.2 points [26]. The eHEALS scores in this study were relatively lower than those reported in all previous studies. It was assumed that participants in this study were highly health conscious because they wanted to participate in this study and monitor their physical fitness and health status. But, they had lower eHEALS scores. The reason for this lower eHealth literacy level was unknown, but the possibility that the "digital divide" due to age had an influence cannot be denied. The Japanese government is concerned about the negative impact of the digital divide on older adults [53], so it will be necessary to continue research on this issue.

5.2. Association between eHEALS and Social Activity

eHealth literacy was associated with two types of social activities. Firstly, eHealth literacy was associated with cultural activities ("cultural activities at least once a week" and "no cultural activity"). Cultural activity is often related to hobbies and may involve using the Internet to obtain information on materials and methods for tackling new tasks. Using the Internet and other means of signing up for new classes may also be related to eHealth literacy. Although it is unclear why there was a significant relationship between eHealth literacy and cultural activity, we hope that future longitudinal studies will explain the mechanisms underlying this relationship.

Secondly, eHealth literacy has also been associated with community activity ("community activity at least once a week" and "no community activity"). Community activity in this study was organizational activities unique to Japan, such as residents' associations and senior citizens' clubs. A residents' association is an organization formed based on the local connections of people between people who live in a specific area within a municipality [54]. A senior citizens' club is an organization that conducts projects to maintain and promote the physical and mental health of older adults based in the community under the "Welfare Law for Older Adults", enacted in 1963 [55]. One possible reason for this may be that community activities facilitate access to various types of information because information from Japanese administrative agencies such as local government welfare departments is actively provided when community activities collaborate with public agencies. Another possible reason may be the impact of social activity on health and health behaviors. Social activity has been reported to prevent frailty and the need for nursing care; in particular, participation in local communities and hobbies was effective [40,46]. Although some aspects remain unclear about the mechanisms that prevent functional impairment in social activity, engaging in social activity may contribute to increasing the activeness and social capital of older adults because social activity encourages older adults to go out and be more active in their daily lives and may increase social support by frequently access to health information and communication with neighbors [46]. Therefore, it is possible that eHealth literacy is related to social activity, such as cultural and community activities, among older adults in the community.

This study showed no significant association between eHealth literacy and sports activity. Sports activity is also an effective health behavior that prevents functional impairment by increasing physical activity [46,56]. A previous study of young people found an association between regular exercise and eHealth literacy [22–25]. eHealth literacy was hypothesized to be related to sports activity, but no association was found. We found that 63.5% of the participants engaged in sports activities at least once a week, which was the most common activity among social activities. In addition, most participants were a highly health-conscious group who attended health classes on their own and engaged in other sports activities. Therefore, it is possible that no association with sports activity was observed.

5.3. Association between eHEALS and Health Behavior or Health Status

This study found no association between eHealth literacy and health behaviors. We examined health behaviors such as smoking, eating, going out at least once a week, and a sitting time of at least 8 h a weekday. The eHEALS scores were not associated with smoking status. These results were consistent with general surveys of Japanese adults [27] and university students [22]. We cannot determine the reason for this, but it may be because there were many nonsmokers, and the mean age was high.

The results of this study showed associations between eHealth literacy and IADL total score and intellectual activity in older adults. But, there was no association with frailty variables in this study. Previous studies have reported that health literacy had association with frailty [57]. Although health literacy is also included in the concept of eHealth literacy, no study has observed the relationship between eHealth literacy and frailty. This study is the first to examine these relationships and can be said to be original.

5.4. Factors Associated with the Lowest eHEALS Score

Five factors significantly associated with having the lowest eHEALS score were cultural activity at least once a week, no cultural activity, no community activity, total IADL score, and intellectual activity.

Engaging in cultural activity at least once a week had a favorable influence (decrease in the risk) and "no cultural activity" had a negative influence (increase in the risk) on having the lowest eHEALS score. These results suggest that cultural activity may be a predictive factor of the lowest level of eHealth literacy.

"No community activity" was found to be associated with having the lowest eHEALS score. Community activity has the advantage of providing social support, such as access to health-related information [46], and eHealth literacy may be affected by the lack of access to such opportunities. "Cultural activity at least once a week" and "no cultural activity" were associated with eHealth literacy, while only "no cultural activity" was associated with community activity after adjusting age and gender. Regarding the difference between cultural activity and community activity, we can also consider that one of the influences is that community activities have negative aspects, such as obligations and burdens to the community [58].

Higher IADL scores had a lower likelihood of resulting in the lowest eHEALS score. Some degree of independence and cognitive function may be required to use the Internet to operate digital technologies. Therefore, higher levels of IADL may have an association with eHealth literacy.

5.5. Comparison with Previous Studies and Key Findings

A new finding of this study was the association between eHealth literacy and social activities (cultural activities and community activities). These results show that (1) participating in community activities at least once a week is the best choice, and (2) not participating in cultural or community activities at all may reduce the risk of having the lowest level of eHealth literacy. To our knowledge, no previous studies have investigated the association between eHealth literacy and social activities in older adults. This study may add a new perspective to eHealth literacy research. In future digitalized society, social activity may be useful in programs that reduce elderly adults' concerns about digital technology and technology. Finding the causal relationship between eHealth literacy and social activities is desired. On the other hand, the relationship between eHealth literacy and health behaviors observed in previous studies was not observed at all [22–25,59], but the reason for the discrepancy between the results of this study and previous studies is unclear. The mean eHEALS score of participants in this study was low, at 12.4 out of 40 (SD 8.2), which may be a contributing factor. Future research will need a longitudinal study to determine whether the initiation of cultural or community activities increases eHealth literacy among participants with low eHealth literacy. The current study also investigated the association between eHealth literacy and health status (IADL, frailty, DVS, etc.) in older adults. Although no association was found in the results of this study, these are items that have not been investigated in previous eHealth literacy studies. Future research will provide basic research for developing public policies, medical practices, and programs for older adults, including improving eHealth literacy among older adults, promoting digital health, and bridging the digital divide.

5.6. Limitations

This study had several limitations. First, the participants were from only one town in a rural area. The results may not be applicable to older adults in other regions. Second, this study did not measure individual characteristics related to socio-economic status or the Internet environment. In particular, the influence of educational background and academic background is important, so future research should evaluate it as much as possible. Third, the causal relationship between eHealth literacy and the variables in this study is unclear because this study was cross-sectional. Finally, this study was limited to those who attended health classes, which may have been influenced by the fact that they were more health conscious than the general older adult population.

6. Conclusions

This study investigated the association between eHealth literacy and social activities among community-dwelling older adults. As a result, eHealth literacy was significantly associated with both cultural activity and community activity. The eHealth literacy level of older adults in this study was relatively very low. Engaging in cultural activity had positive influences on the risk of having the lowest levels of eHealth literacy. Also, interestingly, avoiding "no cultural activity" and "no community activity" had positive influences. This study is one of the first to show the relationship between eHealth literacy and social activity among older adults. The results of this study add a new perspective to previous eHealth literacy research.

Author Contributions: Conceptualization, M.E. and K.Y.; methodology, M.E. and K.Y.; formal analysis, M.E. and K.Y.; investigation, K.Y.; resources, K.Y.; data curation, M.E.; writing—original draft preparation, M.E.; writing—review and editing, M.E. and K.Y.; visualization, M.E. and K.Y.; supervision, K.Y.; project administration, K.Y.; funding acquisition, K.Y. All authors have read and agreed to the published version of the manuscript.

Funding: This research was funded by JSPS KAKENHI, grant number 20K11446 and 23K10763.

Institutional Review Board Statement: This study was conducted in accordance with the Declaration of Helsinki and approved by the Ethics Committee for Human Studies, Faculty of Education, Saga University (registration number SGED0006).

Informed Consent Statement: All the participants provided written informed consent to participate in this study.

Data Availability Statement: The data presented in this study are available on request from the corresponding author.

Conflicts of Interest: The authors declare no conflicts of interest.

References

1. United Nations, Department of Economic and Social Affairs, Population Division. 2022. Available online: https://www.un.org/development/desa/pd/sites/www.un.org.development.desa.pd/files/undesa_pd_2022_wpp_key-messages.pdf (accessed on 20 March 2024).
2. Cabinet Office. Aging Society Report. 2023. Available online: https://www8.cao.go.jp/kourei/whitepaper/w-2023/zenbun/05pdf_index.html (accessed on 20 March 2024).
3. Scott, A.J. The longevity society. *Lancet Healthy Longev.* **2021**, *2*, e820–e827. [CrossRef] [PubMed]
4. Nomura, S.; McEnany, M.; Sugawara, J.; Noritake, R.; Miyata, H. Partnership for Health System Sustainability and Resilience, LSE Consulting. Sustainability and Resilience in Japan's Health System. 2022. Available online: https://www3.weforum.org/docs/WEF_PHSSR_Japan_final_2022.pdf (accessed on 20 March 2024).
5. United Nations, Department of Economic and Social Affairs. World Population Ageing. 2019. Available online: https://digitallibrary.un.org/record/3846855/files/WorldPopulationAgeing2019-Highlights.pdf (accessed on 20 March 2024).
6. Chen, C.; Ding, S.; Wang, J. Digital health for aging populations. *Nat. Med.* **2023**, *29*, 1623–1630. [CrossRef] [PubMed]

7. Ministry of Internal Affairs and Communications. Effects of ICT Use by Olde Adults, Research Report on Evaluation and Dissemination of ICT Utilization for Older Adults and People with Disabilities. 2008. Available online: https://www.soumu.go.jp/main_sosiki/joho_tsusin/b_free/pdf/b_free03_3_07.pdf (accessed on 20 March 2024).
8. Fujiyama, M. The Japan Research Institute Limited. Research Focus Towards Digitalization, 2023. Available online: https://www.jri.co.jp/MediaLibrary/file/report/researchfocus/pdf/14554.pdf (accessed on 24 March 2024).
9. Pan American Health Organization (PAHO); International Telecommunication Union. The Role of Digital Technologies in Aging and Health, Decade of Healthy Aging in the Americas: Situation and Challenges, 2023. Available online: https://iris.paho.org/bitstream/handle/10665.2/57344/9789275126554_eng.pdf?sequence=3&isAllowed=y (accessed on 12 March 2024).
10. Ministry of Internal Affairs and Communications. Results of Telecommunication Usage Trend Survey, 2020. Available online: https://www.soumu.go.jp/johotsusintokei/statistics/data/230529_1.pdf (accessed on 20 March 2024).
11. Anderson, M.; Perrin, A. Tech Adoption Climbs among Older Adults. 2017. Available online: https://www.pewresearch.org/internet/2017/05/17/tech-adoption-climbs-among-older-adults/#fn-18808-1 (accessed on 20 March 2024).
12. Nakagomi, A.; Shiba, K.; Kawachi, I.; Ide, K.; Nagamine, Y.; Kondo, N.; Hanazato, M.; Kondo, K. Internet use and subsequent health and well-being in older adults: An outcome-wide analysis. *Comput. Hum. Behav.* **2022**, *130*, 107156. [CrossRef]
13. Heo, J.; Chun, S.; Lee, S.; Lee, K.H.; Kim, J. Internet use and well-being in older adults. *Cyberpsychol. Behav. Soc. Netw.* **2015**, *18*, 268–272. [CrossRef] [PubMed]
14. Millward, P. The 'grey digital divide': Perception, exclusion and barriers of access to the internet for older people. *First Monday* **2003**, *8*, 4–5. [CrossRef]
15. UNECE. Ageing in the Digital Era. 2021. Available online: https://unece.org/sites/default/files/2021-07/PB26-ECE-WG.1-38_0.pdf (accessed on 20 March 2024).
16. FitzPatrick, M.A.; Hess, A.C.; Sudbury-Riley, L.; Schulz, P.J. A Typology of Patients Based on Decision-Making Styles: Cross-Sectional Survey Study. *J. Med. Internet Res.* **2019**, *21*, e15332. [CrossRef] [PubMed]
17. Veenhof, B.; Clermont, Y.; Sciadas, G. *Literacy and Digital Technologies: Linkages and Outcomes*; Science, Innovation and Electronic Information Division (SIEID) 7-A, R.H. Coats Building; Catalogue No. 56F0004MIE, No. 12; Ministry of Industry: Ottawa, ON, Canada, 2005; ISBN 0-662-42253-8. ISSN 1492-7918.
18. Norman, C.D.; Skinner, H.A. eHealth Literacy: Essential Skills for Consumer Health in a Networked World. *J. Med. Internet Res.* **2006**, *8*, e9. [CrossRef] [PubMed]
19. Norman, C.D.; Skinner, H.A. eHEALS: The eHealth Literacy Scale. *J. Med. Internet Res.* **2006**, *8*, e27. [CrossRef] [PubMed]
20. Kim, K.; Shin, S.; Kim, S.; Lee, E. The Relation Between eHealth Literacy and Health-Related Behaviors: Systematic Review and Meta-analysis. *J. Med. Internet Res.* **2023**, *25*, e40778. [CrossRef] [PubMed]
21. Mitsutake, S.; Shibata, A.; Ishii, K.; Okazaki, K.; Oka, K. Developing Japanese version of the eHealth Literacy Scale (eHEALS). Article in Japanese. *Jpn. J. Public Health* **2011**, *58*, 361–371.
22. Tsukahara, S.; Yamaguchi, S.; Igarashi, F.; Uruma, R.; Ikuina, N.; Iwakura, K.; Koizumi, K.; Sato, Y. Association of eHealth Literacy With Lifestyle Behaviors in University Students: Questionnaire-Based Cross-Sectional Study. *J. Med. Internet Res.* **2020**, *22*, e18155. [CrossRef] [PubMed]
23. Hsu, W.; Chiang, C.; Yang, S. The effect of individual factors on health behaviors among college students: The mediating effects of eHealth literacy. *J. Med. Internet Res.* **2014**, *16*, e287. [CrossRef] [PubMed]
24. Britt, R.K.; Collins, W.B.; Wilson, K.; Linnemeier, G.; Englebert, A.M. eHealth Literacy and Health Behaviors Affecting Modern College Students: A Pilot Study of Issues Identified by the American College Health Association. *J. Med. Internet Res.* **2017**, *19*, e392. [CrossRef] [PubMed]
25. Yang, S.C.; Luo, Y.F.; Chiang, C.H. The Associations Among Individual Factors, eHealth Literacy, and Health-Promoting Lifestyles Among College Students. *J. Med. Internet Res.* **2017**, *19*, e15. [CrossRef] [PubMed]
26. Cui, G.H.; Li, S.J.; Yin, Y.T.; Chen, L.J.; Li, J.Q.; Liang, F.Y.; Liu, X.Y.; Chen, L. The relationship among social capital, ehealth literacy and health behaviours in Chinese elderly people: A cross-sectional study. *BMC Public Health* **2021**, *21*, 45. [CrossRef] [PubMed]
27. Mitsutake, S.; Shibata, A.; Ishii, K.; Oka, K. Associations of eHealth Literacy With Health Behavior Among Adult Internet Users. *J. Med. Internet Res.* **2016**, *18*, e192. [CrossRef] [PubMed]
28. Kumagai, S.; Watanabe, S.; Shibata, H.; Amano, H.; Fujiwara, Y.; Shinkai, S.; Yoshida, H.; Suzuki, T.; Yukawa, H.; Yasumura, S.; et al. Effects of dietary variety on declines in high-level functional capacity in elderly people living in a community. *Nihon Koshu Eisei Zasshi* **2003**, *50*, 1117–1124. [PubMed]
29. Seino, S.; Nofuji, Y.; Yokoyama, Y.; Abe, T.; Nishi, M.; Yamashita, M.; Narita, M.; Hata, T.; Shinkai, S.; Kitamura, A.; et al. Combined Impacts of Physical Activity, Dietary Variety, and Social Interaction on Incident Functional Disability in Older Japanese Adults. *J. Epidemiol.* **2023**, *33*, 350–359. [CrossRef] [PubMed]
30. Vicente, M.R.; Madden, G. Assessing eHealth skills across Europeans. *Health Policy Technol.* **2017**, *6*, 161–168. [CrossRef]
31. Green, G. Seniors' eHealth literacy, health and education status and personal health knowledge. *Digit Health* **2022**, *8*, 20552076221089803. [CrossRef]
32. Honma, Y.; Kagamimori, S.; Naruse, Y. Active Life Expectancy and ADL in Japanese Elderly. *Jpn. J. Public Health* **1998**, *45*, 1018–1029. (In Japanese)
33. Koyano, H. Measurement of competence in the elderly living at home: Development of an index of competence. *Jpn. J. Public Health* **1987**, *34*, 109–114. (In Japanese)

34. Lawton, M.P.; Brody, E.M. Assessment of older people: Self-maintaining and instrumental activities of daily living. *Gerontologist* **1969**, *9*, 179–186. [CrossRef] [PubMed]
35. Arai, H. Significance of Frail. *Geriatr. Gerontol. Int.* **2014**, *51*, 497–501.
36. Satake, S.; Arai, H. The revised Japanese version of the Cardiovascular Health Study criteria (revised J-CHS criteria). *Geriatr. Gerontol. Int.* **2020**, *20*, 992–993. [CrossRef] [PubMed]
37. Ghazi, S.N.; Berner, J.; Anderberg, P.; Sanmartin, B.J. The prevalence of eHealth literacy and its relationship with perceived health status and psychological distress during COVID-19: A cross-sectional study of older adults in Blekinge, Sweden. *BMC Geriatr.* **2023**, *23*, 5. [CrossRef] [PubMed]
38. Fujihara, S.; Miyaguni, Y.; Tsuji, T.; Kondo, K. Community-level social participation and functional disability among older adults: A JAGES multilevel longitudinal study. *Arch. Gerontol. Geriatr.* **2022**, *100*, 104632. [CrossRef] [PubMed]
39. Hikichi, H.; Kondo, N.; Kondo, K.; Aida, J.; Takeda, T.; Kawachi, I. Effect of a community intervention programme promoting social interactions on functional disability prevention for older adults: Propensity score matching and instrumental variable analyses, JAGES Taketoyo study. *J. Epidemiol. Community Health* **2015**, *69*, 905–910. [CrossRef] [PubMed]
40. Ukawa, S.; Tamakoshi, A.; Okada, Y.; Ito, Y.M.; Taniguchi, R.; Tani, Y.; Sasaki, Y.; Saito, J.; Haseda, M.; Kondo, N.; et al. Social participation patterns and the incidence of functional disability: The Japan Gerontological Evaluation Study. *Geriatr. Gerontol. Int.* **2020**, *20*, 765–772. [CrossRef] [PubMed]
41. Noguchi, T.; Kondo, K.; Saito, M.; Nakagawa-Senda, H.; Suzuki, S. Community social capital and the onset of functional disability among older adults in Japan: A multilevel longitudinal study using Japan Gerontological Evaluation Study (JAGES) data. *BMJ Open* **2019**, *9*, e029279. [CrossRef] [PubMed]
42. Aida, J.; Kondo, K.; Kawachi, I.; Subramanian, S.V.; Ichida, Y.; Hirai, H.; Kondo, N.; Osaka, K.; Sheiham, A.; Tsakos, G.; et al. Does social capital affect the incidence of functional disability in older Japanese? A prospective population-based cohort study. *J. Epidemiol. Community Health* **2013**, *67*, 42–47. [CrossRef] [PubMed]
43. Nemoto, Y.; Saito, T.; Kanamori, S.; Tsuji, T.; Shirai, K.; Kikuchi, H.; Maruo, K.; Arao, T.; Kondo, K. An additive effect of leading role in the organization between social participation and dementia onset among Japanese older adults: The AGES cohort study. *BMC Geriatr.* **2017**, *17*, 297. [CrossRef] [PubMed]
44. Sakamoto, A.; Ukawa, S.; Okada, E.; Sasaki, S.; Zhao, W.; Kishi, T.; Kondo, K.; Tamakoshi, A. The association between social participation and cognitive function in community-dwelling older populations: Japan Gerontological Evaluation Study at Taisetsu community Hokkaido. *Int. J. Geriatr. Psychiatry* **2017**, *32*, 1131–1140. [CrossRef] [PubMed]
45. Ishikawa, Y.; Kondo, N.; Kondo, K.; Saito, T.; Hayashim, H.; Kawachi, I.; JAGES Group. Social participation and mortality: Does social position in civic groups matter? *BMC Public Health* **2016**, *16*, 394. [CrossRef] [PubMed]
46. Kanamori, S.; Kai, Y.; Aida, J.; Kondo, K.; Kawachi, I.; Hirai, H.; Shirai, K.; Ishikawa, Y.; Suzuki, K.; JAGES Group. Social participation and the prevention of functional disability in older Japanese: The JAGES cohort study. *PLoS ONE* **2014**, *9*, e99638. [CrossRef] [PubMed]
47. Minister of Health, Labour and Welfare. The Second Term of National Health Promotion Movement in the Twenty First Century (Health Japan 21) Particulars. 2012. Available online: https://www.mhlw.go.jp/www1/topics/kenko21_11/top.html (accessed on 23 March 2024).
48. Suka, M.; Odajima, T.; Okamoto, M.; Sumitani, M.; Igarashi, A.; Ishikawa, H.; Kusama, M.; Yamamoto, M.; Nakayama, T.; Sugimori, H. Relationship between health literacy, health information access, health behavior, and health status in Japanese people. *Patient Educ. Couns.* **2015**, *98*, 660–668. [CrossRef] [PubMed]
49. Ogawa, W.; Hirota, Y.; Miyazaki, S.; Nakamura, T.; Ogawa, Y.; Shimomura, I.; Yamauchi, T.; Yokote, K. Creation Committee for Guidelines for the Management of Obesity Disease 2022 by Japan Society for the Study of Obesity (JASSO). Definition, criteria, and core concepts of guidelines for the management of obesity disease in Japan. *Endocr. J.* 2023; *Epub ahead of print*. [CrossRef] [PubMed]
50. Fried, L.P.; Tangen, C.M.; Walston, J.; Newman, A.B.; Hirsch, C.; Gottdiener, J.; Seeman, T.; Tracy, R.; Kop, W.J.; Burke, G.; et al. Frailty in older adults: Evidence for a phenotype. *J. Gerontol. A Biol. Sci. Med. Sci.* **2001**, *56*, M146–M157. [CrossRef] [PubMed]
51. Kubota, A.; Okamoto, N.; Fukuda, S. Relationship between e-Health literacy and awareness of physical activity and exercise habits in daily life among community-dwelling elderly people. *J. Health Phys. Educ. Recreat.* **2023**, *73*, 641–645.
52. Berkowsky, R.W. Exploring predictors of ehealth literacy among older adults: Findings from the 2020 CALSPEAKS survey. *Gerontol. Geriatr. Med.* **2021**, *7*, 3–4. [CrossRef] [PubMed]
53. Ministry of Internal Affairs and Communications, Japan. Information and Communications in Japan WHITE PAPER. 2022, Section 8 Digital Usage Trends. Available online: https://www.soumu.go.jp/johotsusintokei/whitepaper/eng/WP2022/2022-index.html (accessed on 20 March 2024).
54. Ministry of Internal Affairs and Communications. What Are Residents' Associations, Neighborhood Associations, etc.? 2013. Available online: https://www.soumu.go.jp/main_content/000307324.pdf (accessed on 12 March 2024).
55. Ministry of Health, Labour and Welfare. 2017 Overview of Welfare Administration Report Examples. 2017. Available online: https://www.mhlw.go.jp/toukei/saikin/hw/gyousei/17/dl/gaikyo.pdf (accessed on 12 March 2024).
56. Tak, E.; Kuiper, R.; Chorus, A.; Hopman-Rock, M. Prevention of onset and progression of basic ADL disability by physical activity in community dwelling older adults: A meta-analysis. *Ageing Res. Rev.* **2013**, *12*, 329–338. [CrossRef] [PubMed]

57. Yoshizawa, Y.; Tanaka, T.; Takahashi, K.; Fujisaki-Sueda-Sakai, M.; Son, B.K.; Iijima, K. Impact of health literacy on the progression of frailty after 4 years among community-dwelling older adults. *Int. J. Environ. Res. Public Health* **2021**, *19*, 394. [CrossRef] [PubMed]
58. Rook, K.S. The negative side of social interaction: Impact on psychological well-being. *J. Personal. Soc. Psychol.* **1984**, *46*, 1097. [CrossRef] [PubMed]
59. Arcury, T.A.; Sandberg, J.C.; Melius, K.P.; Quandt, S.A.; Leng, X.; Latulipe, C.; Miller Jr, D.P.; Smith, D.A.; Bertoni, A.G. Older Adult Internet Use and eHealth Literacy. *J. Appl. Gerontol.* **2020**, *39*, 141–150. [CrossRef] [PubMed]

European Journal of
Investigation in Health, Psychology and Education

MDPI

Article

Association between Levels of Loneliness, Laboratory Measurements, and Behavioral Aspects in a Primary Care Setting in Crete, Greece

Panagiotis Volkos [1,*], Manolis Linardakis [2], Panagiotis Stachteas [3], Foteini Anastasiou [4], Athina Tatsioni [5], Marilena Kampa [6] and Emmanouil K. Symvoulakis [7]

1 Fourth Local Health Team—Academic Unit of Heraklion, 71303 Heraklion, Greece
2 Department of Social Medicine, School of Medicine, University of Crete, 70013 Heraklion, Greece
3 Laboratory of Primary Health Care, General Practice and Health Services Research, School of Medicine, Aristotle University of Thessaloniki, 54124 Thessaloniki, Greece
4 Fourth Local Primary Care Team (TOMY), Municipality Practice, Academic Practice of Heraklion, University of Crete, 71303 Heraklion, Greece
5 Research Unit for General Medicine and Primary Health Care, University of Ioannina, 45110 Ioannina, Greece
6 Laboratory of Experimental Endocrinology, School of Medicine, University of Crete, 70013 Heraklion, Greece
7 Clinic of Social and Family Medicine, Faculty of Medicine, University of Crete, 70013 Heraklion, Greece
* Correspondence: medp2012072@med.uoc.gr; Tel.: +30-2811-118853

Abstract: This paper examines potential associations of loneliness with laboratory data and specific psychosocial and behavioral attitudes. The sample collection took place in an urban Primary Health Care unit between May and July 2023, consecutively, and once exclusion criteria were implemented. Participants were aged between 40 and 75 years. Routine laboratory test results upon study initiation and six months before were used. The University of California, Los Angeles (UCLA), Loneliness Scale (Version 3), blood glucose, serum lipids, Fibrosis-4 index, and Creatinine Clearance (CrCl) were assessed through hierarchical multiple logistic regression analysis. Based on full model (3rd) analysis, those who were engaged in an individual sport or activity or had contacts with more friends presented significantly lower odds for increased loneliness levels (odds ratio (OR): 0.28 [95% confidence interval (CI) 0.09–0.91], $p = 0.034$ and OR: 0.76 [95%CI 0.66–0.88], $p < 0.001$, respectively). The consumption of alcohol was associated with increased loneliness (OR: 5.55 [95%CI 1.42–21.63], $p = 0.014$). Elevated triglyceride levels were linked with moderate or no loneliness (OR: 0.20 [95%CI 0.05–0.83], $p = 0.026$), while an increased LDL/HDL atherosclerotic index was related to increased subjective loneliness (OR: 4.50 [95%CI 1.12–18.13], $p = 0.035$). The need for holistic approaches—involving primary care personnel—in understanding and addressing loneliness, recognizing its multifaceted nature as well as the diverse factors that contribute to this issue, is considered challenging.

Keywords: atherosclerotic index; behavior; loneliness; social contacts; triglycerides

1. Introduction

Loneliness is a common feeling; it remains unpleasant and undesirable and many people try to buffer it [1]. As Victor and Yang (2012) reported, loneliness increases among young adults (under the age of 25 years), decreases during middle age, and deteriorates again among older adults aged 65 years and over. Furthermore, it was reported that the "quantity" of social relationships plays an important role in the younger ones, while "quality" is more essential in the elderly [2].

In general, loneliness is related to several health problems, including cardiovascular diseases. The presence of loneliness or social isolation leads to a risk increase of coronary heart disease by 29%, while social isolation is also associated with a higher risk of stroke by 32% [3]. Moreover, individuals who report feeling lonely were found to have higher odds of an increased cholesterol level (1.31 times), the presence of diabetes (1.40 times), and depression (2.78 times) [4]. Additionally, augmented loneliness and limited social participation were linked with a greater risk for dementia, according to the meta-analysis of Kuiper et al. (2015) [5]. From the aforementioned studies, it could be argued that loneliness interplays, in various ways, with health and disease. Therefore, by linking this feeling with laboratory markers, some valuable insights about a neglected health risk might be delivered.

Given that depression and loneliness were previously linked [4], mental health issues should be taken into consideration when studying the impact of loneliness on physical well-being. More specifically, it was reported that higher levels of loneliness are associated with increased odds of metabolic syndrome, although, according to the authors, that relationship was mediated by the occurrence of depression [6]. In addition, loneliness was found to be correlated with a greater risk of metabolic syndrome, a higher level of triglycerides, and lower levels of high-density lipoprotein cholesterol (HDL-C) for people with psychotic disorders [7]. According to the above, it appears that mental health issues are, somehow, related to loneliness and several physical conditions, without having specific knowledge about the exact operating mechanism.

In the literature, loneliness was studied alongside social inclusion (or exclusion) and social isolation, and given the fact that these social terms are content and effect-connected, they may be positively or negatively predictive for loneliness. According to the study of Dahlberg et al. (2022), social exclusion indicators such as participation in the community, social relationships, material resources, and the neighborhood are associated with an increased likelihood of loneliness in Nordic countries [8]. Other than that, social exclusion may cause feelings of lower self-esteem, anger, depression, anxiety, and self-destructive behavior [9]. The effects of social inclusion and isolation on physical health have been investigated, showing that higher levels of social inclusion are linked with lower blood glucose and low-density lipoprotein (LDL) [10]. Greater social isolation was correlated with two-fold increased odds of deterioration in renal function and the presence of chronic kidney disease [11]. According to the review of Holt-Lunstad (2022), it is concluded that social connections should be addressed as a public health issue [12].

All of the above are showing that loneliness is a feeling that can influence health to a great extent and needs to be taken into account for both prevention and treatment purposes, especially when considering that several societies tend to become more individualistic than collective [13]. Relating laboratory data to an easy-in-use tool for loneliness may provide critical information to a health professional team, in order to take preventive action at a psychosocial, behavioral, and physical level.

The primary objective of this study is to examine potential associations of loneliness with laboratory findings within a primary care setting. The secondary aim was to triangulate scale scores—detecting loneliness—with routine laboratory results and other meanings of psychosocial and behavioral attitudes.

2. Materials and Methods

This study followed an observational, cross-sectional design and took place in the 4th TOMY (Topiki Monada Ygeias—Local Health Unit) of Heraklion, Crete, Greece, which is an urban Primary Health Care (PHC) unit. The study population targeted all of the registered adults of the unit between 40 and 75 years of age. The participants had to be able to read, write, and comprehend the Greek language, with Body Mass Index (BMI) ≤ 29.9 kg/m^2, without major head trauma or major psychiatric disorder, and those who were not pregnant or breastfeeding during the study period. The sample was collected between May and July 2023 and 120 participants were included, from 288 scheduled appointments during two morning sessions weekly, in a consecutive manner, after exclusion criteria were applied. Routine laboratory test results upon study initiation and six months before were used. Patients were asked to provide further information whenever needed. STROBE checklist for cross-sectional studies was strictly followed.

2.1. Data Collection

A sheet to collect information was designed for the purposes of the present study. It contained information regarding age, gender, marital status, level of education, occupation, height, weight, smoking habits, consumption of alcohol, chronic diseases, prescribed medications, existence of any psychiatric diagnosis, the number of friends they came into contact with, either face-to-face or via electronic means, during the last six months, level of individual physical activity or sport during the last year, and experience of a dramatic event in the family during the last year. For the purposes of this study, blood glucose (mg/dL), total cholesterol (mg/dL), triglycerides (TG) (mg/dL), HDL-C (mg/dL), LDL-C (mg/dL), aspartate aminotransferase (AST) (U/L), alanine aminotransferase (ALT) (U/L), platelet count, and creatinine (mg/dL) were tabulated. Also, Fibrosis-4 (Fib-4) score, modified Creatinine Clearance (CrCl) (mL/min/1.73 m^2), and HDL-C/LDL-C index were calculated.

2.2. University of California, Los Angeles (UCLA), Loneliness Scale (Version 3)

The feeling of loneliness was measured using UCLA Loneliness Scale, Version 3 [14]. The scale assesses feelings of perceived loneliness and comprises 20 items (11 with negative and 9 with positive meanings). Answers are based on a 4-point Likert-type scale, with never = 1, rarely = 2, sometimes = 3, and always = 4. To measure the outcome of the scale, 9 items need to be reversed (items 1, 5, 6, 9, 10, 15, 16, 19, and 20) and then all of the items need to be summed up. The final score range is 20–80. Higher score indicates greater feelings of subjective loneliness. The cut-offs used were those reported by Lee and colleagues (2021): total score < 28 as absence or low sense of loneliness, 28 to 43 as moderate feeling, and >43 as high feeling of loneliness [15,16]. The scale was validated in Greek [17]. Cronbach α was estimated at 0.880.

2.3. Cut-Offs for Laboratory Variables

The following cut-offs were used to separate normal and abnormal findings: in total cholesterol > 200 mg/dL or receiving medication, in TG > 150 mg/dL or receiving medication, in LDL > 160 mg/dL or receiving medication, in HDL <40 and <50 mg/dL for men and women, respectively, in blood glucose 100+ mg/dL or receiving medication, in Fib-4 1.45+ [18], and in CrCl < 90 mL/min/1.73 m^2 [19,20]. For the atherosclerotic index LDL-C/HDL-C, the cut-off was 2.517 [21].

2.4. Ethics

The approval to conduct the study, for the needs of an ongoing PhD thesis, was obtained from the Ethics and Deontology Committee of the University of Crete (protocol number: 166/11.11.2022). The research protocol was additionally approved by the 7th Health Regional Authority of Crete (protocol number: 6460) and the study was performed in accordance with the Helsinki Declaration. Written informed consent was obtained by the participants.

2.5. Statistical Analysis

Data analysis was implemented using the SPSS program (IBM Corp. Released 2019, IBM SPSS Statistics for Windows, v.25.0, Armonk, NY, USA: IBM Corp.). Frequency of absolute and relative distributions and measures of location and dispersion of descriptive and laboratory features of the participants were estimated. Score levels of UCLA scale, blood glucose, serum lipids, Fibrosis-4 index, and CrCl were also estimated, as well as the frequencies of their higher levels. Hierarchical multiple logistic regression analysis was implemented in higher levels of loneliness and in relation to basic characteristics, health habits, blood glucose, serum lipids, Fibrosis-4 index, and CrCl of 120 patients–attendees. Acceptable level of significance was set at 0.05.

3. Results

The mean age of participants was 59.8 (standard deviation (SD) = 9.5) years, and most were women (73.3%, n = 88). Table 1 presents the baseline characteristics of the 120 patients–attendees within the PHC setting of the current study. Regarding the educational level, 25% (n = 30) of the participants reported tertiary education, whereas MSc or PhD degrees were found to be held in 2.5% (n = 3) of the patients.

Table 1. Basic characteristics of 120 patients–attendees within primary care setting of current study.

		n	%
Gender	male/female	32/88	26.7/73.3
Age, years	mean ± stand. dev.(min, max)	59.8 ± 9.5 [40, 75]	
Family status	unmarried, divorced, widow	39	32.5
	married	81	67.5
Children	none	17	14.2
	1	11	9.2
	2+	92	76.6
Education level	Primary school	24	20.0
	Junior high school	13	10.8
	High school	34	28.3
	Technical education	19	15.9
	University/Technological School	27	22.5
	MSc, PhD	3	2.5
Occupation	employed	51	42.5
	unemployed, retired	69	57.5

Regarding the behavioral risk factors of the participants, current smokers represented the 30% (n = 36), while the alcohol consumption of one or more drinks per week was equally prevalent (30%, n = 36). The mean BMI was 26 (SD = 2.9) kg/m^2, and remarkably, only 34.2% (n = 41) of patients–attendees had a BMI bellow 25 kg/m^2. With regards to chronic medical conditions, only 13.3% (n = 16) of the participants reported having no chronic disease, whereas the prevalence of mental health disorders was accounted for by 37.5% (n = 45). Nevertheless, hyperlipidemia (30%, n = 36) was the most prevalent physical medical condition followed by diabetes mellitus (28.3%, n = 34) (Table 2).

Table 2. Health habits and characteristics of 120 patients–attendees within primary care setting of current study.

		n	%
Body Mass Index, kg/m^2	mean ± stand. dev.(min, max)	26.0 ± 2.9 (18.6, 29.8)	
	normal	41	34.2
	overweight	79	65.8
Smoking	yes	36	30.0
Alcohol consumption, drinks per week	none	84	70.0
	1+	36	30.0
Conditions, chronic diseases [a]	yes	104	86.7
	mental disorder	45	37.5
	hyperlipidemia	36	30.0
	diabetes mellitus	34	28.3
	hypothyroidism	21	17.5
Routine contacts or meetings with friends during the last 6 months	mean number (median) [min, max]	8 (6) [0, 25]	
Personal sport/activity during the last year	yes	49	40.8
Recent dramatic event in family during the last year	yes	44	36.7

[a] Some participants displayed co-morbidity.

Among the 120 participants, the perceived feeling of loneliness was found with a mean score of 41 (SD = 10.1), as assessed with the UCLA Loneliness Scale, Version 3. More particularly, 109 (90.8%) participants reported moderate or high levels of subjective loneliness, while only 11 (9.2%) participants reported the absence or low feeling of loneliness (Table 3). Laboratory tests revealed impaired renal function and decreased levels of creatinine clearance (mean = 77.4, SD = 21.8) and a good lipid profile with normal levels of total cholesterol (mean = 188.5 mg/dL, SD = 37.9), HDL-C (mean = 59.5 mg/dL, SD = 18.4), LDL-C (mean = 108 mg/dL, SD = 29.9), and triglycerides (mean = 110.3 mg/dL, SD = 58.6), and a mildly impaired glucose metabolism (mean = 104.4 mg/dL, SD = 25.3).

Table 3. Levels of University of California Los Angeles Loneliness Scale (UCLA), blood glucose, serum lipids, Fibrosis-4 index, and Creatinine Clearance (CrCl) of 120 patients–attendees within primary care setting of current study.

	Mean	Stand. Dev.	Median	Min	Max
University of California Los Angeles Loneliness Scale [a]	41.0	10.1	39.5	21	69
absence or low sense of loneliness (<28.0)	n = 11 or 9.2%				
moderate sense (28.0–43.0)	n = 63 or 52.5%				
high sense (>43.0)	n = 46 or 38.3%				
Blood glucose, mg/dL	104.4	25.3	100.0	46	258
100+ or medication	n = 68 or 56.7%				
Total cholesterol, mg/dL	188.5	37.9	186.5	115	278
>200 or medication	n = 70 or 58.3%				
Triglycerides, mg/dL	110.3	58.6	97.0	39	319
>150 or medication	n = 46 or 38.3%				
HDL-C, mg/dL	59.5	18.4	56.0	26	144
<40/50 or medication	n = 24 or 20.0%				
LDL-C, mg/dL	108.0	29.9	107.4	47	186
>160 or medication	n = 40 or 33.3%				
LDL-C: HDL-C index	1.966	0.744	1.838	0.403	4.545
>2.517	n = 31 or 25.8%				
Fibrosis-4 index	1.193	0.489	1.165	0.350	3.090
1.45+	n = 28 or 23.3%				
Creatinine Clearance (CrCl), mL/min/1.73 m^2	77.4	21.8	74.0	31	167
<90	n = 90 or 75.0%				

[a] Score ranges between 20 and 80 as higher score indicates greater sense of subjective loneliness.

Table 4 presents the association of the increased levels of loneliness assessed by the UCLA Loneliness Scale with participants' demographic and laboratory characteristics after using hierarchical multiple logistic regression. Initially, according to the first model, married people seemed to have significantly lower odds for an increased sense of loneliness (odds ratio (OR): 0.39 [95% confidence interval (CI) 0.17–0.91] p = 0.030). In the second model, personal characteristics were not significantly related to the feeling of loneliness, while participants who were engaged in an individual activity or sport during the last year seemed to have significantly lower odds for an increased feeling of loneliness (OR: 0.29 [95%CI 0.10–0.84], p = 0.023). Moreover, the number of social contacts (each additional friend with whom any participant routinely came into contact with (either face-to-face or via electronic means) was strongly related to significantly lower odds for feeling lonely (OR: 0.82 [95%CI 0.73–0.93], p = 0.001). Likewise, in the third model of hierarchical multiple logistic regression, where the laboratory results (glucose, blood serum lipids, fibrosis index, and creatinine clearance) were incorporated, participants with elevated triglyceride levels were associated with moderate or no loneliness (OR: 0.20 [95%CI 0.05–0.83], p = 0.026), while those with an increased LDL/HDL atherosclerotic index had an increased subjective feeling of loneliness (OR: 4.50 [95%CI 1.12–18.13], p = 0.035). Interestingly, participants who were engaged in an individual sport or activity or had more social contacts with friends presented significantly lower odds for an increased feeling of loneliness (OR: 0.28 [95%CI 0.09–0.91], p = 0.034 and OR: 0.76 [95%CI 0.66–0.88], p < 0.001, respectively). Finally, the consumption of alcoholic beverages within the week was associated with an increased feeling of loneliness (OR: 5.55 [95%CI 1.42–21.63], $p = 0.014$).

Table 4. Hierarchical multiple logistic regression analysis of higher levels of loneliness in relation to basic characteristics, health habits, blood glucose, serum lipids, Fibrosis-4 index, and Creatinine Clearance (CrCl) of 120 patients–attendees within primary care setting of current study.

	University of California Los Angeles Loneliness Scale (UCLA) (High Sense of Loneliness vs. Moderate/Low Sense)		
	1st Model	**2nd Model**	**3rd Model**
	Odds Ratio (95%CI) [*p*-Value]		
Gender (female vs. male)	0.77 (0.32, 1.85) [0.553]	0.63 (0.20, 2.02) [0.440]	0.87 (0.22, 3.42) [0.845]
Age (for every 5 year change)	1.09 (0.82, 1.46) [0.538]	1.21 (0.85, 1.71) [0.301]	1.31 (0.85, 2.03) [0.227]
Family status (married vs. unmarried, divorced, widow)	**0.39** (0.17, 0.91) [0.030]	0.38 (0.14, 1.07) [0.066]	0.34 (0.10, 1.10) [0.071]
Children (for each additional child)	0.61 (0.34, 1.08) [0.088]	0.66 (0.34, 1.27) [0.214]	0.67 (0.31, 1.44) [0.302]
Education (for each level of increase)	0.94 (0.71, 1.26) [0.695]	1.06 (0.75, 1.50) [0.731]	1.12 (0.75, 1.68) [0.578]
Occupation (unemployed, retired vs. employed)	0.50 (0.19, 1.31) [0.156]	0.36 (0.11, 1.17) [0.090]	0.39 (0.11, 1.35) [0.136]
Body Mass Index (overweight vs. normal)		0.51 (0.19, 1.39) [0.186]	0.47 (0.14, 1.60) [0.229]
Smoking (yes vs. no)		1.35 (0.48, 3.77) [0.568]	2.44 (0.77, 7.77) [0.130]
Alcohol consumption, drinks per week (yes vs. no)		2.63 (0.85, 8.20) [0.095]	**5.55** (1.42, 21.63) [0.014]
Individual sport/activity during the last year (yes vs. no)		**0.29** (0.10, 0.84) [0.023]	**0.28** (0.09, 0.91) [0.034]
Recent dramatic event in family during the last year (yes vs. no)		1.94 (0.73, 5.17) [0.185]	2.58 (0.83, 8.02) [0.101]
Routine contacts or meetings with friends during the last 6 months (for each additional person)		**0.82** (0.73, 0.93) [0.001]	**0.76** (0.66, 0.88) [<0.001]
Mental disorder (yes vs. no)		1.11 (0.42, 2.93) [0.826]	1.41 (0.47, 4.22) [0.540]
Blood glucose (100+ vs. <100 mg/dL)			1.04 (0.33, 3.26) [0.942]
Total cholesterol (>200 vs. ≤200 mg/dL)			0.45 (0.13, 1.58) [0.213]
Triglycerides (>150 vs. ≤150 mg/dL)			**0.20** (0.05, 0.83) [0.026]
LDL-C: HDL-C index (>2.517 vs. ≤2.517)			**4.50** (1.12, 18.13) [0.035]
Fibrosis-4 index (≥1.45 vs. <1.45)			1.19 (0.32, 4.38) [0.791]
Creatinine Clearance (<90 vs. ≥90)			0.83 (0.21, 3.30) [0.787]
R^2 Negelkerke	0.146	0.380	0.507

Bold indicates the odds with *p*-value < 0.05.

4. Discussion

The present study focused on assessing the levels of loneliness in primary care attendees and exploring potential associations with demographic, behavioral, and routine laboratory test results. Among participants, mental health disorders were prevalent in 37.5%

of participants and the most frequent physical medical conditions were hyperlipidemia (30%) and diabetes mellitus (28.3%), while laboratory tests overall showed an impaired renal function, acceptable lipid profile, and mildly impaired glucose metabolism. The perceived feeling of loneliness was moderately reported, while nine out of ten participants reported moderate or high levels of subjective loneliness. The association of loneliness with demographic and behavioral characteristics showed that married individuals had lower odds of feeling lonely; however, this association diminished in the subsequent models of analysis. Engagement in individual activities or sports, a higher number of social contacts reported, and a lack of weekly alcohol consumption were found to be related with decreased loneliness. Regarding the laboratory tests, elevated triglyceride levels were associated with moderate or no loneliness, while an increased LDL/HDL atherosclerotic index was linked to increased levels of loneliness.

The finding that a consistent proportion of primary care attendees report moderate or high levels of loneliness aligns with the existing literature, indicating that loneliness is becoming a growing community health issue and a prevalent subject for discussion in healthcare settings [22]. Loneliness and social isolation are both linked to negative health consequences, such as a diminished health status, poor quality of life, increased utilization of healthcare services, and increased morbidity and mortality [23–25]. According to a cross-sectional study conducted in Colorado, USA, the prevalence of loneliness was estimated to be about 20% among adults visiting outpatient primary care facilities [26]. Nevertheless, especially among the elderly, social isolation and loneliness are so frequent that they are currently considered to be the new geriatric 'giants' [27]. However, according to a multistate study, one third of respondents under the age of 25 reported that they had experienced loneliness, in contrast to one out of ten within the group aged over 65 years [26]. Therefore, attention to detecting signs of loneliness should be paid regardless of a person's age.

Furthermore, the initial observation that married participants had lower odds of feeling lonely is consistent with some previous studies, suggesting that their marital status can influence feelings of loneliness and perceived social support [28]. In a sample with older individuals, divorced and widowed persons described higher levels of loneliness, in comparison with the married ones [29]. Also, gender should be taken into account, since the utilization of outpatient health care was positively correlated with loneliness in women but not in men [30]. Additionally, the protective role of engagement in individual activities or sports and the reported social contacts are consistent with previous research, emphasizing the positive impact of social engagement and connections on mental well-being in general [31–33]. Both the present study's results and the existing literature underline the importance of the aforementioned behavioral factors that may play a protective role against the adverse effects of loneliness. Furthermore, previous studies have shown that, at an individual level, social interaction, social support, and behavioral interventions which concentrate on enhancing social skills and addressing maladaptive social cognition have been noted to effectively alleviate loneliness [25,34], while in seniors, taking care of their grandchildren or undertaking volunteering activities may show similar results [35]. This suggests that promoting and facilitating such initiatives may have positive implications for mitigating loneliness.

According to our findings, the consumption of alcoholic beverages weekly was associated with a fivefold increased feeling of loneliness, although the association between alcohol consumption and loneliness is not well established in terms of cause or consequence. It is known that experiencing loneliness, conversely approached, has the potential to compromise self-regulatory abilities, leading to an increased susceptibility to noxious behaviors such as excessive alcohol consumption [36]. However, within a cohort of community-based adults aged 50 and above, loneliness was associated with a decreased frequency of alcohol consumption [37]. When studying loneliness and health behaviors, micro- or macro-circumstances, at a personal, cultural, or social level, can influence an already complex phenomenon, whereas the demand for variables or methodologies, toward this purpose, remains challenging [38]. Therefore, additional research is needed in order to understand how loneliness and alcohol are related and identify the possible mediating factors, taking into consideration gender, ethnicity, culture, social status, and personal motivations.

Incorporating routine laboratory data into the analysis provided novel insights into the comprehensive assessment of the relationship between physical health and loneliness. This is particularly noteworthy as a limited body of the literature has delved into the direct correlation between specific laboratory parameters and the subjective experience of loneliness. Elevated triglyceride levels [6,7,39] and diminished HDL-C levels [6,7] have been previously observed in individuals experiencing loneliness. However, there was no discernible correlation between total cholesterol, LDL-C, and non-HDL-C levels with loneliness [40]. Notably, in our study, participants with elevated triglyceride levels were associated with lower odds of feeling lonely. It could be hypothesized that people who feel less lonely may make diet choices as part of a more active social life. In our sample, obese participants were not included and this design peculiarity may be related to our finding about elevated triglycerides presented. However, further investigation is needed to establish solid conclusions. On the contrary, an increased LDL/HDL atherosclerotic index was linked to increased loneliness. This finding is important since the overall lipid profile within study participants was initially assessed as good. The aforementioned information suggests a potential interplay between the lipid metabolism and subjective feelings of loneliness, indicating a need for the further exploration and understanding of the latent mechanisms. Future research could focus on mental health issues and how they are related to physical and lifestyle factors.

Apart from the connection between loneliness and laboratory results, several studies have linked loneliness directly to chronic conditions. For example, both greater loneliness [41] and impaired social health (which includes loneliness) [42] have been associated with cardiovascular disease. Additionally, individuals reporting the occurrence of chronic obstructive pulmonary disease demonstrated a higher incidence of social isolation and loneliness in comparison with the rest of the participants [43]. There is also some evidence showing an association between loneliness and dental health or even tooth loss [44]. Dental health is a neglected issue that deserves more attention as a public health priority and it is noteworthy to mention such an association for many reasons. Furthermore, loneliness may have a pluripotent burden on human lives since, apart from its impact on physical well-being, it was reported to be related with mental health issues, as mentioned earlier. More specifically, loneliness was linked with depression [45,46], anxiety [47], eating disorders [48], or even mortality caused by suicide [49]. By 'Puzzling' the mentioned 'pieces of knowledge', it can be understood that loneliness appears to influence many dimensions of physical and mental health with a direct manner, without being able to precisely assess its multiple impact on life, when more than one dimension are synchronically affected overtime.

Understanding the factors associated with loneliness within primary care attendees has significant implications for healthcare interventions. Tailoring interventions to address not only behavioral aspects, but also considering laboratory data may enhance knowledge integration. Strategies that promote social engagement and support networks may be proved valuable in mitigating feelings of loneliness [25,34]. The healthcare system constitutes a pivotal yet underutilized partner in endeavors aimed at discerning, averting, and alleviating the negative consequences of social isolation and loneliness [50,51]. Concerning primary care, a better quality of the offered services may lead to decreased loneliness scores among attendees [52]. Therefore, family physicians and other healthcare providers, simultaneously with screening for conventional risk factors (like smoking, physical inactivity, alcohol consumption, and diet), should systematically screen to detect individuals who may be experiencing isolation, loneliness, or social vulnerability [27]. Subsequently, they should suggest evidence-based and patient-centered interventions aiming at fortifying social connections for such patients [24]. In fact, there is evidence that group interventions implemented by primary care professionals have shown promising results in addressing loneliness [53]. Although with another, and reversed, meaning, primary care and loneliness deal with health and social dimensions of life, in terms of magnitude and mutual interference. For this reason, developing a primary care ability to detect and manage loneliness goes beyond a conventional debate. However, additional research is imperative to furnish conclusive guidance regarding the specific effectiveness of interventions designed for distinct populations and underlying mechanisms [24,27,54], or to determine whether social resources are useful in alleviating loneliness. For example, surveys could focus on the design and intergenerational implementation of educational programs for both older adults [55] and adolescents and young adults [56]. These initiatives might be tailored and adopted in the context of the community to gain loneliness coping skills as individuals.

Strengths and Limitations

The combination of laboratory measurements and the identification of novel associations bring a fresh perspective to the understanding of loneliness within primary care attendees, at least in terms of the medical perception. While this study provides some valuable insights, several limitations should be acknowledged. This study sample is relatively small and may not be representative of broader population groups, so findings should be discussed with caution. Small or moderate samples may lead to an overestimation of the effect measure, although this phenomenon also depends on the data structure [57]. However, in the present study, structure issues did not appear. This overestimation, in samples above 100, might be tolerable as it does not appear to have any relevance for the interpretation of the results in the context of a single study since it is much lower than the standard error of the estimate, and this eventuality should be assessed when small studies are pooled together [57].

Nevertheless, the present survey did not intend to project these finding with any generalization for the entire primary care population. On the other hand, the application of the criteria, such as a certain range of age (40–75) and BMI ($\leq$29.9/m^2), led to obtaining less uncertainty with the emerged associations. For example, it is not well established how Millenials perceive loneliness [58] or how obesity interacts with loneliness and social isolation [59]. In this way, the detected levels of loneliness do not appear to be overestimated and all the associations which have emerged show a socio-behavioral linkage (alcohol consumption, sport activity, routine contacts, and lipid profile).

In addition, the cross-sectional nature of the study restricts the founding of causation, while the self-reported nature of the information on behavioral aspects may introduce bias. Additionally, a different source, time, and process occurring within the laboratory tests included, from a period of six months, may lead to a further limitation. However, in our opinion, this asynchronous integration of information, for research meanings, that bridge social with clinical inputs, may be interesting since many of the variables socially or behaviorally investigated might have a retrospectively longitudinal projection with loneliness.

Furthermore, it is imperative to note that loneliness could be correlated with the diminished utilization of healthcare services and attenuated solicitation for medical interventions. Therefore, it is conceivable that our study may not accurately capture the exact prevalence of loneliness at a unit coverage level. Finally, the prevalence of mental and physical health conditions may differ from existing epidemiological or local community data. Future research should consider longitudinal designs and provide useful insights into the dynamic nature of loneliness and its associations with socio-demographic and behavioral characteristics and laboratory markers over time, incorporating a broader and more representative sample from multiple primary care settings. This can contribute to extrapolating more solid observations regarding loneliness, moving towards the interface between health and disease.

The present study did not include individuals with obesity or morbid obesity. In an interesting systematic review, focusing on obesity and loneliness or social isolation, while some studies point to an association between increased loneliness and obesity, the authors recognized that mixed observations occur [59]. Moreover, the rationale of including participants between 40 and 75 years of age was based on previous findings from primary care settings in Crete that used a similar population group—above 40 years of age—investigating local trends of cardio-metabolic morbidity [60]. Also, a different impact of loneliness may occur among younger adult generations, as has been shown in a study that included different age groups during the early COVID-19 pandemic period [58].

5. Conclusions

In conclusion, involvement in individual activities or sports, higher numbers of social contacts reported, and a lack of weekly alcohol consumption and elevated triglyceride levels were associated with moderate or no loneliness, while an increased LDL/HDL atherosclerotic index was linked to increased levels of loneliness. This preliminary analysis offers some new information on socio-demographic, behavioral, and routine laboratory test results and how these variables interplay with perceived loneliness among primary care attendees. This study's findings underscore the need for open-minded approaches and variable selection when addressing meanings of loneliness, recognizing its pluripotent effect, as well as the different aspects that may contribute to its pervasive complexity. Primary care may offer promising attributes in terms of research findings that emerge from a mixed methodology and socio-iatrogenic thinking. Further research aiming at understanding similar associations may discuss tailored interventions for loneliness and neglected mental and physical circumstances or discussions within primary care settings.

Author Contributions: Conceptualization, P.V. and E.K.S.; methodology, P.V. and E.K.S.; validation, M.L.; formal analysis, M.L.; data curation, P.V.; writing—original draft preparation, P.V. and P.S.; writing—review and editing, E.K.S., M.L., P.S., F.A., A.T. and M.K.; visualization, F.A., A.T. and M.K.; project administration, P.V. and E.K.S. All authors have read and agreed to the published version of the manuscript.

Funding: This research received no external funding.

Institutional Review Board Statement: The approval to conduct the study, for the needs of an ongoing PhD thesis, was obtained by the Ethics and Deontology Committee of the University of Crete (protocol number: 166/11.11.2022). The research protocol was additionally approved by the 7th Health Regional Authority of Crete (protocol number: 6460) and the study was performed in accordance with the Helsinki Declaration.

Informed Consent Statement: Informed consent was obtained from all subjects involved in the study.

Data Availability Statement: Datasets are available from the first author upon reasonable request.

Conflicts of Interest: The authors declare no conflicts of interest.

References

1. Perlman, D.; Peplau, L.A. Toward a Social Psychology of Loneliness. In *Personal Relationships in Disorder*; Duck, S., Gilmour, R., Eds.; Academic Press: London, UK, 1981; pp. 31–56.
2. Victor, C.R.; Yang, K. The Prevalence of Loneliness among Adults: A Case Study of the United Kingdom. *J. Psychol. Interdiscip. Appl.* **2012**, *146*, 85–104. [CrossRef]
3. Valtorta, N.K.; Kanaan, M.; Gilbody, S.; Ronzi, S.; Hanratty, B. Loneliness and Social Isolation as Risk Factors for Coronary Heart Disease and Stroke: Systematic Review and Meta-Analysis of Longitudinal Observational Studies. *Heart* **2016**, *102*, 1009–1016. [CrossRef]
4. Richard, A.; Rohrmann, S.; Vandeleur, C.L.; Schmid, M.; Barth, J.; Eichholzer, M. Loneliness Is Adversely Associated with Physical and Mental Health and Lifestyle Factors: Results from a Swiss National Survey. *PLoS ONE* **2017**, *12*, e0181442. [CrossRef]
5. Kuiper, J.S.; Zuidersma, M.; Oude Voshaar, R.C.; Zuidema, S.U.; van den Heuvel, E.R.; Stolk, R.P.; Smidt, N. Social Relationships and Risk of Dementia: A Systematic Review and Meta-Analysis of Longitudinal Cohort Studies. *Ageing Res. Rev.* **2015**, *22*, 39–57. [CrossRef] [PubMed]
6. Henriksen, R.E.; Nilsen, R.M.; Strandberg, R.B. Loneliness as a Risk Factor for Metabolic Syndrome: Results from the HUNT Study. *J. Epidemiol. Community Health* **2019**, *73*, 941–946. [CrossRef] [PubMed]
7. Badcock, J.C.; Mackinnon, A.; Waterreus, A.; Watts, G.F.; Castle, D.; McGrath, J.J.; Morgan, V.A. Loneliness in Psychotic Illness and Its Association with Cardiometabolic Disorders. *Schizophr. Res.* **2019**, *204*, 90–95. [CrossRef] [PubMed]
8. Dahlberg, L.; McKee, K.J.; Lennartsson, C.; Rehnberg, J. A Social Exclusion Perspective on Loneliness in Older Adults in the Nordic Countries. *Eur. J. Ageing* **2022**, *19*, 175–188. [CrossRef]

9. Abrams, D.; Hogg, M.A.; Marques, J.M. *The Social Psychology of Inclusion and Exclusion*; Psychology Press: New York, NY, USA, 2005.
10. Floyd, K.; Veksler, A.E.; Mcewan, B.; Hesse, C.; Boren, J.P.; Dinsmore, D.R.; Pavlich, C.A. Social Inclusion Predicts Lower Blood Glucose and Low-Density Lipoproteins in Healthy Adults. *Health Commun.* **2017**, *32*, 1039–1042. [CrossRef]
11. Zhou, W.; Li, Y.; Ning, Y.; Gong, S.; Song, N.; Zhu, B.; Wang, J.; Zhao, S.; Shi, Y.; Ding, X. Social Isolation Is Associated with Rapid Kidney Function Decline and the Development of Chronic Kidney Diseases in Middle-Aged and Elderly Adults: Findings From the China Health and Retirement Longitudinal Study (CHARLS). *Front. Med.* **2021**, *8*, 782624. [CrossRef]
12. Holt-Lunstad, J. Social Connection as a Public Health Issue: The Evidence and a Systemic Framework for Prioritizing the "Social" in Social Determinants of Health. *Annu. Rev. Public Health* **2022**, *43*, 193–213. [CrossRef]
13. Hamamura, T. Are Cultures Becoming Individualistic? A Cross-Temporal Comparison of Individualism-Collectivism in the United States and Japan. *Personal. Soc. Psychol. Rev.* **2012**, *16*, 3–24. [CrossRef] [PubMed]
14. Russell, D.W. UCLA Loneliness Scale (Version 3): Reliability, Validity, and Factor Structure. *J. Pers. Assess.* **1996**, *66*, 20–40. [CrossRef] [PubMed]
15. Lee, C.; Cho, B.; Yang, Q.; Chang, S.J.; Ryu, S.I.; Noh, E.Y.; Park, Y.H. A Psychometric Analysis of the 20-Item Revised University of California Los Angeles Loneliness Scale Among Korean Older Adults Living Alone. *Res. Gerontol. Nurs.* **2021**, *14*, 306–316. [CrossRef]
16. Lee, E.E.; Depp, C.; Palmer, B.W.; Glorioso, D.; Daly, R.; Liu, J.; Tu, X.M.; Kim, H.C.; Tarr, P.; Yamada, Y.; et al. High Prevalence and Adverse Health Effects of Loneliness in Community-Dwelling Adults Across the Lifespan: Role of Wisdom as a Protective Factor. *Int. Psychogeriatr.* **2019**, *31*, 1447–1462. [CrossRef] [PubMed]
17. Pikea, P.; Parpa, E.; Tsilika, E.; Galanos, A.; Mystakidou, K. Psychometric Properties of the Greek-University of California, Los Angeles Loneliness Scale-Version 3 in a Sample of People with Human Immunodeficiency Virus. *World J. AIDS* **2016**, *06*, 157–168. [CrossRef]
18. Sterling, R.K.; Lissen, E.; Clumeck, N.; Sola, R.; Correa, M.C.; Montaner, J.; Sulkowski, M.S.; Torriani, F.J.; Dieterich, D.T.; Thomas, D.L.; et al. Development of a Simple Noninvasive Index to Predict Significant Fibrosis in Patients with HIV/HCV Coinfection. *Hepatology* **2006**, *43*, 1317–1325. [CrossRef]
19. Arakawa, K.; Saeki, A.; Ide, R.; Matsushita, Y. Presepsin Cut-off Value for Diagnosis of Sepsis in Patients with Renal Dysfunction. *PLoS ONE* **2022**, *17*, e0273930. [CrossRef]
20. Park, E.Y.; Kim, T.Y. Where Are Cut-off Values of Serum Creatinine in the Setting of Chronic Kidney Disease? *Kidney Int.* **2010**, *77*, 645–646. [CrossRef]
21. Sun, T.; Chen, M.; Shen, H.; PingYin; Fan, L.; Chen, X.; Wu, J.; Xu, Z.; Zhang, J. Predictive Value of LDL/HDL Ratio in Coronary Atherosclerotic Heart Disease. *BMC Cardiovasc. Disord.* **2022**, *22*, 273. [CrossRef]
22. Sirois, F.M.; Owens, J. A Meta-Analysis of Loneliness and Use of Primary Health Care. *Health Psychol. Rev.* **2023**, *17*, 193–210. [CrossRef]
23. Gerst-Emerson, K.; Jayawardhana, J. Loneliness as a Public Health Issue: The Impact of Loneliness on Health Care Utilization Among Older Adults. *Am. J. Public Health* **2015**, *105*, 1013–1019. [CrossRef]
24. Kanbay, M.; Tanriover, C.; Copur, S.; Peltek, I.B.; Mutlu, A.; Mallamaci, F.; Zoccali, C. Social Isolation and Loneliness: Undervalued Risk Factors for Disease States and Mortality. *Eur. J. Clin. Investig.* **2023**, *53*, e14032. [CrossRef] [PubMed]
25. Sharma, T.; Padala, P.R.; Mehta, J.L. Loneliness and Social Isolation: Determinants of Cardiovascular Outcomes. *Curr. Cardiol. Rev.* **2021**, *17*, e051121190873. [CrossRef] [PubMed]
26. Mullen, R.A.; Tong, S.; Sabo, R.T.; Liaw, W.R.; Marshall, J.; Nease, D.E.; Krist, A.H.; Frey, J.J. Loneliness in Primary Care Patients: A Prevalence Study. *Ann. Fam. Med.* **2019**, *17*, 108–115. [CrossRef] [PubMed]
27. Freedman, A.; Nicolle, J. Social Isolation and Loneliness: The New Geriatric Giants: Approach for Primary Care. *Can. Fam. Physician* **2020**, *66*, 176–182. [PubMed]
28. Kislev, E. Aging, Marital Status, and Loneliness: Multilevel Analyses of 30 Countries. *Res. Ageing Soc. Policy* **2022**, *10*, 77–103. [CrossRef]
29. Liu, H.; Copeland, M.; Nowak, G.; Chopik, W.J.; Oh, J. Marital Status Differences in Loneliness Among Older Americans During the COVID-19 Pandemic. *Popul. Res. Policy Rev.* **2023**, *42*, 74. [CrossRef] [PubMed]
30. Boehlen, F.H.; Heider, D.; Schellberg, D.; Hohls, J.K.; Schöttker, B.; Brenner, H.; Friederich, H.C.; König, H.H.; Wild, B. Gender-Specific Association of Loneliness and Health Care Use in Community-Dwelling Older Adults. *BMC Geriatr.* **2023**, *23*, 502. [CrossRef] [PubMed]
31. Eime, R.M.; Young, J.A.; Harvey, J.T.; Charity, M.J.; Payne, W.R. A Systematic Review of the Psychological and Social Benefits of Participation in Sport for Children and Adolescents: Informing Development of a Conceptual Model of Health through Sport. *Int. J. Behav. Nutr. Phys. Act.* **2013**, *10*, 1–21. [CrossRef]
32. Fong, P.; Cruwys, T.; Robinson, S.L.; Haslam, S.A.; Haslam, C.; Mance, P.L.; Fisher, C.L. Evidence That Loneliness Can Be Reduced by a Whole-of-Community Intervention to Increase Neighbourhood Identification. *Soc. Sci. Med.* **2021**, *277*, 113909. [CrossRef]
33. Liu, N.; Zhong, Q. The Impact of Sports Participation on Individuals' Subjective Well-Being: The Mediating Role of Class Identity and Health. *Humanit. Soc. Sci. Commun.* **2023**, *10*, 544. [CrossRef]
34. Masi, C.M.; Chen, H.Y.; Hawkley, L.C.; Cacioppo, J.T. A Meta-Analysis of Interventions to Reduce Loneliness. *Pers. Soc. Psychol. Rev.* **2011**, *15*, 219–266. [CrossRef] [PubMed]

35. Akhter-Khan, S.C.; Hofmann, V.; Warncke, M.; Tamimi, N.; Mayston, R.; Prina, M.A. Caregiving, Volunteering, and Loneliness in Middle-Aged and Older Adults: A Systematic Review. *Aging Ment. Health* **2023**, *27*, 1233–1245. [CrossRef]
36. Paul, E.; Bu, F.; Fancourt, D. Loneliness and Risk for Cardiovascular Disease: Mechanisms and Future Directions. *Curr. Cardiol. Rep.* **2021**, *23*, 1–7. [CrossRef] [PubMed]
37. Canham, S.L.; Mauro, P.M.; Kaufmann, C.N.; Sixsmith, A. Association of Alcohol Use and Loneliness Frequency Among Middle-Aged and Older Adult Drinkers. *J. Aging Health* **2016**, *28*, 267–284. [CrossRef] [PubMed]
38. Volkos, P.; Linardakis, M.; Stamati, M.; Symvoulakis, E.K. *Exploring Loneliness, Trust, and Psychosocial Meanings among Primary Care Attendees: Findings from a General Practice Setting in Crete, Greece*; 2024.
39. Abdellaoui, A.; Sanchez-Roige, S.; Sealock, J.; Treur, J.L.; Dennis, J.; Fontanillas, P.; Elson, S.; Nivard, M.G.; Ip, H.F.; Van Der Zee, M.; et al. Phenome-Wide Investigation of Health Outcomes Associated with Genetic Predisposition to Loneliness. *Hum. Mol. Genet.* **2019**, *28*, 3853–3865. [CrossRef]
40. Kobos, E.; Szewczyk, A.; Świątkowska, T.; Kryczka, T.; Sienkiewicz, Z. Relationship between Loneliness and Blood Glucose Control in Diabetes. *BMC Public Health* **2020**, *20*, 1140. [CrossRef]
41. Wang, X.; Ma, H.; Li, X.; Heianza, Y.; Fonseca, V.; Qi, L. Joint Association of Loneliness and Traditional Risk Factor Control and Incident Cardiovascular Disease in Diabetes Patients. *Eur. Heart J.* **2023**, *44*, 2583–2591. [CrossRef] [PubMed]
42. Teshale, A.B.; Htun, H.L.; Hu, J.; Dalli, L.L.; Lim, M.H.; Neves, B.B.; Baker, J.R.; Phyo, A.Z.Z.; Reid, C.M.; Ryan, J.; et al. The Relationship between Social Isolation, Social Support, and Loneliness with Cardiovascular Disease and Shared Risk Factors: A Narrative Review. *Arch. Gerontol. Geriatr.* **2023**, *111*, 105008. [CrossRef]
43. Suen, A.O.; Iyer, A.S.; Cenzer, I.; Farrand, E.; White, D.B.; Singer, J.; Sudore, R.; Kotwal, A. National Prevalence of Social Isolation and Loneliness in Adults with Chronic Obstructive Pulmonary Disease. *Ann. Am. Thorac. Soc.* **2023**, *20*, 1709–1717. [CrossRef]
44. Takahashi, S.; Naganuma, T.; Kurita, N.; Omae, K.; Ohnishi, T.; Yoshioka, T.; Ito, F.; Takeshima, T.; Fukuma, S.; Hamaguchi, S.; et al. Social Isolation/Loneliness and Tooth Loss in Community-Dwelling Older Adults: The Sukagawa Study. *Innov. Aging* **2023**, *7*, igad065. [CrossRef] [PubMed]
45. Zhang, Y.; Kuang, J.; Xin, Z.; Fang, J.; Song, R.; Yang, Y.; Song, P.; Wang, Y.; Wang, J. Loneliness, Social Isolation, Depression and Anxiety among the Elderly in Shanghai: Findings from a Longitudinal Study. *Arch. Gerontol. Geriatr.* **2023**, *110*, 104980. [CrossRef] [PubMed]
46. Moustakopoulou, L.; Adamakidou, T.; Plakas, S.; Drakopoulou, M.; Apostolara, P.; Mantoudi, A.; Mastrogiannis, D.; Zartaloudi, A.; Parissopoulos, S.; Koreli, A.; et al. Exploring Loneliness, Fear and Depression among Older Adults during the COVID-19 Era: A Cross-Sectional Study in Greek Provincial Towns. *Healthcare* **2023**, *11*, 1234. [CrossRef] [PubMed]
47. Trtica, L.M.; Volarić, M.; Kurevija, T.; Mihaljević, S.; Dupan, Z.K.; Wittlinger, T. Psycho-Social and Health Predictors of Loneliness in Older Primary Care Patients and Mediating Mechanisms Linking Comorbidities and Loneliness. *BMC Geriatr.* **2023**, *23*, 801. [CrossRef] [PubMed]
48. Bellapigna, C.; Kalibatseva, Z. Psychosocial Risk Factors Associated with Social Anxiety, Depressive and Disordered Eating Symptoms during COVID-19. *AIMS Public Health* **2023**, *10*, 18. [CrossRef] [PubMed]
49. Alothman, D.; Lewis, S.; Card, T.; Tyrrell, E.; Fogarty, A.W. The Association between Living Alone, Loneliness and Suicide Mortality and Effect Modification by Age: A Case:Control Study. *J. Affect. Disord.* **2024**, *352*, 278–280. [CrossRef] [PubMed]
50. Holt-Lunstad, J. Loneliness and Social Isolation as Risk Factors: The Power of Social Connection in Prevention. *Am. J. Lifestyle Med.* **2021**, *15*, 567–573. [CrossRef] [PubMed]
51. Committee on the Health and Medical Dimensions of Social Isolation and Loneliness in Older Adults; Division of Behavioral and Social Sciences and Education; Health and Medicine Division; Board on Behavioral Cognitive and Sensory Sciences; Board on Health Sciences Policy; Committee on the Health and Medical Dimensions of Social Isolation and Loneliness in Older Adults. *Social Isolation and Loneliness in Older Adults: Opportunities for the Health Care System*; The National Academies Press: Washington, DC, USA, 2020.
52. Kaneko, M.; Shinoda, S.; Nakayama, I.; Xu, J.; Yagome, S.; Goto, A. Usual Source and Better Quality of Primary Care Are Associated with Lower Loneliness Scores: A Cross-Sectional Study. *Fam. Pract.* **2023**, cmad049. [CrossRef]
53. Agudelo-Hernández, F.; Guapacha-Montoya, M.; Rojas-Andrade, R. Mutual Aid Groups for Loneliness, Psychosocial Disability, and Continuity of Care. *Community Ment. Health J.* **2024**, *60*, 608–619. [CrossRef]
54. Fakoya, O.A.; McCorry, N.K.; Donnelly, M. Loneliness and Social Isolation Interventions for Older Adults: A Scoping Review of Reviews. *BMC Public Health* **2020**, *20*, 129. [CrossRef]
55. Kobylarek, A.; Madej, M.; Roubalová, M.; Maturkanič, P. Holistic Education of Seniors in the Eastern European Model of the U3A. *Acta Missiologica* **2022**, *16*, 87–98.
56. Králik, R. The Influence of Family and School in Shaping the Values of Children and Young People in the Theory of Free Time and Pedagogy. *J. Educ. Cult. Soc.* **2023**, *14*, 249–268. [CrossRef]
57. Nemes, S.; Jonasson, J.M.; Genell, A.; Steineck, G. Bias in Odds Ratios by Logistic Regression Modelling and Sample Size. *BMC Med. Res. Methodol.* **2009**, *9*, 56. [CrossRef] [PubMed]
58. Grelle, K.; Shrestha, N.; Ximenes, M.; Perrotte, J.; Cordaro, M.; Deason, R.G.; Howard, K. The Generation Gap Revisited: Generational Differences in Mental Health, Maladaptive Coping Behaviors, and Pandemic-Related Concerns During the Initial COVID-19 Pandemic. *J. Adult Dev.* **2023**, *30*, 381–392. [CrossRef] [PubMed]

59. Hajek, A.; Kretzler, B.; König, H.H. The Association between Obesity and Social Isolation as Well as Loneliness in the Adult Population: A Systematic Review. *Diabetes, Metab. Syndr. Obes. Targets Ther.* **2021**, *14*, 2765–2773. [CrossRef]
60. Anastasaki, M.; Papadakis, S.; Linardakis, M.; Anyfantakis, D.; Symvoulakis, E.K.; Lionis, C. Burden of Metabolic Syndrome among Primary Care Patients in Crete, Greece: A Descriptive Study. *Eur. J. Gen. Pract.* **2020**, *26*, 166–174. [CrossRef]

MDPI AG
Grosspeteranlage 5
4052 Basel
Switzerland
Tel.: +41 61 683 77 34

European Journal of Investigation in Health, Psychology and Education Editorial Office
E-mail: ejihpe@mdpi.com
www.mdpi.com/journal/ejihpe

www.ingramcontent.com/pod-product-compliance
Lightning Source LLC
LaVergne TN
LVHW070448061126
851858LV00011B/185
9783725882816